XXX. *Extract of a letter from Mr.* Lambert, *surgeon at Newcastle upon Tyne, to Dr.* Hunter; *giving an Account of a new Method of treating an* Aneurysm. *Read* June 15, 1761.

… I confidered the coats and motions of arteries, and compared their wounds with the wounds of veins and other parts. I reflected upon the procefs of nature in the cure of wounds in general, and…Upon the whole, I was in hopes that a future of the wound in the artery might be fuccefsful; and if fo, it would certainly be preferable to tying up the trunk of the veffel.

If it fhould be found by experience, that a large artery, when wounded, may be healed up by this kind of future, without becoming impervious, it would be an important difcovery in furgery. It would make the operation for the Aneurysm ftill more fuccefsful in the arm, when the main trunk is wounded; and by this method, perhaps, we might be able to cure the wounds of fome arteries that would otherwife require amputation, or be altogether incurable.

Atlas of
VASCULAR SURGERY

Second edition

Atlas of
VASCULAR SURGERY

Falls B. Hershey, M.D., F.A.C.S.

*Associate Professor of Clinical Surgery, Washington University School of
Medicine, St. Louis, Mo.; Area Consultant in Surgery, United States
Veterans Administration, St. Louis, Mo.; formerly Director, St. Louis
Heart Association Artery Bank; formerly Chairman, Department of Surgery,
Michael Reese Hospital and Medical Center, Chicago, Ill.; Diplomate,
American Board of Surgery*

Carl H. Calman, M.D., F.A.C.S.

*Formerly Assistant in Clinical Surgery, Washington University
School of Medicine, St. Louis, Mo.; Diplomate, American Board of Surgery*

Illustrated by Kathryn Murphy Masterson and William R. Schwarz

The C. V. Mosby Company

Saint Louis   1967

To our wives, Julie and Marty, *and the patient, loyal, and loving wives of surgeons everywhere*

F. B. H. and C. H. C.

Preface

This book was written to instruct residents as well as practicing surgeons in the methods and techniques of vascular surgery. It is dedicated to them, with the hope that it will be a guide to successful and safe technique, sound judgment, and an understanding of the scope, applications, and limitations of vascular operations.

In addition to surgical procedures, short descriptions of disease patterns, both pathological and physiological, together with outlines of the various diagnostic procedures, are included. The discussions of surgical technique emphasize only those matters that are peculiar to the vascular system, avoiding the repetition of that already familiar to the general surgeon.

The chapter on arteriography outlines the major techniques that find frequent application. In addition to the methods presented herein, numerous additional basic methods and variations are available. With a little experience, innovation in this field is not difficult. Radiography frequently provides structural anatomical information for vascular reconstructive procedures. Since the vascular surgeon will usually perform and interpret his own angiograms, knowledge of these procedures is essential.

Accurate preoperative diagnosis and careful postoperative management are an integral part of the surgical procedures described and are essential to success. However, since the amount of such information that can be included in an atlas is necessarily limited, the reader must add his own knowledge of pathology, physiology, and surgery, his own evaluation of new techniques and results reported in the surgical literature, and his own personal observations and experiences.

If this atlas is successful in communicating to the experienced vascular surgeon some helpful idea or in guiding a resident more safely through his first vascular operation, it will have justified our efforts.

In the four years since the first edition was published, a great deal of practical and experimental work, as well as a great deal of clinical experience in vascular surgery, has been accumulated by many groups throughout the country. In this second edition we observe more standardization and better definition of procedures and indications. A number of ingenious innovations in technique, such as use of the Fogarty balloon catheter and the partial occluding Teflon clip for the vena cava, have been devised. As a result, vascular surgery in all of its facets has been more widely accepted and applied. Morbidity rates, as well as mortality rates, have decreased.

A number of unsolved or poorly solved problems remain. The greatest of these is possibly the problem of inadequate arterial circulation below the bifurcation of the common femoral artery. The very number of procedures proposed, such as onlay vein grafts and in situ saphenous vein transplantation, all attest to the difficulties in restoring arterial flow in this area.

We have reviewed a great deal of experimental and clinical published work, as well as our own experiences, in this edition. It has been encouraging indeed to note that a great many of the suggestions advanced four years ago are now in wide use. The continued work of many skilled surgeons in this field will assure continued progress.

We are permanently indebted to many teachers and friends. A partial list must include Dr. Robert H. Linton, whose rigorous admonition, "You've got to do it *right*," still echoes to former residents, and Dr. Michael E. DeBakey, whose bold attack and elegant and simple techniques for aneurysm and occlusive disease have been inspiring examples.

Our own early arterial replacements would not have been possible without the inspiration, encouragement, and financial support of Dr. Carl A. Moyer, formerly Bixby Professor of Surgery, Washington University School of Medicine, who helped us establish the St. Louis Heart Association Artery Bank. This organization supplied arterial homografts until satisfactory synthetic prostheses were developed. Dr. Cyril A. Costello was also most helpful.

Dr. Eric Carlsson and Dr. Hokan Arvidsson devised or introduced many arteriographic techniques during their tenures at Barnes Hospital. These contributions include the Seldinger apparatus and the "up-and-around" retrograde injection of the femoral artery.

The technique of transmetatarsal amputation is that of Dr. Leland S. McKittrick. His unparalleled success with transmetatarsal amputation is due to experience and surgical judgment not completely communicable in an atlas.

These surgeons will recognize some of their precepts and techniques but are in no way responsible for deficiencies or shortcomings.

We are grateful to Dr. Thomas Sheridan for the description of the Nakayama stapler and to Dr. Norman Brill and Dr. Gonzalo Magsaysay for assistance with the discussions on phlebography, the vein eraser, and brachiocerebral arteriography.

The usefulness of this book is due in large part to the fine drawings of Mrs. Kathryn Murphy Masterson and William R. Schwarz. Some new drawings have been made by Michael K. Meyers and Wesley Bloom.

Falls B. Hershey
Carl H. Calman

Contents

Atlas of
VASCULAR SURGERY

Chapter 1

Introduction

HISTORICAL REVIEW*

Paré published his views on the use of ligatures in amputations in 1564 and Harvey his great work on the circulation in 1638. The earliest recorded arterial suture is that of the brachial artery by Hallowell in 1759. The story of this event as recorded by Lambert is interesting. Lambert apparently had developed the method of suture after consideration of the "union of divided parts—in the operation of the harelip and in horses' necks that are bled by farriers." Hallowell, who had a patient with a bleeding arterial wound (Lambert refers to it as an aneurysm), performed the suture by winding a ligature around the ends of a small steel pin, slightly more than ¼ inch long, passed through the lips of the arterial wound. The patient was hospitalized approximately one month. It is recorded that his pulse was little altered immediately after the operation and apparently continued so. Lambert stated that it might be possible to "cure the wounds of some arteries," thus avoiding amputations.

The advent of general anesthesia and of antiseptic and aseptic surgical technique permitted surgeons to extend their art. An early improvement was repair rather than ligation of injured vessels. Another milestone was portacaval anastomosis by Eck in 1879. Schede in 1882 reported a successful suture repair of the femoral vein. Other reports followed. In 1899 Jassinowski announced his technique for repairing vascular lacerations with interrupted fine silk sutures that did not penetrate the intima. Publications dealing with variations and applications of this technique followed in large numbers.

Circular suture of the entire blood vessel was experimentally performed by Briau and Joboulay in 1896. They anastomosed the carotid artery with everting

---

*Yamanoüchi, H.: Über die zirkulären Gefässnähte und Arterienvenenanastomosen, sowie über die Gefässtransplantationen, Deutsche Ztschr. Chir. **112**:1-118, 1911; Carrel, A.: The suture of blood vessels, Bull. Hopkins Hosp. **18**:18-28, 1907; Watts, S. H.: The suture of blood vessels. Implantation and transplantation of vessels and organs, an historical and experimental study, Bull. Hopkins Hosp. **18**:153-177, 1907; Lambert: Letter to Dr. Hunter, Medical observations and inquiries, vol. 2, London, 1762; Bernheim, B. W.: Surgery of the vascular system, Philadelphia, 1913, J. B. Lippincott Co.; Guthrie, C. G.: Blood vessel surgery and its applications, New York, 1912, Longmans, Green & Co. (reprinted in 1959 by University of Pittsburgh Press).

sutures that also approximated the intima. Murphy in 1897 announced both a suture and a metallic prosthesis. Dörfler in 1899 advocated the use of fine needles, fine silk, and a continuous suture through all layers of the vessel. Publications became so numerous that by 1911 Yamanoüchi cited a bibliography of 133 references, mostly in German. The problems of autotransplantation, homotransplantation, heterotransplantation, and preservation of vessels were investigated. Carrel was a prominent figure in this work in the United States, and the method of triangulation of a blood vessel developed by Carrel and Guthrie is still useful. Guthrie's book, published in 1912, provides an excellent historical review and a summary of the methods and experimental results of that time.

SURGICAL PRINCIPLES AND BASIC TECHNIQUES
General surgical principles and their applications in vascular surgery

The successful outcome of vascular operations depends upon thorough understanding and conscientious application of the principles of general surgery and upon careful diagnosis and preoperative and postoperative care. It must be recognized, for example, that the most meticulous repair of a gunshot wound of the femoral artery may fail because of insufficient debridement of damaged muscle, improper fixation of an associated fracture, inadequate blood replacement, etc.

Infection is one of the most serious complications that can occur in vascular surgery. The infected arterial wall becomes soft and friable so that suture lines leak or disrupt, and the surgeon may be compelled to ligate a blood vessel or to sacrifice a limb.

When synthetic materials are used, the problems of infection are somewhat different. These materials are, of course, unaffected by the infectious process itself and can function as conduits in the presence of infection. However, like other foreign bodies, prosthetic grafts maintain an infectious process that otherwise might be eradicated. Ultimately, if infection extends to the anastomosis, disruption results.

Treatment of such infections is always difficult, and the prosthesis finally must be removed. Whenever possible, a new bypass vein graft or prosthesis should be placed through uncontaminated tissue planes. Vein grafts resist infection and are preferable in potentially contaminated wounds.

Because of the catastrophic consequences of infection in vascular surgery, prevention is of the utmost importance. All the details of aseptic technique should receive meticulous attention. Hematomas or fluid collections invite abscess formation, and drains should be employed when necessary. Careful closure eliminates dead space in the wound and about prosthetic materials.

The surgeon has usually mastered these problems and is able to secure adequate exposure and hemostasis. Experience demonstrates that skill and practice in general or traumatic surgery do not, in themselves, confer the knowledge needed to master the problems of vascular reconstructive procedures. Vascular surgery is, however, not obscure or unusually difficult—it is merely different.

The axioms in vascular surgery are adequate exposure, proximal and distal control of blood vessels prior to arteriotomy, and prevention of thrombosis. With good technique, it should not be necessary to rely on anticoagulants to obtain good results from vascular procedures. Use of anticoagulants will be discussed later in this chapter.

Experience has shown that it is generally unwise to attribute poor results to arterial spasm. When the results of reconstructive procedures are poor and pulses do not return as expected, thrombosis is a more likely explanation than is severe arterial spasm.

It is essential at the end of a surgical procedure to be certain that the blood vessels are open distally. Arteriograms at the end of an operation are frequently helpful and permit a prompt correction.

The use of Fogarty balloon catheters to clear blood vessels distally before final closure of a bypass or anastomosis is becoming frequent.

Perivascular dissection

Perivascular dissection is a basic technique in vascular surgery. The easiest and clearest plane of dissection is close to the blood vessel. The procedure is begun by picking up the perivascular tissue with fine forceps and cutting it. The plane along the vessel is developed by sharp and blunt dissection with Metzenbaum scissors. Curved Metzenbaum scissors modified by grinding the points to resemble the Stevens tenotomy scissors are very useful.

Small rolls of umbilical tape held in a hemostat are used to dissect about the complete circumference of a thin-walled vessel. They can be employed in pairs, one to hold the vessel aside and the other to roll the perivascular areolar tissue away. The same method may be used to dissect longitudinally along the blood vessel. When dissecting longitudinally, all dissection and application of tension should follow the long axis of the vessel. Tapes under the vessel aid in handling and in exposure and are relatively atraumatic. Experience teaches the amounts of tension that are necessary and safe. However, intimal tears with consequent thrombosis are produced by overstretching thin blood vessels.

Anastomosis of small vessels requires meticulous techniques. At the site of anastomosis even the finest shreds of adventitia should be trimmed from the edge. After transection, retraction of the tissues will often produce new shreds of tissue that should be removed. Removal of the adventitia facilitates anastomosis of small vessels, for if this is not excised the mobility of the outer layer can leave the operator in some doubt about piercing the intima of the vessel with each stitch. When suturing large vessels, adventitia is needed for a secure closure. In small vessels, however, an overly thick adventitial layer will slide back and forth, making each passage of the needle a problem in visualization. Fragments of adventitial tissue falling into the suture line or being carried into the lumen of the vessel by the suture increase the danger of postoperative thrombosis. In diseased vessels it may be impossible to distinguish the usual anatomical layers.

Suture techniques

The currently preferred suture material for vascular surgery is braided Dacron in sizes ranging from 3-0 to 7-0. This material is available commercially,* and one brand is coated with Teflon for lubrication, eliminating the need for any

---

*Mersiline and Tevdec (latter is coated with Teflon).

3

supplemental lubrication. Dacron maintains its strength in the tissues throughout years of implantation. Since no true healing occurs between prosthetic implants and the host artery, such a material is essential to prevent disruption at the suture line between the prosthesis and the artery.

These suture materials are supplied with swaged-on atraumatic needles. Previously, in the direct suture of blood vessels, lubrication of the suture material has been employed, primarily as an anticoagulation measure. Lubrication also makes passage of the suture material through atherosclerotic blood vessel walls easier and prevents the suture from sawing the arterial wall. Silicone oil and mineral oil are excellent lubricants. However, Teflon-coated Dacron may be used as supplied without further lubrication.

Monofilament polyethylene suture is now available and is preferred for vein grafts since it slips through the thin vein wall very easily with minimal trauma and will not catch the adventitia by friction and pull it through. Polypropylene* suture materials will probably be subjected to more clinical testing within the next few years. They have excellent knot-tying capability.

In medium-sized vessels the sutures are placed about 1 mm. apart and about 1 mm. back from the edge of the vessel. This distance should be lessened for small vessels and when using 7-0 silk. When suturing aneurysms of the aorta, sutures may be widely spaced (that is, 2 or 3 mm. apart) without leakage. The physical properties of the arterial wall may make accurate placement of sutures difficult. Sutures can be guided into place and the edge of the vessel everted with a long right-angle nerve hook or a sharp-pointed skin hook.

A number of techniques of anastomosis are illustrated throughout this book. Veins are most efficiently handled by the technique of triangulation of the ends of the vessels with three separate stay sutures. These are used to steady the vessel while end-to-end approximation with a continuous simple suture through all layers is accomplished. For larger vessels it is more secure to evert a cuff of artery (Fig. 1, A and B) that will allow intima-to-intima approximation with less suture material exposed to the bloodstream. Such suture lines eliminate leakage, but they have the disadvantages of requiring slightly more artery and of producing moderate constriction. Mattress sutures, therefore, should be avoided in small blood vessels. End-to-side anastomosis is illustrated in Fig. 2.

The technique of suture depends on the age of the patient. In children growth is expected. Therefore, a continuous suture should not be used. Such a suture will first straighten out with growth and subsequently migrate through the wall of the vessel toward the intima. Dissection occurs with an internal constricting septum. The septum fenestrates and the suture, now on the inside of the artery, sloughs internally with a thrombus attached. In growing children, therefore, interrupted mattress sutures should be used instead of a continuous suture (Fig. 1, B), or the continuous suture may be used for one-half the circumference of the anastomosis and interrupted mattress sutures for the remainder.

A well-constructed suture line will leak very little after the vascular clamps are released. Some leakage usually will be observed as the tensions of continuous suture lines readjust to the intervascular pressure. Small openings will close spontaneously. It is wise first to remove the distal clamp, exposing the anastomosis to an initially lower pressure. Experience will teach the surgeon which

---

*Supplied by C. DeWitt Lukens Suture Mfg. Co., St. Louis, Mo.

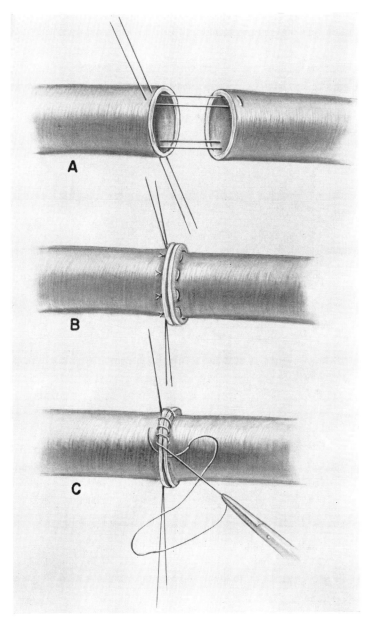

Fig. 1. Anastomosis of a moderate-sized artery. **A,** Placement of mattress sutures to begin anastomosis. **B,** Completion of end-to-end anastomosis with interrupted mattress sutures. **C,** Completion of end-to-end anastomosis with continuous everting suture. (Adapted from Linton, R. R.: Surgery **38:**817, 1955.)

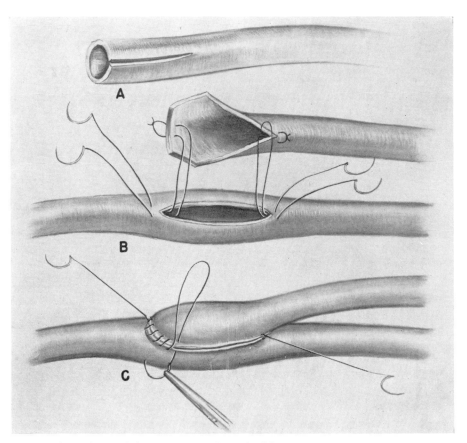

Fig. 2. End-to-side arterial anastomosis. **A,** End of blood vessel slit and shaped. **B,** Two everting mattress-type sutures inserted to begin closure. **C,** Closure completed with over-and-over technique. (Adapted from Linton, R. R.: Surgery **38:**817, 1955.)

leaks are self-sealing and which require correction. In aortic anastomoses some small leaks are repaired by sutures through the adventitia only. Blood flow should be shut off momentarily when an extra suture is to be placed. Sutures placed in an artery carrying blood under pressure or under full tension can only be placed in the cuff of the anastomosis. Otherwise more bleeding results from the new hole in the vessel. Tears may result when a needle is passed through a pulsating vessel. Patched anastomoses are less satisfactory. There is little substitute for precision and perfection of technique in anastomosis of small vessels. Suture lines in diseased or large arteries require sturdy wide cuffs and tight approximation of the edges.

Microsuture and microsurgical techniques

Microsuture techniques have been developed by Jacobson, employing a binocular dissecting microscope with magnifications of from 6× to 40×. An essential for this work is an objective lens of long working distance—eight to twelve inches. A rest is used to stabilize the hands and the blood vessels being operated upon. The instruments are modifications of those devised for ophthalmic surgery, and suture materials are very fine (7-0) silk or ultrafine monofilament nylon with a diameter of 0.001 inch.

Attempts to reconstruct arterial vessels and veins less than 4 mm. in diameter have been complicated by a high rate of thrombosis. The work of Jacobson and associates has illustrated that the basic principles of surgical technique necessary for successful primary vascular surgery are entirely applicable to small vessels. Using microscopic techniques, anastomoses can be accomplished in vessels as small as 1 mm. Sutures are placed much more closely than for larger work.

To date, the insertion of small prostheses has not proved practical because of the lining that forms within the prosthesis.

When microsurgical methods are perfected, many practical applications, particularly in the field of organ transplantation, can be foreseen. Under ordinary circumstances the surgeon may not have immediate access to the instruments and equipment necessary for microsurgical procedures. In dealing with smaller vessels in the 4 mm. to 6 mm. range, there should be no hesitancy to employ the long-focus binocular loupe used for ophthalmic surgery, which is usually readily available.

Nonsuture techniques

Various nonsuture techniques of vascular repair have been used recently. Perhaps the most familiar of these employs stapling instruments, a number of which are now available. With the exception of the Japanese (Nakayama) stapler, all are confined to use for end-to-end anastomoses. The Nakayama stapler, with which we have had considerable laboratory experience, may be used for both end-to-end and end-to-side anastomoses, as illustrated on pp. 5 and 6. All of these instruments promise to be useful in the union of small vessels in the 2 mm. to 4 mm. range. In general, however, there is not yet any wide clinical application. The instruments have long handles and are awkward to manipulate. A length of normal blood vessel is necessary to thread within the cuffs and anvils of their machinery, and atherosclerotic blood vessels cannot be handled easily. We do not, therefore, anticipate that such instruments will replace ordinary suture methods for large and/or diseased blood vessels. Indeed, with the help of a binocular operating microscope of long working distance, the human hand can probably surpass these instruments in precision, if not in speed.

Recently, rapid-setting amide-glue materials (2-methylcyanoacrylate) have been proposed to repair skin, bronchus, and blood vessels without the aid of sutures. Circumferential union of both arteries and veins has been accomplished with these materials, but with a high incidence of early thrombosis and late aneurysm formation. This technique of vascular repair continues to be experimental, and, like the stapling technique, does not possess the dependability, versatility, or precision of suture techniques.

Prevention of thromboses

Thrombosis after anastomosis in large arteries results mainly from turbulence and/or distal obstruction. In small vessels, however, other factors are also important, and refined techniques become more necessary. The clotting process is catalytic and is initiated by release of thromboplastin from injured intimal or other cells. In large arteries a thin layer of clot forms on the internal raw surface after removal of the intima by endarterectomy or after insertion of a prosthesis. There is no obstructive thrombosis if flow is rapid and if there is no narrowing or turbulence. The mechanical problems and also the release of thromboplastin initiated by injury are more troublesome in smaller vessels. Blood vessels should not be overstretched, and the intima should be disturbed or handled as little as possible. Occluding arterial clamps should be noncrushing. Guide sutures are helpful during anastomosis to hold vessels together with a minimum of instrumental handling. Cuffed types of anastomoses expose less suture material to the bloodstream than do those that have no cuff everted. Well-placed sutures are not significant causes of thrombosis.

Successful suture of small arteries requires atraumatic technique, lubrication of sutures, or the use of nonwetting sutures such as Teflon-coated Dacron or monofilament polyethylene, along with exclusion of adventitial tissue from the suture line. These techniques minimize the release of thromboplastin and thus the initiation of clotting. When a vessel is first opened, all blood should be immediately washed out with physiological saline solution. Washing out the blood before clotting minimizes the production of thrombin. Instillation of heparin solution into the vessel proximal and distal to the occluding clamps is advisable. Another hazard is formation of fibrin clot in areas of turbulent blood flow through rough or constricting anastomoses. These faulty anastomoses are always undesirable.

When a plastic prosthesis has been inserted, there is no intima, and it is necessary to depend on the clotting mechanism to seal the prosthesis and on rapid, unobstructed, smooth blood flow to prevent thrombosis on the interior of the prosthetic graft. The thin layer of fibrin is slowly replaced by flat lining tissue that resembles intima.

Ligation of major blood vessels

Sacrifice of major blood vessels produces disabling symptoms. Occasionally after a large artery has been ligated, gangrene does not develop, but arterial insufficiency may be disabling. The symptoms of such insufficiency are coldness, claudication, atrophy of the skin and muscles, pain, decrease in strength, sensory and motor disturbances, edema, and chronic cyanosis. All these unfavorable sequelae of ligation of major vessels can be avoided by restoration of vascular continuity. The aims of vascular surgery are to preserve and to restore blood flow when possible.

When ligation of a major blood vessel is unavoidable, selection of the best site is important. In general, ligation between proximal and distal collateral channels minimizes disability and the occurrence of gangrene. Ligation of certain arteries is known from experience to be relatively safe. The external carotid, the hypogastric, and the profunda femoris are examples of vessels that are ligated with impunity. Usually ligation of such vessels as the axillary, the external iliac, or the femoral artery below the exit of the profunda is severely disabling but is not accompanied by gangrene. Ligation of the subclavian artery, the femoral artery above the profunda or in the adductor canal, the internal carotid artery, or the common iliac artery is frequently catastrophic.

The surgical principles for ligation of major arteries are as follows:

1. Arteries should be divided and not ligated in continuity.
2. A transfixion ligature distal to the tie is advisable on large blood vessels to prevent dislodgment of the ligature by arterial pulsations.

3. Tensile strength and size of ligatures and suture ligatures must be sufficient so that there is little danger of breakage.
4. The ligatures should be tied squarely across the vessel with a secure square knot. Several extra "throws" are desirable for the utmost in security.
5. Ligatures should be tied close to the vessel wall, without including any surrounding tissue. Failure to isolate the vessel and the inclusion of peri-vascular areolar tissue and fat allow the ligature to slip off easily.

When large arteries are atherosclerotic, encircling ligatures may fragment and tear the brittle and calcific wall. It is sometimes better to close the vessel with a continuous everting suture over the open end. If the wall of the vessel is extremely hard, an endarterectomy may be necessary before closure can be accomplished. This suture technique also preserves collateral vessels that arise just proximal to the site of proposed ligation and that would otherwise be sacrificed to have sufficient cuff distal to the ligature.

Back bleeding from the distal portion of the ligated vessel is evidence of good collateral flow. In no case should distal ligature of the artery be omitted. It is not necessary to ligate veins accompanying arteries, as once suggested. Venous ligation increases the possibility of venous insufficiency and will not improve the arterial blood flow in the involved extremity.

Preoperative, operative, and postoperative use of anticoagulants

As a rule, use of anticoagulants postoperatively is unnecessary and unwise. The major exception is in patients who have undergone an extensive endarterectomy in the leg. If arterial prostheses are needed during emergency operations on patients who have received anticoagulants, the finest mesh prosthesis must be used even though its impervious fabric may lead to complications after months or years. Such complications (stenosis, septum formation, calcification, thrombosis, occlusion) are more troublesome and more frequent in prostheses of smaller diameters, particularly 8 mm. or smaller.

Regional heparinization is safer and much more useful than systemic administration of anticoagulants during vascular operations. When it is necessary to completely occlude a blood vessel, heparin (0.01%) is injected just prior to closure of the occluding arterial clamp. Similarly, a weak solution of heparin may be used to rinse the ends of arteries prior to suture and inhibit formation of thrombin clots.

It may be advisable to use heparin systemically in patients who have had extensive endarterectomy on the peripheral arteries of the leg. Doses of 50 to 75 mg. of heparin may be given while the patient is on the operating table and intermittently thereafter. Following embolectomy, anticoagulants may be indicated for prophylaxis of subsequent emboli. Regional heparinization is not so convenient as systemic anticoagulation. However, infusion of diluted heparin into the saphenous vein at the foot is recommended following iliofemoral thrombectomy.

Occasionally it is necessary to operate on a patient who is already receiving anticoagulants. In such instances, surgery may be undertaken with safety if prothrombin levels are within the range of 30% to 50%. If heparin has been the anticoagulant used, only a short waiting period is necessary, or rapidly acting antagonists such as protamine or hexadimethrine bromide (Polybrene) may be administered. When anticoagulation treatment is commenced in a patient who may need operation, heparin, of course, is preferred over the long-acting antiprothrombin type of anticoagulant.

INSTRUMENTS FOR VASCULAR SURGICAL PROCEDURES

A large number of especially designed clamps are now available for use in vascular surgery. This discussion illustrates the general characteristics and applications of diverse types of arterial clamps and instruments.

For popliteal, brachial, and similar small arteries, delicate clamps with spring handles and fine teeth, such as DeBakey peripheral vascular clamps (Fig. 3, A), are desirable. For larger arteries, the aorta, and aneurysms, clamps with wider jaws, deeper teeth, and grooves (Fig. 3, B) are more desirable.

A large selection of shapes and sizes of vascular clamps should be available to fit various arteries through any incisions. Handles of different shapes and lengths should also be available to permit the selection of one that will not be in the way when the artery is manipulated. Bulldog clamps may be useful for temporary occlusion of small arteries, but these clamps slip readily. Such clamps equipped with Potts teeth are more secure.

Special shaped clamps with arterial teeth are available and are suitable for various special procedures. The Satinsky clamp (Fig. 3, C) is useful for partially occluding the vena cava in portacaval anastomosis. Derra auricular clamps (Fig. 3, D) are useful to draw up and hold the subclavian artery.

Curved Metzenbaum scissors with the tips ground to resemble the Stevens tenotomy scissors are useful for perivascular dissection. The Potts-Smith angled scissors (Fig. 3, E) are necessary for longitudinal arteriotomies. Narrow smooth-tipped thumb forceps are customarily used to handle the artery in order to avoid intimal damage. A blunt right-angled nerve hook or a sharp-pointed skin hook (Fig. 3, F) is also useful as a retractor to separate the edges of an arterial anastomosis and to guide the suture as it is tightened.

Atraumatic vessel clamps can be improvised from rubber-shod, right-angled clamps or by tying rubber tubing or gauze about large blood vessels, or small [-shaped laboratory clamps may be used (Fig. 3, G and H).

LAWS OF FLUID FLOW AND THEIR APPLICATION TO VASCULAR SURGERY

Liquids flowing through conduits such as the vascular system flow in two fashions, laminar flow or turbulent flow.

Laminar flow

In laminar or streamline flow (Fig. 4, A) the liquid may be visualized as moving in infinitesimally thin and concentric cylindrical layers, parallel to the wall of the containing vessel. The basic law of laminar fluid flow is that of Poiseuille, a physician whose interest in the circulation of the blood led him to

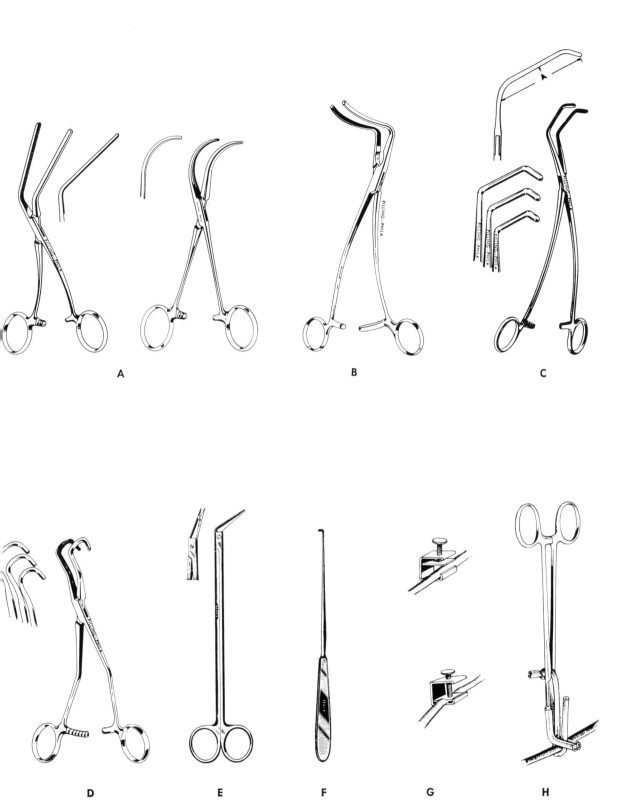

Fig. 3. Types of instruments employed in vascular surgical procedures. **A,** DeBakey peripheral vascular clamps, angled and curved. **B,** Aortic occlusion clamp. **C,** Satinsky clamps. **D,** Derra auricular clamps. **E,** Potts-Smith angled scissors. **F,** Nerve hook. **G,** Laboratory clamp. **H,** Improvised clamp. (**A-D,** Courtesy George P. Pilling & Son Co., Philadelphia, Pa.; **E-F,** courtesy Storz Instrument Co., St. Louis, Mo.)

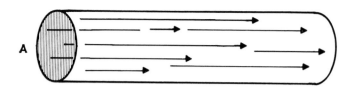

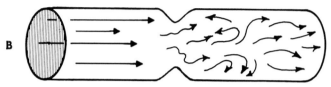

Fig. 4. A, Laminar flow. **B,** Turbulent flow.

study and quantitate the dynamics of fluid flow. His findings can be expressed mathematically as follows:

$$P = \frac{8\ L}{\pi\ R^4}\ V\ Q \tag{1}$$

P = Pressure difference (dynes/cm.²)
L = Length of tube in centimeters
R = Radius of tube in centimeters
V = A constant, the coefficient of viscosity, in poises
Q = Volume rate of flow (ml./sec.)

It can be seen from the equation that the change in pressure necessary to deliver a constant quantity of fluid varies directly with the length of the tube and inversely with the *fourth power* of the radius.

Laminar flow and a rigid straight tube are basic assumptions in deriving Poiseuille's law, either experimentally or theoretically. The law is not strictly applicable (1) to conditions of turbulent flow, (2) to colloidal or particulate suspensions, or (3) to elastic tubes.

With regard to the physiological systems, Poiseuille's law does indeed apply experimentally to viscous fluids in the blood vascular system, and hindrance in such systems remains constant through a wide range of pressures. Pulsatile instead of steady pressure does not alter the results. It is possible that the vessels both elongate and dilate to produce this result. At any rate, the behavior is analogous to a rigid system. Blood, however, is not a strictly viscous fluid but a pseudoplastic liquid that flows disproportionately faster as the propelling forces are increased. It is generally assumed that flow in the human arterial system is of the laminar nature when there is no deformity or disease.

Application of Bernoulli's theorem demonstrating pressure change when there is a change in tubular size with constant flow is graphically illustrated in Fig. 5. As shown, application of this theorem yields for P a figure of 1.16 p for the small increase 0.1 unit in radius (exaggerated in Fig. 5). Such considerations have been used to explain, for instance, poststenotic dilatation of a blood vessel. It is probable, however, that in poststenotic dilatation at least three influences are at work: (1) conversion of kinetic energy of motion into static energy avail-

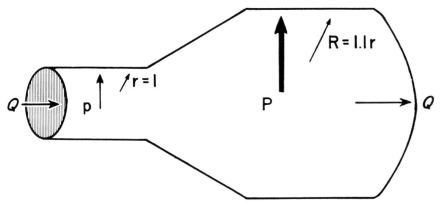

Fig. 5. Bernoulli's theorem, illustrating change in pressure with change in radius. Q = Q. R = 1.1 r (radius). P = 1.16 p (pressure).

able for lateral pressure on, and elastic deformation of, the blood vessel wall (Fig. 5), (2) conversion of kinetic energy of laminar or streamlined flow into static pressure as the result of turbulence just distal to the stenotic area in the blood vessel, and (3) fatigue phenomena that allow gradual weakening of the arterial walls where they are subjected to increased lateral pressure.

In poststenotic areas where turbulent flow has been created, small fibrin thrombi can be precipitated from the blood as the result of the localized area of turbulence, this being analogous to the familiar process of defibrinating blood by agitation with a wire stirring device.

Turbulent flow

Turbulent flow is the other major form of internal motion in moving fluids. In contrast to laminar flow, the fluid particles move in irregular paths at different angles to the main direction of motion (Fig. 4, *B*). Such flow is not so efficient as laminar flow. When turbulence is created in a streamlined system, pressure decreases secondary to the increased dissipation of energy in the form of internal frictional losses.

Conditions for turbulent flow can be determined from the following equation:

$$\text{Re} = \frac{2 \text{ VRP}}{\text{vis}} \qquad (2)$$

Re = Reynold's number (a dimensionless number)
V = Average velocity
R = Radius of conduit
P = Density
vis = Viscosity

When the right side of the equation exceeds the Reynold number for the fluid in question, streamlined flow becomes turbulent.

For human blood the Reynold number is approximately 970. Eliminating the constants of viscosity, density, and the number 2, it will be seen that flow velocity and the radius of the blood vessel determine the conditions necessary for turbulent flow and that turbulence would be difficult with a small velocity

13

or in a vessel of very small radius. Turbulence can also be influenced or created by the following:

1. Change in size of tube
2. Change in direction of tube
3. Irregularity of inner surface of tube
4. A branching system of tubes

Turbulence is more likely to be created by sudden changes in the diameter or direction of a tube or by sudden changes in flow velocities than by gradual changes in these factors. The points in the vascular system where such changes occur seem to be more susceptible to formation of arteriosclerotic plaques than the remainder of the vascular system.

Application

Vascular reconstruction, although bridging anatomical defects, does not necessarily produce an adequate physiological or functional conduit for the blood. It has been demonstrated at times that even though a pulse be present where none was present before, total blood flow is not materially increased.

Szilagyi and associates* have made extensive studies of grafting procedures and their effects upon blood flow. The experiments were conducted with a bubble flowmeter inserted into each femoral blood vessel of the experimental animal, with one side serving as a control. End-to-end anastomoses of a blood vessel reduced flow to 87% of control values. Replacement of a segment of vessel reduced blood flow to approximately 82% of control values. Comparison of a bypass graft with a linearly inserted graft as a control revealed a 20% reduction in flow through the bypass.

Increasing the internal diameter of bypass grafts allows an increase in blood flow until the graft has reached a diameter almost double that of the control vessel. After this there is again a decrease in flow, with further increases in size of the bypass graft. This phenomenon is possibly the result of the creation of turbulence as the product of V and R increases in equation 2.

When various plastic prosthetic materials are compared to intimal-lined homografts, flow is found to be 10% or 20% less through the prosthetic devices. This is a result of the internal surface irregularities of the prosthetic materials.

Practical applications resulting from consideration of the laws of fluid flow and from experimental measurements are as follows:

1. Avoid constricting anastomoses.
2. Optimum size for a prosthesis is somewhat larger, that is, 1.4 to 1.6 the diameter of the host vessel.
3. End-to-side anastomoses should be made bell mouthed when possible (Fig. 2).
4. Bypass prostheses should take off and enter the parent artery at oblique angles, simulating normal arterial bifurcations.

Critical stenosis

Recently a great deal of attention has been focused on the question of the factors influencing flow through a stenotic area in an artery. When measurements

---

*Szilagyi, D. E., and others: The laws of fluid flow and arterial grafting, Surgery **47**:55, 1960.

are made, it is at once apparent that a large diminution in arterial cross section is necessary before a significant reduction in flow can be observed. Obviously in such experiments adjustment in the totality of the circulation must also be considered. The results have clinical significance in two separate situations: (1) in determining if an observed narrowing is the cause of symptoms and (2) if an asymptomatic stenosis exists, in determining the effect of hypotension upon flow through it.

In experimental work, the results are different in those experiments that have retained the usual peripheral resistance of a perfused limb or brain rather than shunting blood into an adjacent vein. The former type of experiment has tended to demonstrate that a stenosis of as much as 80% may be necessary before flow is decreased. Such a stenosis is analogous to narrowing of a vessel by a localized plaque and not similar to the long rough area of stenosis in advanced atherosclerosis. When peripheral resistance is decreased by work, sympathectomy, or direct shunting to the venous system, less stenosis will produce a reduction in flow. The notion of a necessary "critical stenosis" elaborated by work of this type indicates some caution in attributing symptoms to relatively small alterations in the diameter of blood vessels, particularly in the carotid system.

An almost necessary corollary is that ischemic symptomatology such as stroke or myocardial infarct may be produced by a "critical combination" of stenosis, perfusion pressure reduction, and decreasing peripheral resistance.

SYNTHETIC ARTERIAL GRAFTS

Suitable vascular grafts fashioned of synthetic fabric materials have been made from a large number of different basic yarns. The fiber should be nontoxic, nonallergenic, and mechanically strong and durable. Other desirable properties depend upon the method of manufacture rather than upon the material. Knitted and crimped grafts behave better mechanically when flexed and also lengthen with pulsation in a manner similar to elastic arteries.

The suture materials used to insert arterial prostheses should also have long-lasting qualities. A number of patients in whom early prostheses were used developed aneurysms at the host-prosthesis suture line because the silk employed lost strength in the tissues over the years. Since no true healing takes place at the host artery-prosthesis junction, suture material must remain strong, and fraying and raveling at the cut edge of the prosthesis must not occur. Materials known to be stable over long periods are Dacron, Teflon, and polyethylene. Raveling depends upon the knit or weave. Woven fabrics and those constructed of Teflon tend to fray and ravel more than Dacron fabrics and knitted fabrics.

Porosity of the fabric also affects the long-term performance of prostheses by determining their degree of incorporation into the surrounding tissues and allowing fibroblasts to migrate through the porous walls and attach the neo-intimal lining of the graft to connective tissue surrounding the prosthesis. When a graft must be inserted in the thoracic cavity or in a patient who has been heparinized, considerations of porosity are set aside, and tightly woven fabrics must be chosen because of their lack of leakage. Otherwise, a porous graft will prove superior. Currently, preclotting the graft by allowing it to be momentarily distended with blood under pressure and then allowing time for clot to form before blood flow is reestablished is the most widely employed and most practical method of minimizing blood loss through porous grafts. Experimentation with the so-called compound prosthetic graft, using some absorbable agent such as gelatin to seal the graft temporarily or an absorbable fiber interwoven with the Dacron, has not yet yielded a practical graft.

The highest practical porosity and the best handling qualities may currently be found in a knitted Dacron material* that offers a combination of lightness, strength, and porosity, random small crimping, and freedom from raveling at the edges not equaled by other available materials.

When implanted, an arterial prosthesis becomes lined with fibrin which permeates the pores and prevents leakage. It becomes surrounded by a fibrous tissue capsule that becomes adherent as fibroblasts grow through the interstices of the fabric. Fibroblasts gradually replace the fibrin lining by growing through the pores and growing in from each end. This process of neointima formation, which may take place with relative dependability and rapidity in experimental animals, can be slow or incomplete in human beings. As implantation time lengthens, atheromas and calcification can develop in both homografts and synthetic fabric grafts.

If a graft material lacks porosity, the fibrin lining detaches with some ease, leading to septum formation and thrombosis with ultimate occlusion. Because of the lack of adherence to surrounding tissues, hematoma, serum collections, and infections dissect along low-porosity and nonwettable materials more easily. Secure and rapid healing is therefore facilitated by using a material with some porosity and by covering it with living tissue as a source of fibroblasts.

Several factors are involved in the prevention of thromboses in prosthetic materials. In addition to the firm attachment of the fibrinous lining of the graft, as detailed previously, desirable factors are (1) rapid blood flow through the prosthetic segment, (2) lack of distal obstruction so that rapid flow through the prosthesis is possible, and (3) avoidance of constricting or irregular anastomoses on which fibrin thrombi can form secondary to turbulent blood flow.

Because of the healing process within the lumen of prosthetic arterial grafts, the irregularities of the interior of the tube are soon smoothed over. Also, because the fibrin lining may thicken before healing occurs, the use of prostheses smaller than 8 mm. in diameter are inadvisable, and the incidence of immediate and late occlusion rises when prostheses of smaller diameters are used. Vein grafts have many advantages for long-term replacement of small arteries.

Infected arterial prostheses

Sepsis occurring in or about synthetic arterial prostheses is a dreaded complication. Arterial thrombosis and hemorrhage are the usual sequels when infection involves a host artery-prosthesis suture line. In these cases the prostheses must be removed and blood flow rerouted through new prostheses implanted in uncontaminated areas, bypassing the infected area completely.

When a host artery-prosthesis anastomosis is not involved, infected areas may be opened, drained, irrigated with antibiotics, and closed secondarily with some degree of success and without interruption of blood flow through the prosthesis. Consistent, intense and long-continued use of antibiotics adjusted to

---

*Wesolowski Weaveknit (Meadox) or fine-denier DeBakey prostheses.

the sensitivities of the infecting organisms is essential for success by this method.

When infection involves an anastomosis between a prosthesis and the host artery, disruption of the suture line and hemorrhage are inevitable if the infection is neglected. It is necessary to remove the prosthesis and ligate the host artery. The arterial tissue at the infected anastomosis will be friable.

Once an infected prosthesis has been removed and the danger of bleeding from the host artery has been eliminated, the question of further reconstruction arises. Individualization is obviously necessary in these cases. However, the general solution is that of operating with great care and inserting a longer bypass through tissue that has not been invaded by infection. In the femoral area, iliofemoral bypass may be accomplished from the terminal aorta or iliac artery using the obturator foramen as a passageway for the new prosthesis. Bypasses have been accomplished from as far proximal as the axillary artery for infected aortic bifurcation prostheses, and bypass from the opposite iliac or femoral artery is possible when infection is confined in the iliac region.

Chapter 2

Arteriography

INTRODUCTION AND GENERAL COMMENTS

Progress in vascular surgery has been dependent in many instances upon the development and improvement of angiographic techniques. Such techniques provide essential pathological and anatomical information prior to operation. Opacification of blood vessels for radiographic study was first performed only eleven weeks after Roentgen's discovery. However, refinements in equipment and techniques and improvement in the opacity and safety of contrast media have greatly advanced the clinical application of angiography.

Techniques suitable for visualizing the carotid, subclavian, vertebral, and femoral arteries and their branches, as well as the thoracic and abdominal aorta, are described. It is not unusual that special modifications to meet special circumstances must be devised and employed. Incorrect arterial puncture is the commonest cause of failure of angiographic techniques. When an area is inaccessible to arterial puncture or when it is advisable to make repeated x-ray films or to move the patient, retrograde catheterization is a useful technique.

In recent years contrast media for arteriography have been significantly improved. Meglumine iothalamate (Conray) has proved to have relatively low nephrotoxicity and neurotoxicity, both of which had previously been problems, particularly in direct translumbar aortography. Also, with its use there has been an acceptably low incidence of irritation to blood vessels, although it can cause some discomfort in unanesthetized patients. Several concentrations are available, and viscosity is low in the less concentrated solutions. The most concentrated solutions may be advantageously warmed to body temperature before injection.

When angiography is done under local anesthesia, patients always experience momentary pain in the area perfused by the radiopaque medium, with the sensation of heat, prickling, or burning. A transient flush may be observed, particularly in the extremities, and may last for several minutes. The combination of sensations may be extremely unpleasant, and patients should be warned and reassured prior to injection. Children and patients who are unable to cooperate will need general anesthesia to prevent motion during exposure of the films.

Roentgenograms of quality adequate for diagnosis can usually be obtained with a single injection of contrast medium. A rapid cassette changer is essential to obtain the finer details of filling and flow. To some extent, these details may also be obtained by using relatively long exposures on a single film. In femoral arteriography a single film will adequately delineate the common femoral artery and its branches, but a second injection and sequential films may be necessary to delineate the details of popliteal filling.

A simple apparatus, such as the Amplatz injector, is a very useful adjunct for the rapid-pressure injection of contrast media and is quite essential for transbrachial arch aortography and angiocardiography. For femoral arteriograms, adequate pressure through an 18-gauge needle may be obtained with a hand-held syringe, a 20 ml. syringe with finger grips being particularly effective. For translumbar aortograms, the medium can be rapidly injected using a large syringe with a 12-gauge outlet (Robb syringe) and a finger-grip attachment. When the material is injected by hand and a single film is used, a long exposure (1 second) should be employed.

CEREBRAL ARTERIOGRAPHY
Indications

Both the internal carotid and the vertebral arteries may be sites of obliterative lesions that cause cerebral arterial insufficiency. Symptoms of basilar artery insufficiency require radiographic examination of the vertebral arteries. Techniques employed for detection of extracranial obliterative lesions are not identical to those used for detection of intracranial disease.

An almost complete examination of the cerebral circulation is accomplished by percutaneous right transbrachial-cerebral arteriography combined with left percutaneous common carotid arteriography. Both common carotid arteries and their bifurcations, the internal carotid arteries, and the anterior and middle cerebral vessels should be visualized. When occlusive disease in the neck is suspected, lateral views are possibly more revealing than anteroposterior projections, but anteroposterior and Towne projections should be utilized to adequately visualize intracranial circulation, and particularly any intracranial crossover.

Preoperative care

Cerebral arteriography may be done under local anesthesia in cooperative patients. Preoperative medication should be generous, including a barbiturate.

Percutaneous transbrachial-cerebral arteriography

The use of percutaneous brachial artery puncture, together with pressure injection, is currently the best routine method of visualizing the proximal aortic arch, the right vertebral and common carotid arteries and their branches, and the innominate artery. Slightly delayed films will show the descending thoracic aorta and even the abdominal aorta. As a rule, the left carotid and left vertebral arteries are not well visualized, and to complete examination of the cerebral circulation an arteriogram of the left carotid artery must also be done. It is not necessary to visualize both vertebral arteries if there is adequate flow in one of them and no symptoms of basilar artery insufficiency. As a rule, therefore, transbrachial-cerebral angiography is performed on the right side in combination with an arteriogram of the left common carotid artery. When necessary to visualize the basilar circulation on the left in more detail, transbrachial-cerebral arteriograms may be made from the left side.

Occasionally, brachial puncture as described below may be used for simple visualization of the brachial artery, particularly when following up procedures for occlusive disease, congenital malformations, embolism, or suspected injury involving the brachial artery, the forearm, or the hand. In such cases, a tourniquet, digital pressure, or a blood pressure cuff over the proximal brachial artery will assure distal injection, and a pressure injector is not necessary.

Procedure—Percutaneous right transbrachial-cerebral arteriography

1. Place the patient in the supine position, with the upper portion of the chest, the neck and the head positioned over the automatic cassette-changing device. The Sanchez-Perez automatic seriograph that takes a sequence of six to twelve films at intervals of ½ to 1 second is quite satisfactory. Several views may be necessary. If available, simultaneous biplane x-ray films with two seriographic machines are desirable.

In those patients in whom buckling, tortuosity, or compression by osteophytes or by the transverse processes of the vertebras is suspected, cineradiography with rotation of the head and neck during injection may be necessary to demonstrate the suspected difficulty.

Place the right arm on a long arm board that will stabilize the entire arm, shoulder, and wrist. Place a pad about 1½ inches thick beneath the right elbow to secure hyperextension.

Comment: *Correct position of the arm is essential for safe and easy percutaneous puncture. Hyperextension at the elbow makes the brachial artery more superficial and prevents it from rolling. At times a small incision over the brachial artery may be needed. The best position of the wrist is variable, but usually the neutral position with the thumb toward the ceiling is satisfactory. In some patients the brachial artery is more readily palpable with the hand in full supination or pronation.*

2. Prepare and drape the antecubital region. Inject a small wheal of local anesthetic just distal to the most prominent pulsation of the brachial artery.

3. Transfix the brachial artery with a quick vertical thrust of a Seldinger No. 160 or similar type of arterial needle. During the puncture, compress and hold the artery with the opposite hand.

4. Remove the obturator from the arterial cannula and withdraw is slowly until a strong jet of arterial blood appears. Advance the cannula its full length into the lumen of the artery, tape it into position, and again insert the obturator.

5. Prepare the contrast medium. Remove the obturator from the arterial needle, and connect the needle securely to the pressure tubing filled with saline solution or contrast medium. Tape the tubing securely to the forearm.

6. Connect the pressure tubing to the automatic pressure injector, warn the patient regarding the sensations that he may soon feel, and rapidly inject about 60 ml. of Conray 600.* The automatic cassette changer may be started either

---

*Recently we have observed that Conray 400 is equally satisfactory for most purposes.

manually or by the automatic contacts built into some types of pressure injectors. No more than three injections should be made. Do not exceed a total dose of 150 ml. of Conray 600.

7. Irrigate the needle and maintain it in position until the films have been checked. On withdrawal, maintain light pressure over the puncture site for a few minutes with an alcohol sponge.

Left transbrachial-vertebral arteriography

The technique for left transbrachial-vertebral arteriography is the same as that described for right transbrachial-cerebral arteriography except that the left arm is used. An injection of 30 ml. of radiographic contrast medium is sufficient to show the left subclavian and vertebral arteries.

Left transbrachial aortography

Left transbrachial aortography may be used to visualize the descending thoracic aorta and occasionally the abdominal aorta. Use of the transbrachial route eliminates catheterization. A relatively large quantity of radiopaque material (about 100 ml. of Conray 600) should be used. Otherwise, the only modifications of technique are in the positioning of the patient, the film, and the x-ray tube.

The descending aorta is best visualized in the left anterior oblique view. Since timing may be somewhat difficult in abdominal aortography, a rapid cassette changer is necessary. In general, the translumbar route is superior for visualization of the abdominal aorta, but this approach is contraindicated in patients with aneurysms.

Procedure—Percutaneous carotid arteriography

1. Hyperextend the patient's head by placing a rolled towel or sandbag between the shoulders (Fig. 6, A). Excessive hyperextension is undesirable.

2. Make a wheal with a local anesthetic over the carotid pulsation at the anterior edge of sternocleidomastoid muscle and at about the level of the lower border of the thyroid cartilage, which marks the carotid bifurcation. Infiltrate the subcutaneous tissues with the anesthetic agent.

3. Turn the patient's head slightly away from the side of injection to stretch the artery and move it medial to the sternocleidomastoid. Insert a No. 18 Cournand needle almost vertically over the arterial pulsation, and when it is against the artery, transfix it quickly. Withdraw the obturator. Lower the hub of the needle, and withdraw the needle slowly. As the needle withdraws into the artery, a pulsatile stream of bright red blood will spurt from it. Now advance the needle about 1 cm. into the lumen of the vessel, depressing the hub to do so (Fig. 6, B). Connect plastic tubing and a syringe of saline solution. Inject saline solution slowly to keep the needle open.

4. For lateral views, straighten the head, remove the towels or other support from beneath the shoulders, and prepare a large (14″ × 17″) grid-front cassette to visualize both the head and neck. Allow blood to fill the tubing and drive out any bubbles. Connect a syringe containing 50% Hypaque or Conray 600. Caution the patient, and then rapidly inject 8 to 10 ml. of contrast medium, exposing the film toward the end of the injection. The needle may now be connected to a

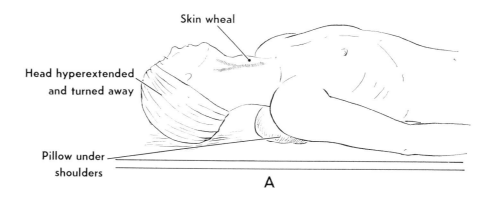

Skin wheal

Head hyperextended
and turned away

Pillow under
shoulders

A

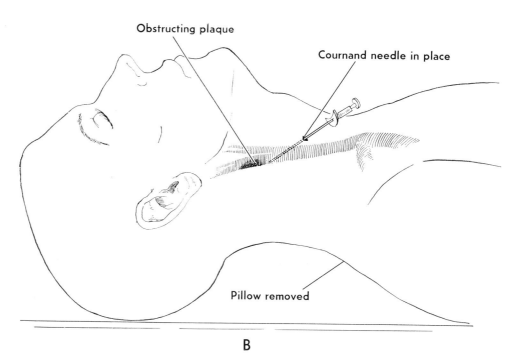

Obstructing plaque

Cournand needle in place

Pillow removed

B

Fig. 6. Position and landmarks for carotid arteriography. **A,** Position of head, neck, and shoulders for puncture. **B,** Position during exposure of radiographs.

syringe filled with saline solution or be plugged with the obturator until the films are developed and inspected.

The Towne view with the axial ray 20 to 30 degrees from the vertical will show the intracranial portion of the internal carotid artery projected away from the base of the skull. A rapid cassette changer, set to take four large ($11'' \times 14''$) films at 1-second intervals, is desirable. Both carotid arteries may be examined on the same day. However, no more than two injections are advisable on each side.

Postoperative care

Keep gentle pressure over the puncture site for a few minutes and apply a small bandage. An ice collar and mild analgesics are usually sufficient to control pain.

FEMORAL ARTERIOGRAPHY
Introduction

Examination of the arteries in the lower extremities via the femoral artery is one of the most frequently employed angiographic procedures. The indication for such examinations is usually arterial insufficiency associated with atherosclerotic occlusive disease. Careful evaluation is essential to choose the proper position of the leg and appropriate injection rates and exposure timing.

If disease of the iliac artery is suspected, the iliac arteries can be visualized by rapid injection into the common femoral artery in a retrograde fashion as described on p. 26. When a hand-held syringe is used, increased pressure for injection may be obtained by using a 20 ml. syringe with finger grips. The ipsilateral iliac artery and the aortic bifurcation and run-off into the opposite iliac and femoral arteries frequently can be visualized with a single injection.

In the presence of obstruction in the superficial femoral artery, popliteal filling from collateral vessels is a most significant preoperative finding. When searching for such information, sequential films produced by a rapid cassette changer are most desirable, if not essential, to catch the short, but delayed, filling phase.

Anatomy

The femoral artery is most superficial immediately distal to the inguinal ligament. Puncture at this level is technically easy, since the pulse is readily palpable and the vessel can be kept from rolling.

Procedure

1. Place the patient in the supine position. The entire leg is positioned over a specially constructed tunnel or over separate films, using separate x-ray machines.

2. Prepare and drape the inguinal region. Infiltrate the skin just over the femoral pulsation and just below the inguinal ligament with local anesthetic.

3. Place a finger on either side of the femoral pulsation to prevent the artery from moving (Fig. 7). Insert a small (No. 160) Seldinger, Cournand, or similar (disposable, 18 gauge, short bevel) needle at an angle of about 45 degrees to the skin. Direct the needle along the course of the femoral artery, roughly toward

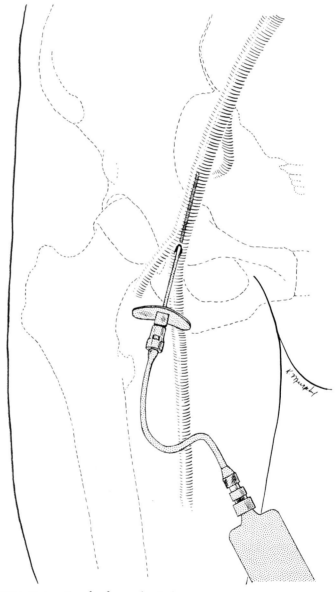

Fig. 7. Percutaneous puncture for femoral arteriogram.

Table 1. Techniques of femoral arteriography

Indication	Position	Needle	Injection time (sec.)	Repeat films	Comment
1. Unilateral occlusive disease of leg					
(a) Mild arterial insufficiency (intermittent claudication)	Anteroposterior with internal rotation of foot	18 gauge or 160	5-10	1 or 2	Prolonged injection avoids reflux of dye up into pelvis
(b) Moderate arterial insufficiency	Anteroposterior with internal rotation of foot	18 gauge or 160	12	1 or 2	To see block and outflow
(c) Severe femoral block (rest pain, gangrene)	Anteroposterior with internal rotation of foot	18 gauge or 160	15	Several films at 3-sec. to 5-sec. intervals	Circulation time to calf is slow and variable
2. Bilateral occlusive disease of legs and one iliac artery	Anteroposterior with internal rotation of foot	17 gauge, thin wall, or 205	5	Several films at 3-sec. to 5-sec. intervals	Visualize iliac arteries and terminal aorta by retrograde reflex; use 14" × 34" cassette first, then 14" × 17" films
3. Visualization of popliteal artery	Maximum internal rotation of foot	17 gauge, thin wall, or 205	5	Use multiple films in cassette changer	This position widens interosseous space and outflow can be seen without overlying bone
(a) Outflow					
(b) Popliteal aneurysm	Lateral				
4. Visualization of calf or fine details of thigh					
(a) Arteriovenous fistula	According to location	17 gauge, thin wall, or 205	5	6 films at 0.5-sec. intervals	Rapid circulation time and rapid dilution of dye require rapid injection
(b) Congenital anomalies	According to location	17 gauge, thin wall, or 205		6 films at 0.5-sec. intervals	To visualize small vessels in capillary and venous phases
(c) Tumors of bone or soft tissue	According to location	17 gauge, thin wall, or 205	5	6 films at 0.5-sec. intervals	To visualize small vessels in capillary and venous phases
(d) Arterial injuries	According to location	17 gauge, thin wall, or 205		6 films at 0.5-sec. intervals	Techniques according to findings in 1, 2, or 3 under Indications

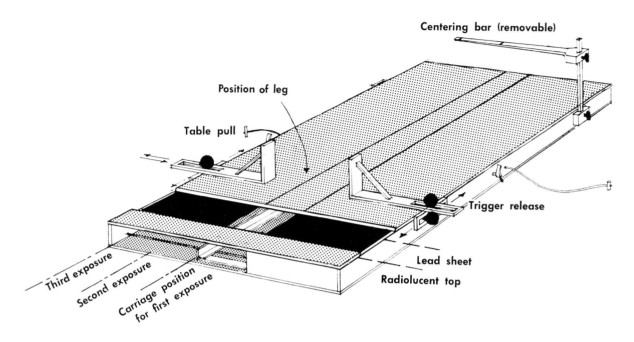

Fig. 8. Radiographic tunnel for multiple exposures of entire leg. (Courtesy Dr. Noah Susman, St. Louis, Mo.)

the umbilicus. Advance the needle until the arterial pulsation can be felt. Now penetrate the artery quickly, transfixing it if necessary. Withdraw the obturator and inner needle. Withdraw the cannula slowly until a pulsatile flow of bright red blood appears. Now depress the hub of the cannula toward the skin. Advance the cannula within the artery for about 1 to 2 cm. Connect plastic tubing and a syringe filled with saline solution (Fig. 7).

4. Details of position, needle size, volume of injection, concentration of medium, and exposure may vary according to the indications for angiography (Table 1).

Two or three exposures may be made on the same 14″ × 34″ film in a specially constructed tunnel (Fig. 8). With this device the cassette is held in a tunnel that shields the remainder of the film. The radiolucent portion of the cover is moved sidewise at appropriate intervals for consecutive exposures. For arteriovenous fistula, a rapid cassette changer positioned below the fistula should be employed because of the rapid circulation time. Occasionally, multiple films obtained with the rapid changer under the knee and calf show additional desirable details of the popliteal artery and its branches.

Retrograde aortogram and bilateral femoral arteriogram

If one femoral pulse is palpable, the terminal aorta and both iliac and femoral arteries may be visualized by the percutaneous femoral route, injecting the medium up and around by forceful hand injection. This technique has supplanted the translumbar aortogram and retrograde catheterization except for special purposes.

Procedure

1. Anesthesia, preparation, and draping are identical with those for angiography of the leg by the femoral route. Have the patient practice the Valsalva maneuver with your command to "shoot" on the count of 10.

2. Make the femoral puncture with a large (No. 205) Seldinger needle. Connect to a 50 ml. syringe of 60% contrast medium in a large-bore (Robb) syringe or to a syringe-pressure injector mechanism.

3. Position the patient over a large film to show the terminal aorta. After injection, expose several 14" × 17" films beneath the thigh and leg to demonstrate the pattern of flow through the extremities. Inject contrast medium as rapidly as possible after the Valsalva maneuver has been held for 10 seconds. Expose the abdominal film, using a long exposure time (1 second) just before the completion of the injection.

Postoperative care

Withdraw the needle after inspecting the films. Hold firm pressure over the puncture site for five minutes. When using a large-bore needle, compression for ten minutes may be necessary. Pain is usually minimal, and complications are rare.

Discussion

A complete map of the arteries from the terminal aorta to the midcalf area may be obtained by the percutaneous femoral route. Thorough investigation is mandatory prior to any elective operation, since one of the more common causes of failure to restore blood flow after operation is unrecognized and uncorrected narrowing of vessels proximal or distal to the site of surgery. Retrograde catheterization of the iliac arteries may be difficult if the patient has occlusive disease and unnecessary if reflux injection via the cannula is successful. If neither femoral pulse is palpable, the retrograde method cannot be employed and translumbar aortography becomes necessary.

TRANSLUMBAR AORTOGRAPHY

Translumbar aortography is performed to investigate occlusive disease of the abdominal aorta, the aortic visceral branches, the iliac arteries, and the proximal portion of the common femoral arteries. It is unwise to use this method for the investigation of possible aneurysm of the abdominal aorta. For lateral views of the renal, superior mesenteric, and celiac arteries, a long needle with a Teflon cannula fitted over it may be employed, the patient being turned after withdrawal of the metallic portion of the needle.

Contraindications to the use of translumbar aortography are hemorrhagic disease, severe hypertension, renal disease, and suspected aneurysm of the abdominal aorta. In aneurysm a central channel surrounded by atheromatous material may give a false picture of the pathology. In addition, the point of entrance of the needle is at the usual site of rupture, so that this catastrophic emergency may be precipitated by attempted aortography. Alternative techniques for visualization of the aorta and its branches are intravenous aortography and selective retrograde catheterization of the aorta and its branches. The latter technique is described later in this chapter.

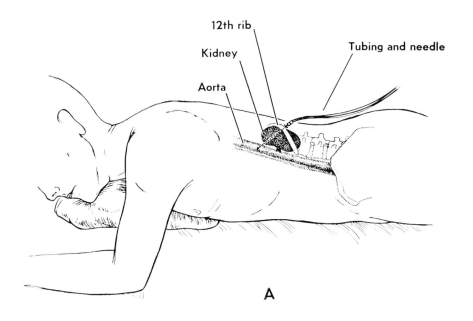

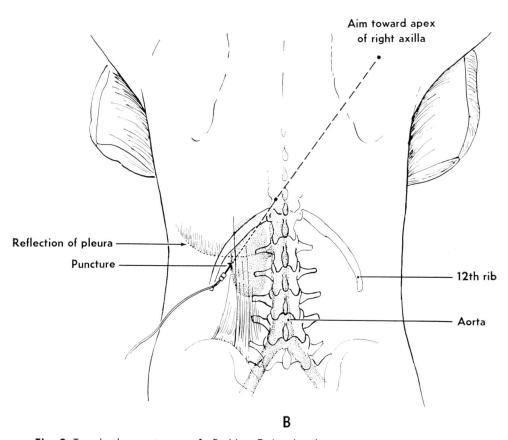

Fig. 9. Translumbar aortogram. **A,** Position. **B,** Landmarks.

Adequate hydration should be maintained. When impaired renal function may be due to vascular insufficiency, and this is the reason for aortography, the translumbar aortogram should be performed during mannitol diuresis induced by the infusion of 500 ml. of 5% to 10% mannitol solution (Osmitrol).

Anesthesia

Either local or general anesthesia is satisfactory. Local anesthesia is preferred unless the patient is extremely apprehensive and restless.

Position

Place the patient in the prone position (Fig. 9, A). A pillow may be placed under the shoulders and upper chest but not under the abdomen. A pillow under the abdomen places the aorta at a greater distance from the skin.

Procedure

1. Administer an intravenous dose of contrast medium to test sensitivity, using 4 or 5 ml.

2. Prepare and drape the skin of the back on the left side. The site of injection is 2 cm. below the twelfth rib on the left and 5 or 6 cm. to the left of the midline (Fig. 9, B). Infiltrate the site of injection with local anesthetic. Advance the needle along the line that will be followed by the long aortographic needle, and infiltrate a small amount of anesthetic agent into the sacrospinalis muscle mass.

3. Make a small stab wound in the skin at the anesthetized site. Introduce a 17-gauge 7-inch Touhy thin-wall needle, directing it toward the apex of the right axilla. The side of the vertebral body is usually encountered. When this happens, withdraw the needle slightly and redirect it at a somewhat more acute angle with the midsagittal plane.

4. A brisk pulsating stream of bright red blood will spurt out when the needle has punctured the aorta. Test the patency of the connection with a small amount of saline solution. Flow should be without significant resistance and without pain if the patient is awake. Do not inject contrast medium if the flow of blood is slow, if it is dark in color, or if it is not definitely pulsatile. When the needle is introduced, the tip should lie within the abdominal aorta, at the level of the eleventh or twelfth thoracic vertebra, and well above the visceral branches of the aorta.

5. Connect the needle to a syringe filled with Conray 600 and plastic connecting tubing. Rapidly inject 10 ml. of contrast medium and immediately expose the first film. The film will confirm that the needle is properly placed and is not opposite or in the orifice of the renal artery or other vital visceral branches. Keep the needle open with small injections of saline solution until the test film has been developed. When all is satisfactory, inject 30 to 50 ml. of contrast medium by pressure injection. Expose the abdominal film immediately. A second exposure may be arranged at a lower level to show the femoral arteries.

6. Withdraw the needle. If the initial films are unsuccessful, do not make another attempt at translumbar aortography on the same day. Second injections have proved dangerous.

Complications

Complications are rare when suitable precautions are taken and safe routines enforced.

Retroperitoneal extravasation

Retroperitoneal extravasation of contrast medium usually causes no ill effects. X-ray films show the contrast medium spreading along the vertebral column. Temporary back pain and warmth in the left leg due to increased blood flow rapidly subside.

Hemorrhage

Minor leakage from the puncture site causes no difficulty. Aortography is contraindicated for patients with hemorrhagic diathesis and for those receiving anticoagulant therapy. The Touhy needle makes a smaller puncture wound than needles with conventionally tapered points. Multiple punctures should be avoided, and translumbar aortography should not be employed if there is any suspicion of aortic aneurysm.

Renal damage

Renal damage is a frequent serious complication of translumbar aortography. Significant renal disease is consequently a contraindication unless stenosis or occlusion of a renal artery is suspected. Trial radiographs after injection of 10 ml. of contrast medium are recommended to avoid accidental injection of large amounts of contrast medium directly into the renal arteries. Normally, the tip of the aortographic needle will lie well above the origin of the renal arteries and the trial dose will be delivered directly into the aorta. The volume of contrast medium injected at any day's examination should be limited to about 50 ml. Multiple and repeated injections must be avoided, even though the contrast material is not directed exclusively into the renal arteries. Patients should be well hydrated at the time of examination. Mannitol diuresis is advisable during renal arteriograms if renal function is borderline.

Intramural dissection of aorta

Dissection of the aortic wall by contrast medium has been observed without harmful effects. However, it causes pain and discomfort. This complication is avoided by not injecting contrast medium unless there is a free pulsatile flow of blood and by testing the position of the needle with a small trial injection of 10 ml. of contrast medium. Intramural dissection occurs if the tip of the needle lies partly in the aortic wall during the injection of contrast medium. Such dissection might tear or occlude the origins of small branches, causing ischemia of the spinal cord or other organs.

Paraplegia

Paraplegia is one of the rarer but most feared complications of translumbar aortography. The incidence of paraplegia is reduced by using less toxic contrast media, by employing smaller amounts of medium, and by insisting on correct placement of the needle. The toxicity of contrast agents increases with repeated injections, and more than half of the patients with paraplegia received more than one injection during the same examination.

This tragic complication is fortunately rare, the incidence being estimated at 0.2%. Fear of the complication has encouraged more frequent employment of other methods to visualize the aorta and its branches, such as intravenous aortography and percutaneous retrograde catheterization of the aorta.

SELECTIVE PERCUTANEOUS RETROGRADE AORTIC CATHETERIZATION

Selective retrograde catheterization is a valuable and rather universally applicable technique for visualization of many portions of the arterial tree. Selective retrograde techniques employing long catheters have been extended to visualize the renal, coronary, and bronchial arterial circulations in detail in combination with cinefluoroscopic roentgenographic techniques.

Retrograde aortography has several advantages over the translumbar method, including better visualization, greater scope in visualization, and freedom in positioning the patient. The method described may also be employed in conjunction with retrograde pyelograms. Intravenous aortography is employed when iliac vessels are occluded or when aneurysms of the aorta preclude safe and accurate passage of retrograde catheters.

Selective retrograde aortography can usually be performed by the cutaneous route, via the femoral vessels in adults. Open operation is preferable for the brachial artery and also for the small femoral vessel in infants and children.

The most versatile material for special aortic catheters to visualize particular locations, such as mesenteric, renal, or hepatic vessels, is the soft but relatively firm and thick-walled x-ray-opaque polyethylene (Ödman-Leden*) tubing. Special tips may be formed by heating the material at relatively low temperatures, facilitating catheterization of various branches of the aorta. This soft material has the disadvantage of requiring cold sterilization in bactericidal solution or by gas. When retrograde aortography is to be done, catheters of proper length, and with whatever curved tips may be necessary, should be designed and carefully prepared in advance.

Anesthesia

General anesthesia may be employed. However, local infiltration with adequate preoperative medication, including a barbiturate, is quite satisfactory.

Seldinger technique

Retrograde aortography was originally performed by introducing a needle into the femoral artery and passing a small polyethylene catheter through it. Hematomas occurred frequently because the hole in the artery was considerably larger than the catheter within it. With the Seldinger technique larger catheters can be passed through small punctures by using a flexible metal guide.

The Seldinger technique employs three basic pieces of apparatus: a thin-walled pointed needle, a blunt outer cannula that cannot injure the arterial wall (Fig. 10, B), and a flexible metal guide. The cannula is introduced into the ar-

---

*Similar materials are now available from Becton-Dickinson & Co., Rutherford, N. J.

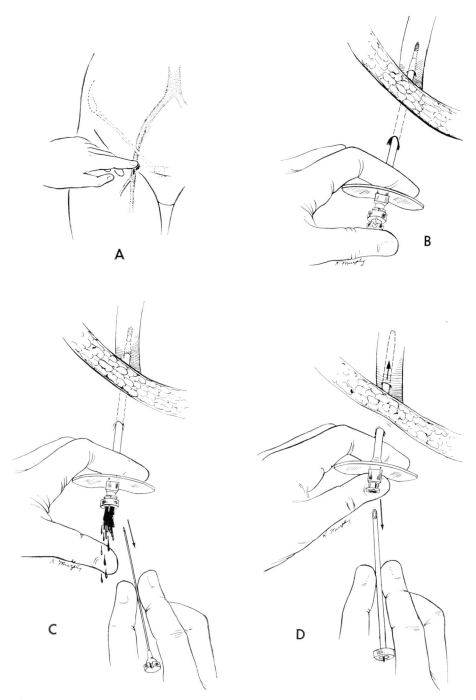

Fig. 10. Percutaneous retrograde catheterization of aorta. **A** and **B,** Insert needle just below inguinal ligament. **C,** Withdraw stylet and observe pulsatile bleeding. **D,** Withdraw sharp obturator and advance cannula.

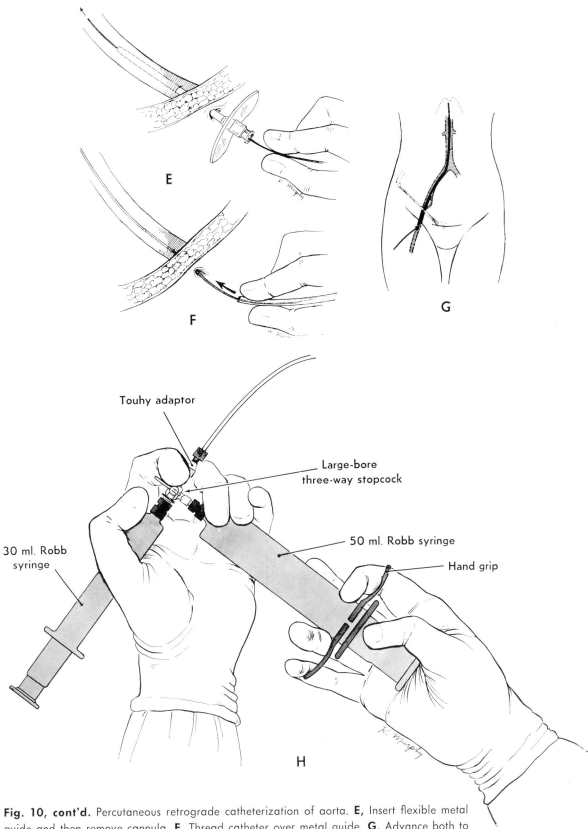

Fig. 10, cont'd. Percutaneous retrograde catheterization of aorta. **E,** Insert flexible metal guide and then remove cannula. **F,** Thread catheter over metal guide. **G,** Advance both to desired location in artery. **H,** Arrangement of equipment for rapid injection by hand.

33

tery with the pointed needle within it. The needle is withdrawn to permit introduction of a flexible guide through the cannula instead of the needle. The cannula is withdrawn, leaving the guide in the artery. Finally, the angiographic catheter is threaded over the guide and thence into the artery. Positioning is done fluoroscopically, after which the guide is withdrawn to permit the injection of contrast medium.

Procedure

The skin of the groin has been previously shaved and prepared. The catheters used in this procedure may be several feet long and must not touch an unsterile field. Consequently, the operators should wear sterile gowns, and the operative area should be draped widely.

1. Infiltrate the area overlying the femoral pulse and just below the inguinal ligament with a local anesthetic. Make a small vertical ¼-inch incision through the skin. (See Fig. 10, A.)

2. Introduce a Seldinger needle, slowly, until the arterial pulsation is felt. Pierce the arterial wall with a quick motion. The artery is usually transfixed. (See Fig. 10, B.)

3. Remove the stylet. If the artery has been transfixed, withdraw the needle slowly. When the tip is in the artery, there will be a pulsatile flow of bright red blood from the needle. (See Fig. 10, C.)

4. Remove the sharp inner needle, leaving the blunt cannula in the artery. Advance the blunt cannula proximally for 1 to 2 cm. (See Fig. 10, D.)

5. Insert the flexible wire guide (Fig. 10, E). Guides are available in several lengths, and the length of the guide is chosen to reach the site for radiological examination. When the flexible guide has been introduced several centimeters beyond the tip of the needle, withdraw the blunt cannula.

6. Now pass the catheter over the guide (Fig. 10, F). This catheter must be of known length and always shorter than the total length of the guide.

When the catheter reaches the skin, advance it and the arterial guide together until the catheter is several inches within the artery. Withdraw the flexible guide partially until it protrudes only slightly from the plastic tubing. This is determined by measurement of both prior to insertion. Now advance the guide and catheter together to the desired injection site.

7. Scout films, fluoroscopy, or image intensification fluoroscopy is employed to check the location of the catheter. The flexible metal guide should be retained within the catheter during the introduction in order to prevent bending or kinking of the tubing. (See Fig. 10, G.)

8. When the position of the catheter is satisfactory, withdraw the guide. Connect the plastic tubing to the coupling and the combination of syringes and three-way stopcock illustrated (Fig. 10, H). The arrangement of syringes makes a convenient handle and allows considerable pressure to be placed on the injecting syringe. Inject the contrast medium by hand under as much pressure as possible or, preferably, in 0.5 to 1.5 seconds with a mechanical injector. The amount and other details vary somewhat, depending upon the area to be visualized (Table 2). A small trial injection of 10 ml. of contrast medium is usually advisable to check the position of the catheter.

Table 2. Retrograde catheterization of the aorta

Purpose	Puncture	Seldinger needle	Position of catheter	Volume	Films and position
Aortic arch arteriogram	Femoral	No. 205	Arch of aorta	100 ml. mechanically	Biplane changer with carotid compression
Aortic-renal arteriogram	Femoral	No. 160 or 205	Twelfth thoracic vertebral level	10-30 ml.	Supine; changer or single film
Superior mesenteric arteriogram	Femoral	No. 205	Twelfth thoracic vertebral level	50 ml.	Supine and lateral; single films
Terminal aorta and bilateral femoral arteriogram	Femoral	No. 205	Catheter usually unnecessary	50 ml.	Supine; single film

Special catheters are available for special purposes. Tips are sometimes bent to go around the arch or into selected orifices. Radiopaque catheters have thick walls and small lumens. Side holes at the tips prevent recoil of the tip during brisk injection.

OPERATIVE ARTERIOGRAMS

Emergency situations occasionally arise wherein arteriograms must be obtained on the operating room table. Such situations most frequently arise when operative findings in patients with traumatic injuries or embolism suggest distal arteriosclerosis, thrombosis, or distal embolism that was unsuspected before operation.

In vascular operations on an extremity it is always wise to prepare and drape the entire limb, since this will facilitate distal exploration or arteriography when necessary.

The x-ray grid-front cassette is placed in a sterile pillowcase and positioned under the limb or other part to be investigated. The artery, vein, or prosthesis is then punctured for injection of contrast medium. Alternatively, a small or tapered catheter may be held in place by a Javid clamp for the arteriogram. From 10 to 30 ml. of contrast medium is then injected in the same way as for any other arteriographic procedure, using relatively long exposures and injection times. Immediately afterward, the artery should be flushed with about 100 ml. of dilute heparin solution in normal saline solution to prevent excessive arterial irritation and possible spasm.

Operative arteriography should be used routinely after reconstructive procedures in the lower extremity and after embolectomy or at any other time that operative findings suggest or operative procedures depend upon distal obstruction. After femoral bypass, operative arteriograms are useful to check the distal anastomosis and may occasionally reveal a distal dissection or flap formation otherwise unsuspected.

Chapter 3

Aneurysms of the abdominal aorta

EXPLORATION OF ABDOMINAL AORTA

Aneurysm, localized occlusive disease, and embolic disease are conditions of the abdominal aorta that are correctable by surgical operation with highly satisfactory results and modest risk.

Surgical anatomy and physiology

The infrarenal portion of the aorta and the iliac arteries are readily uncovered by incisions in the posterior parietal peritoneum and dissection in an avascular retroperitoneal plane. The duodenum, small bowel, and sigmoid colon may be readily mobilized. The only important structures overlying the lower portion of the abdominal aorta are the sigmoid colon and its mesentery and, retroperitoneally, the ureters. Lymphatic vessels appear anterior to the aorta as fibrous bands and are divided without danger. Aneurysms of the aorta are frequently adherent to the vena cava or to the iliac veins, especially the right, and may make resection difficult and dangerous.

Although most of the pathological conditions of the abdominal aorta are centered below the renal arteries, the visceral branches of the upper abdominal aorta may develop aneurysmal or atherosclerotic disease that can be surgically corrected. Details for exposure of these vessels are presented elsewhere (Chapter 9).

Occlusion time is not especially critical when the aorta is clamped below the renal arteries. However, prolonged occlusion should be avoided. Flow through the aorta and one leg can usually be reestablished within forty-five minutes to one hour. Prolonged cross clamping leads to complications and may result in poor renal function following aortic surgery. Experimental evidence regarding noxious reflexes arising from clamping the aorta is conflicting, but complications from embolism by atherosclerotic sludge and from prolonged hypotension are more frequent. Methods that avoid such complications are described in this chapter.

36

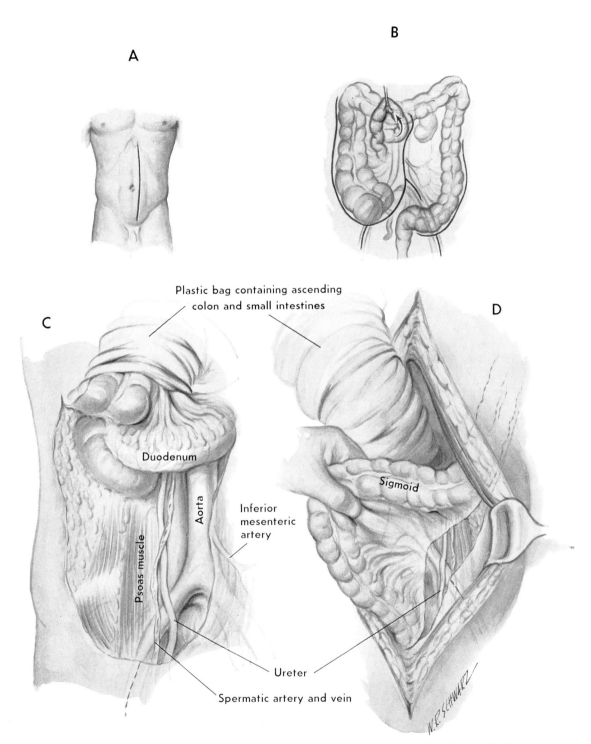

A

B

C

D

Plastic bag containing ascending
colon and small intestines

Duodenum

Aorta

Psoas muscle

Inferior
mesenteric
artery

Sigmoid

Ureter

Spermatic artery and vein

W.P.SCHWARZ

Fig. 11. Exploration of abdominal aorta. **A,** Incision. **B,** Peritoneal incisions. **C,** Retro-peritoneal structures on right side after delivery of ascending colon and small bowel out-side abdomen. **D,** Exposure of left external iliac artery by reflection of sigmoid colon.

Surgical exploration

1. Make an incision from the xiphoid to the pubis (Fig. 11, *A*). Shorter incisions usually prove inadequate, and the long incision is necessary even though only the lower aorta is to be explored. The paramedian route is illustrated, but midline incisions are now preferred.

2. Retract the small intestine to the right. Incise the posterior parietal peritoneum overlying the aorta. This is medial to the mesentery of the small bowel. The incision is expedited by delicately elevating the peritoneum alone, sliding the dissecting scissors underneath it, and then dividing the isolated leaflet of peritoneum. Fig. 11, *B*, shows this incision extended to mobilize the ascending colon, a procedure that may be necessary in obese persons (Fig. 11, *C*). Further upward exposure of the aorta is obtained by upward extension of the peritoneal incision, division of the ligament of Treitz, and retraction of the third portion of the duodenum to the right.

3. When delivery of the small intestine and ascending colon outside the abdomen is necessary, the intestine should be protected with pads soaked in warm saline solution and enclosed in a Lahey bag or plastic sheet. Thus protected, the entire intestine supplied by the superior mesenteric artery may be delivered from the abdomen. Helpful adjuncts in obtaining adequate exposure are oversized retractors made in extra depths (5 inches and 7 inches) and similar widths for this purpose.

4. For access to the left iliac artery, extend the incision over the aorta downward along the left iliac artery and make an additional incision in the posterior parietal peritoneum lateral to the lower portion of the descending colon and the upper sigmoid colon (Fig. 11, *B*). Elevate the sigmoid colon (Fig. 11, *D*). The left ureter can be identified readily to the left of the sigmoid mesentery and may be allowed to remain in situ. Isolation and retraction of the ureter with a tape is usually unnecessary.

RESECTION OF ANEURYSMS OF ABDOMINAL AORTA
Introduction

Resection of aneurysms of the abdominal aorta can be performed with reasonable risk but requires more than average surgical skill. Resection of the entire sac is unnecessary and frequently hazardous. Usually we leave some of the sac and use it to cover the prosthesis (Figs. 16 and 17). Surgery is almost always advisable because arteriosclerotic aneurysms that cause symptoms usually continue to enlarge and rupture within a year. Operation is advised for patients with large aneurysms, aneurysms observed to increase in size, and aneurysms that cause other symptoms. Because of the magnitude of the procedure, operation is contraindicated in patients with serious medical diseases who already have a poor prognosis. Operation is not advised for extremely elderly patients or those who present an excessively high surgical risk. Such patients are poor risks and complications are usually catastrophic. However, in experienced hands, the mortality of elective resection should not exceed 10%.

Preoperative preparation and anesthesia

Aortograms, particularly lumbar aortograms, are unnecessary and may even be dangerous. Aneurysmal sacs are filled with laminated clot, so that the channel may appear normal on the arteriograms. The only certain way to determine operability, size, and location of the aneurysm is surgical exploration.

We advise prophylactic digitalization for this and all other major arterial surgery in elderly patients.

Bowel preparation with neomycin and succinylsulfathiazole (Sulfasuxidine) is essential. Sigmoid or rectal ischemia can occur because sacrifice of the inferior mesenteric artery is always necessary and the collateral circulation to the colon may be barely sufficient.

Light general and endotracheal anesthesia should be supplemented by muscle relaxants when necessary. Begin an infusion of 500 ml. of 10% mannitol* in patients with large aneurysms or with borderline renal function. The anesthesiologist must prevent hypotension by proper blood replacement. Usually two or three pints of blood will be required, but at least 6 units should be on hand before operation. Before the aortic clamp is released, blood must be running at a rapid rate in a large vein. Rapid transfusion requires a cannula and, if necessary, surgical cutdown is performed before the operation is begun.

Procedure

1. Place the patient in the supine position. Palpate and mark the pedal pulses for future reference. Insert a urethral catheter for measurement of urine output during and after surgery. Prepare and drape the groin as well as the abdomen so that this area will be accessible if necessary.

2. Make a long midline or paramedian incision extending from the xiphoid to the pubis (Fig. 12, A). Explore the abdominal cavity for evidence of other disease. Retract the small intestine to the right, uncovering the aorta. If necessary, the small intestine may be displaced from the abdomen. Incise the peritoneum at the left side of the mesentery of the small bowel and divide the ligament of Treitz to permit retraction of the duodenum and small bowel farther to the right. Incise the peritoneum over the left common iliac artery and retract the sigmoid mesentery to the left to uncover the left common iliac artery as far as its bifurcation. Usually the left ureter cannot be seen from the medial side. To retract the sigmoid mesentery farther to the left, ligate and divide the inferior mesenteric artery at its origin from the aorta. Do not disturb the connection between the left colic and sigmoid branches.

Comment: *Good exposure and thorough exploration are essential for safety. The incision must be long, and the small bowel must be retracted well out of the way. We have never regretted delivery of the small intestine outside the abdomen. Keep the intestine moist, covered, and warm. This is accomplished by protecting the bowel with a large piece of gauze moistened with saline solution and covering it with a piece of plastic sheet or a Lahey bag. (See pp. 36-38 for more details regarding exploration of the aorta.)*

3. Determine the operability of the lesion as follows. Identify the left renal vein as it crosses the aorta. Find the inferior mesenteric vein in the edge of the left mesocolon, crossing the aneurysm and vanishing beneath the pancreas to join the splenic vein. Dissect around the sides of the aorta at the level of the

---

*Solutions of mannitol are commercially available (Osmitrol), or 12.5 or 25 Gm. may be added to 800 ml. of 5% dextrose in water.

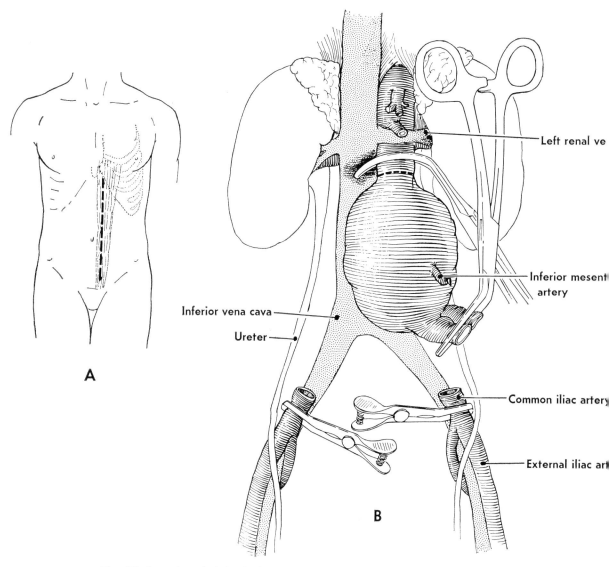

Left renal ve

Inferior mesent
artery

Inferior vena cava

Ureter

Common iliac artery

External iliac ar

Fig. 12. Resection of abdominal aneurysms. **A,** Incision. **B,** Resection. *Continued.*

left renal vein. The aorta is most likely to be free from the inferior vena cava at this high level.

Comment: *The neck of the aneurysm always appears wide and anterior in position. Dissection posteriorly reveals that the aneurysmal sac has lifted the posterior wall of the proximal aorta forward, leaving a triangular space between the proximal aorta and the spine. There is 1 inch or more of relatively normal aorta between the left renal artery and the aneurysm. The availability of a variety of prostheses permits reconstruction even though the diameter of the aorta at this level may exceed 25 mm. Almost all abdominal aneurysms have been operable since appropriate sizes of prostheses have been available and since we have learned to find the "free angle" between the proximal aorta and the spine.*

4. Obtain proximal control of the aorta above the aneurysm. Dissect around the back of the aorta, using Semb forceps. Make maximum use of the free space

already mentioned between the posterior aortic wall and the spine just proximal to the aneurysmal sac. Pass an umbilical tape about the aorta. Select an aortic clamp of appropriate size and angulation. Usually a straight clamp is applied vertically. A Glover or DeBakey aortic clamp applied transversely fits well also.

5. Obtain control of the iliac arteries distal to the aneurysm. Dissect the iliac arteries free from the underlying veins distal to the aneurysm and pass umbilical tape about them. This assures distal control of the aneurysm. Avoid the ureters.

Comment: *Secondary aneurysms can be present in one or both common iliac arteries. Save at least one hypogastric artery for blood supply to the pelvic organs. Coincidental occlusive disease may be present and may require local endarterectomy. Long occlusions may be bypassed by connecting the end of the graft to the side of the iliac artery distal to the occlusion.*

6. Proximal and distal control is now assured. With the aortic clamp in position, but with the jaws open, rapidly inject into the aorta through a No. 18 needle 30 mg. of heparin in 30 ml. of saline solution. Close the aortic clamp immediately. Clamp the iliac arteries with toothed bulldog or other suitable clamps.

Resection of aneurysm

1. Divide the iliac arteries. Hold the ends with occluding clamps, and carefully dissect the iliac arteries from the iliac veins. Lift the clamps in order to visualize the lumbar arteries and the attachments to the vena cava. Carefully continue the dissection upward. (See Fig. 12, *B.*) As the aneurysm is dissected off the vertebral column, clamp and divide the lumbar arteries.

Comment: *It is unwise to lift, roll, or retract the aneurysm. These movements may dislodge emboli from the clotted contents of the aneurysmal sac. Intrasaccular anastomosis and reconstruction is safer than resection because the most dangerous part of the dissection is removal of the sac of the aneurysm from the adherent vena cava. If the aneurysm is large, enter the aneurysm and resect the anterior portion, leaving the aneurysmal sac adherent to the vena cava and leave a cuff of aneurysm proximally and distally. The sac may be sewn over the prosthesis to separate it from bowel (Figs. 16 and 17). Calcium and debris should be removed from the lining of the sac. Tributaries of the vena cava, or small leaks, should be stitched with arterial suture.*

2. Divide the aorta at the neck of the aneurysm, leaving a generous cuff distal to the aortic clamp. The proximal anastomosis can be performed inside the cuff of proximal aorta if the aneurysm is close to the clamp.

Aortic anastomosis

1. Select a prosthesis with a proximal diameter matching that of the severed aorta. Shorten the prosthesis proximally so that the bifurcation will be at the same or at a higher level than that of the excised aorta. Do not cut the iliac ends of the graft at this time.

2. Begin the anastomosis of the aorta and graft with a double-armed 3-0 or 4-0 Tevdec, polyethylene, or polypropylene suture placed at each side (Fig. 12, *C*). Sutures are placed first through the prosthesis and then through the proximal aorta.

To place the posterior row of sutures, turn the handle of the Glover or

DeBakey clamp superiorly, allowing the assistant to suspend the graft (Fig. 12, *D*). Sew the posterior edges together with an everting continuous over-and-over stitch, with the sutures placed 1.5 to 2 mm. apart and 1.5 to 2 mm. from the edge of the aorta. To prevent leakage, pull each stitch snugly as it is placed. It is usually preferable to sew from the prosthesis toward the aorta.

Lower the prosthesis into the abdomen and complete the anterior row of sutures in the same fashion (Fig. 12, *E*).

Comment: *Occasionally the aortic cuff is quite large and requires pleating or a large prosthesis. Double layers of stitches are useless if the artery is very fragile, and a single layer of continuous over-and-over sutures holds the edges*

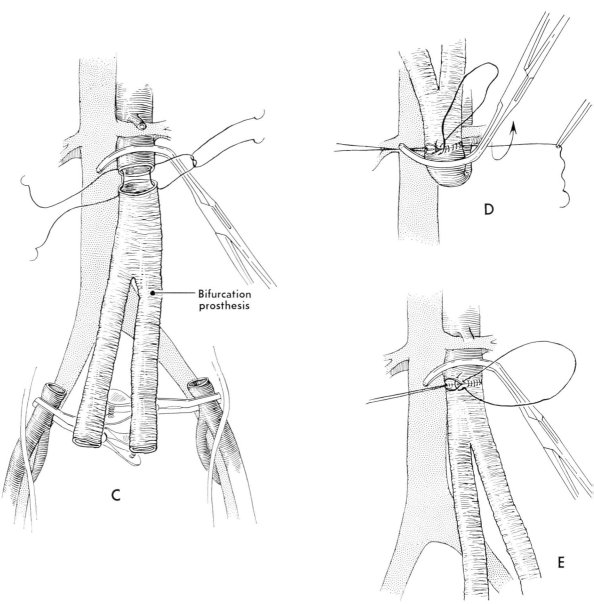

Fig. 12, cont'd. Resection of abdominal aneurysms. **C** to **E**, Aortic anastomosis. **D**, Posterior row of sutures. **E**, Anterior row of sutures.   *Continued.*

well when placed 2 mm. or more from the edge of the artery. The aortic anastomosis may disrupt when the wall has been weakened by removal of a calcific plaque. This problem is met by covering the aortic anastomosis and proximal aorta with a sleeve of prosthetic material fashioned from the remainder of the graft.

3. Preclot the prosthesis as follows. Pinch the ends of the prosthesis with the fingers. Momentarily release the aortic clamp in order to flush out the aorta and to force blood through the pores under pressure. Aspirate excess blood and blood clots from the prosthesis and then cover it with gauze soaked in bacitracin solution. When the correct preclotting procedure is used, there is little leakage from the DeBakey Dacron prosthesis. Sealing of the pores of the prosthesis with gelatin may reduce implantation porosity without impairing healing porosity, but these grafts are not yet commercially available.

Iliac anastomosis

Comment: *The technique of iliac anastomosis may be adapted to the aorta, popliteal artery, or other vessels. The vertical end-to-end anastomosis described below is the most widely applicable type. Special situations will be discussed later. Avoid the common error of leaving the prosthesis too long, and allow for about 10% lengthening when filled under normal blood pressure. If this is not anticipated, the prosthesis may lengthen and bow anteriorly as it is stretched by the pressure of the restored blood flow.*

1. Shorten the iliac limb of the prosthesis. Clamp the iliac limb of the prosthesis vertically, and stretch it to meet the divided iliac artery. Replace the bulldog clamp on the iliac artery with a long-handled arterial clamp also applied vertically, so that the tip of the clamp is at the middle of the posterior wall. The assistant holds the ends of the prosthesis and the artery together with the clamps while the anastomosis is sutured.

Place a double-armed mattress suture of 4-0 polyethylene or Dacron from the prosthesis to the iliac artery, starting at the tips of the clamps posteriorly (Fig. 12, *F*). Tie the mattress suture while the assistant holds the ends in approximation with the clamps. Rotate the clamps sufficiently, about 90 degrees, to gain access to the sutures and begin the medial row (Fig. 12, *G*).

2. Suture the medial side of the prosthesis and the artery together with a continuous over-and-over stitch using one of the needles. Sew from the prosthesis toward the artery. Place the sutures 1 to 2 mm. apart and 1 to 2 mm. from the edge of the vessels and pull them until they are snug.

3. Rotate the arterial clamps to gain access to the lateral side (Fig. 12, *H*) and perform the anastomosis in the same fashion as on the medial (Fig. 12, *I*). Release the distal clamp to check back bleeding before completing the anastomosis. Join the medial and lateral sutures anteriorly and tie them with a secure knot.

Restoration of blood flow to first leg

1. Flush the completed iliac anastomosis in a retrograde direction by momentarily releasing the clamp on the iliac artery (Fig. 12, *J*).

2. Flush the proximal aorta through the uncompleted iliac end as follows. Apply an arterial clamp near the bifurcation on the finished side and release

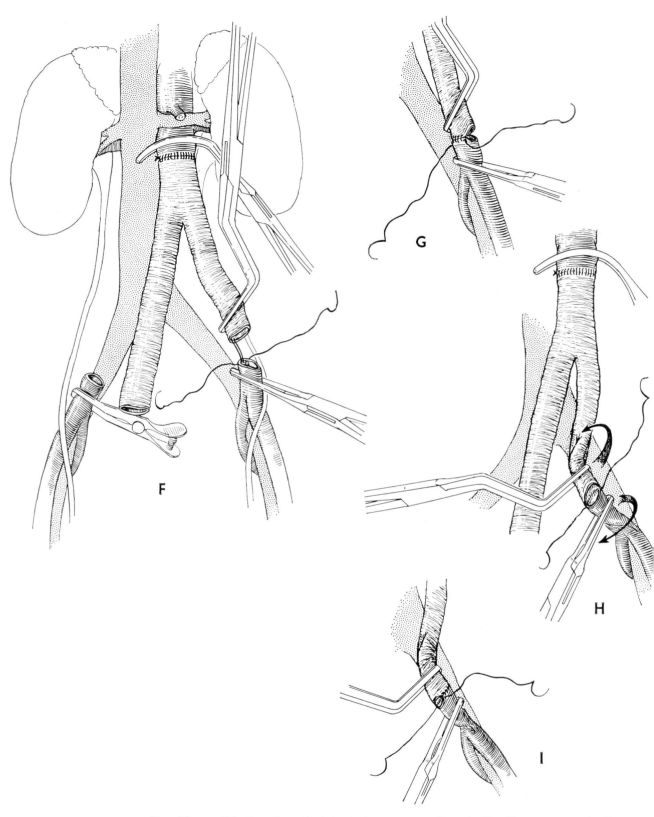

Fig. 12, cont'd. Resection of abdominal aneurysms. **F** to **I**, First iliac anastomosis. **F,** Placement of mattress suture. **G,** Medial row. **H,** Medial row completed. Rotation for lateral row. **I,** Lateral row.

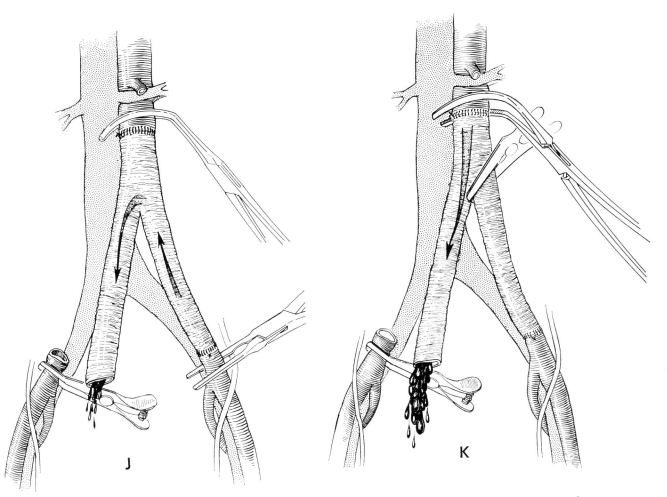

Fig. 12, cont'd. Resection of abdominal aneurysms. **J** and **K,** Restoration of flow to first leg. **J,** Check back bleeding. **K,** Flush proximal aorta.   *Continued.*

the aortic clamp briefly to flush possible clots from the prosthesis (Fig. 12, *K*).

3. Open flow to the first leg as follows. Quickly reapply the clamp to the open limb of the graft. Slowly remove the clamp on the aorta to establish blood flow to the first limb (Fig. 12, *L*).

Comment: *Hypotension may result unless the aortic clamp is released very slowly over a five-minute period. Blood should be running rapidly at this time. Ample intravenous saline solution also helps to prevent this "declamping shock."*

Second iliac anastomosis

1. Cut the remaining iliac limb of the prosthesis to the correct length. Clamp the vessels in a vertical direction. Have the assistant approximate the vessels. Place the mattress suture and tie it securely (Fig. 12, *M*).

2. Suture the medial side of the prosthesis and artery with a continuous over-and-over stitch, repeating step 2 under iliac anastomosis (Fig. 12, *N*).

3. Rotate the arterial clamps (Fig. 12, *O*), and suture the lateral side of the anastomosis in the same fashion as the medial, repeating step 3 under iliac anas-

45

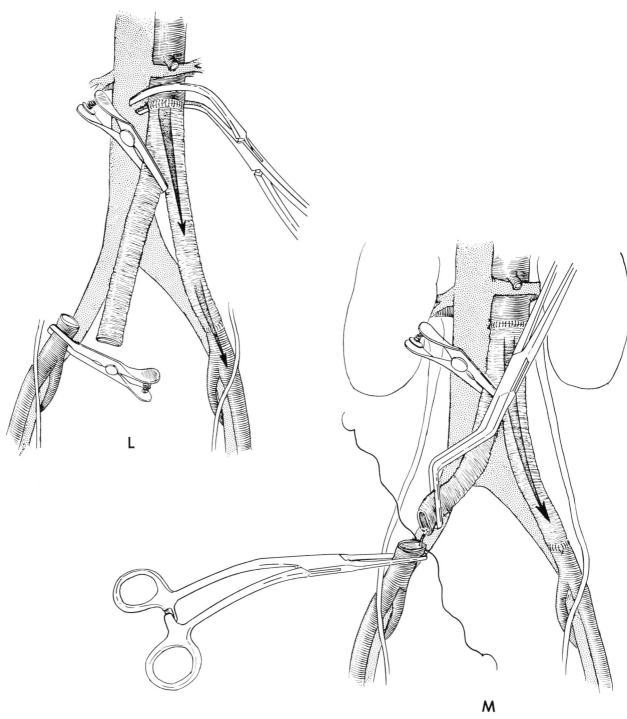

Fig. 12, cont'd. Resection of abdominal aneurysms. **L,** Clamp open limb of graft. Release aortic clamp slowly to restore flow to first leg. **M,** Begin remaining iliac anastomosis.

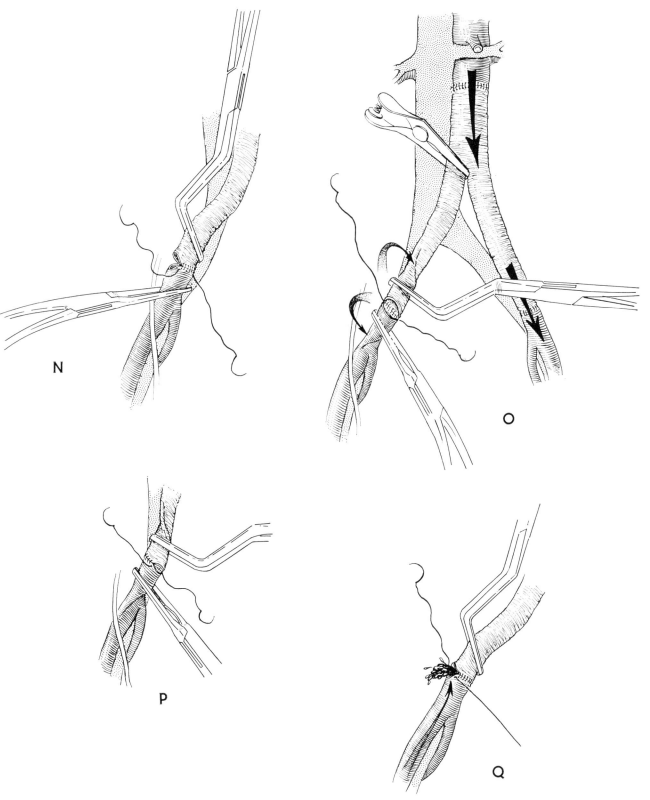

Fig. 12, cont'd. Resection of abdominal aneurysms. **N** to **Q,** Second iliac anastomosis. **N,** Medial row completed. **O,** Rotation of clamps for access to lateral row. **P,** Lateral row of sutures partially completed. **Q,** Check back bleeding from leg by release of distal clamp.

Continued.

tomosis (Fig. 12, *P*). Leave 1 cm. of the front of the anastomosis unfinished until the following flushing procedure is performed.

Restoration of blood flow to second leg

1. Check back bleeding by removing the clamp from the iliac artery (Fig. 12, *Q*). Then reapply the clamp.

2. Briefly release the proximal iliac clamp on the second side and flush out the second iliac limb of the prosthesis (Fig. 12, *R*). Reapply this clamp proximally for a few moments to allow completion of the anastomosis. Now remove the distal clamp and allow the empty artery and prosthesis to be filled with blood. Tie the suture to complete the anastomosis. (See Fig. 12, S.)

3. Remove the proximal clamp slowly to restore pulsatile blood through the new anastomosis and into the second leg. Cover the prostheses and anastomoses

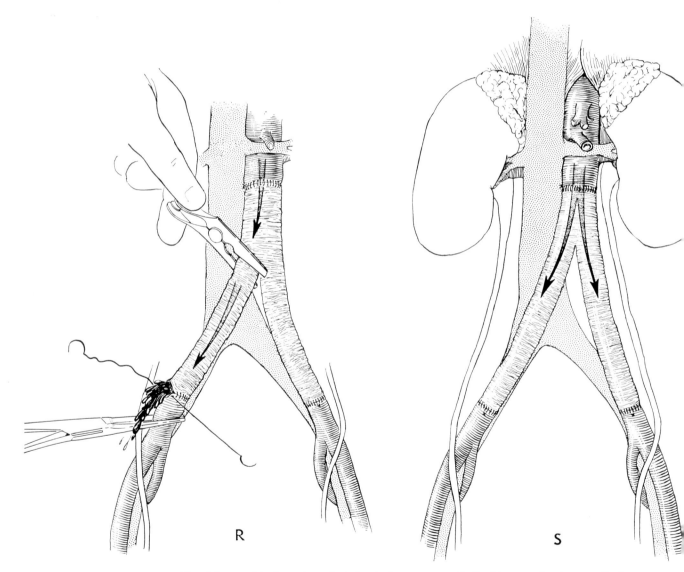

R

S

Fig. 12, cont'd. Resection of abdominal aneurysms. **R,** Flushing proximal aorta. **S,** Anastomosis completed and flow restored.

with gauze soaked in bacitracin. To prevent hypotension at this point, it is usually advisable to transfuse rapidly one or more units of blood.

Comment: *The flushing technique should be done carefully, since it is essential to remove atheromatous debris, clots, and sludge proximal to the aortic clamp. If occlusion time has been prolonged, clots can also form distally, and these must be detected and removed. Back bleeding is encouraged by brisk pressure or massage over the femoral triangle or by a Fogarty or suction catheter. Flushing out the air in the graft prevents air embolism so that pulses in the feet are restored promptly.*

Closure

The prosthesis must be covered with living tissue and must not be permitted to lie against the jejunum or the duodenum. Remnants of the posterior portion of the aneurysm sac, peritoneum, preaortic areolar tissue, and mesentery of the descending colon are available for suturing over the graft. Omentum is rarely needed but may be applied on the top of the graft. If the omentum is short, it may be drawn through a hole in the transverse mesocolon. Coverage of the prosthetic graft with soft tissue is necessary to prevent accumulations of serum or blood and to allow fibroblasts to invade the meshwork and anchor the new intima or pseudointima in place. The ligament of Treitz has been divided and the duodenum and upper jejunum lie to the right of the graft and should be separated from the prosthesis by preaortic tissues and omentum. Otherwise, aortic enteric fistulas from the anastomosis to the duodenum may form. We know of one iliac-cecal fistula. The interposition of soft tissue will prevent this complication.

A tube gastrostomy with a Foley or Hurwitt triple-lumen gastrostomy catheter should be employed to avoid postoperative distention.

Postoperative care

1. Do not use anticoagulants.
2. Observe and chart extremity pulses hourly during the first twenty-four hours.
3. Replace fluids and electrolytes and blood after careful consideration of cardiac status and renal status.
4. Maintain prophylactic digitalization.
5. Give antibiotics for five days to prevent pulmonary infections.
6. Employ gastric suction for several days to prevent abdominal distension.
7. Reoperate immediately if femoral pulses disappear.

Complications

Hemorrhage and embolism are almost always avoidable. Oliguria is infrequent unless the aorta has been occluded for long periods or hypotension occurs during the operation. Multiple small renal emboli and infarcts have been reported in patients with fatal oliguria. We have found pulmonary complications and abdominal distention infrequent since we abandoned the nasogastric tube and substituted gastrostomy for gastrointestinal decompression.

Cardiac and cerebrovascular complications are the most common causes of postoperative deaths.

Interference with the blood supply of the colon, particularly the combination of ligation of the inferior mesenteric and both hypogastric arteries, may result in ischemia or gangrene of the sigmoid colon. Mucosal ulceration of the rectosigmoid colon produces a bloody diarrhea. The severity of this complication is lessened by preparation of the bowel. Fortunately, the collateral blood supply to the colon from the superior mesenteric artery via the marginal artery and the left colic-sigmoid arterial anastomoses as well as from the hemorrhoidal arteries via one hypogastric artery is almost always sufficient. Sigmoid ischemia not sufficient to produce necrosis or ulceration may be manifest as bloating, cramping, and diarrhea. Sigmoidoscopic examination reveals a change from normal pink mucosa to dusky cyanotic mucosa at or just above the rectosigmoid junction.

VARIATIONS IN ANEURYSMS OF ABDOMINAL AORTA

Fig. 13 shows some of the variations in abdominal aneurysms that may be encountered. Tube grafts may be satisfactory for replacement of small aneurysms.

Tube grafts

Bifurcation grafts are not always necessary for abdominal aneurysms. In some cases the operation can be simplified by inserting a tube prosthesis of appropriate diameter into the distal and proximal cuff of the aneurysm. This is illustrated in Fig. 16 and described in detail on p. 58. This simplifies the operation since only two anastomoses are needed instead of three, the aneurysm need not be dissected off the inferior vena cava, and the prosthesis is covered, padded, and separated from the duodenum by use of the sac. After proximal and distal control, boldly open the aneurysm and remove the contents of the sac. The sac is trimmed at the sides and sutured over the prosthesis after debris and lining of the sac are curetted away. The orifices of the lumbar arteries are sutured if they bleed.

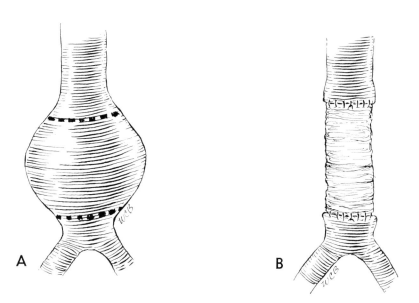

Fig. 13. A, Small abdominal aneurysm. **B,** Tube graft for small abdominal aneurysm.

50

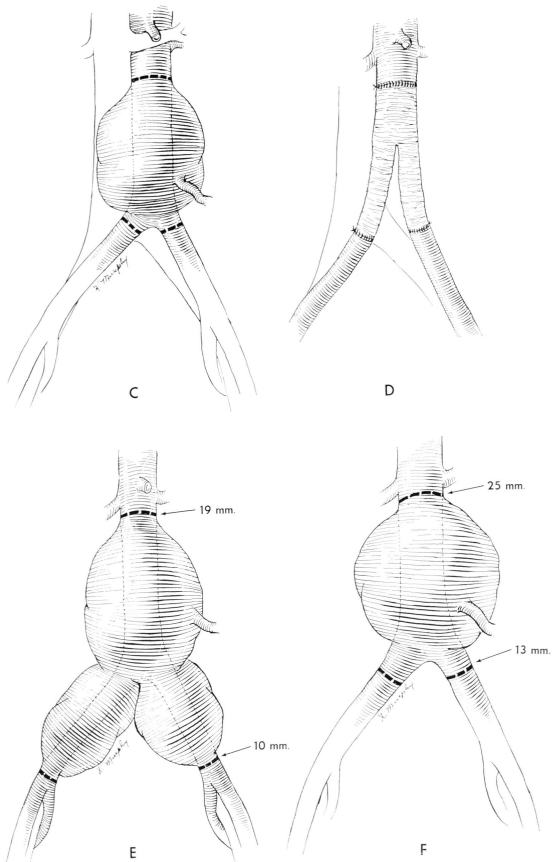

Fig. 13, cont'd. C-F, Alternative methods of iliac anastomosis. **C** and **D,** Higher bifurcation makes iliac anastomoses easier. **E,** Associated iliac aneurysms. **F,** Dilated iliac arteries.

End-to-end anastomosis in presence of iliac aneurysm

At times aneurysmal dilatation of an iliac artery (Fig. 13, *E*) may require division of the artery near the junction of the internal and external iliac arteries. Division of both hypogastric arteries should, ordinarily, be avoided. The iliac arteries cannot now be rotated a full 180 degrees. Therefore, the iliac clamps should be applied vertically and the anastomosis begun posteriorly and carried forward on either side. Because this technique of anastomosis is so convenient, we prefer it to all other techniques and use it most frequently. (See Fig. 12, *F-I.*)

Save at least one hypogastric artery to avoid ischemia to the colon. Restore flow to both hypogastric arteries wherever possible. It is unnecessary to resect the large iliac sacs. The end of the bifurcation graft is sutured into the cuff of the distal end of the iliac artery. After the clot and lining of the aneurysms have been removed, the sac can be trimmed and sutured over the prosthesis.

Comment: *The details of suturing are less important than snug coaptation of the edges through sturdy tissue. During completion of the anastomoses the clamps are released following the maneuvers already detailed to flush out any debris or accumulated clots proximal and distal to the anastomotic sites.*

BLEEDING ANEURYSMS OF ABDOMINAL AORTA
Introduction

The usual terminal event of abdominal aortic aneurysm is bleeding. Once leakage of blood has commenced, further disruption of the wall of the aneurysm, hemorrhage, irreversible shock, and death may be expected. In some instances the rupture and hemorrhage progress slowly. There may be a few hours or even days before death, and in this interval accurate diagnosis and early surgery offer some hope of survival for these patients.

The operation differs from the elective operation because of the need to arrest hemorrhage quickly by clamping the aorta above the aneurysm. Isolation of the aorta below the renal arteries by the elective method described earlier is usually feasible, but at times proximal control of the bleeding may be obtained only by the transthoracic route. Manual compression of the neck of the aneurysm below the renal arteries is unsatisfactory during dissection of that region. Although the transabdominal route is more accessible, the transthoracic route may be necessary when a large amount of intra-abdominal bleeding has occurred.

Operation should not be denied to any patient who is a reasonable risk, since the outlook is hopeless without surgery. Patients who are poor risks for elective resection of an aneurysm are usually beyond any surgical help following rupture.

Diagnosis

A pulsating abdominal mass is usually obvious. Back pain is an early sign of bleeding in some patients. Signs of blood loss may not occur for several hours or until the aneurysm ruptures into the free peritoneal cavity. As a rule, the pulsating hematoma is confined in the retroperitoneal tissues and is more prominent on the left side. Although the aneurysm most often ruptures at the point where it is thinned out by contact with the vertebras, we have observed rupture into the duodenum, and rupture into the inferior vena cava has been reported.

Anesthesia

General anesthesia is essential. Induction should be accomplished rapidly and without straining. Rapid blood replacement as indicated should accompany the anesthetic.

Normal blood pressure may not be obtainable until proximal control of the aorta has been achieved.

Procedure

Proximal control of aorta just below diaphragm

A hematoma, a very high sac, or an anterior sac that covers the left renal vein may prevent a safe approach to the aorta below the renal vein and the renal arteries until proximal control can be obtained at a higher level. In thin patients, the aorta may be identified and clamped as it emerges beneath the diaphragm. In obese patients or when bleeding is very active, transthoracic control is safer and faster.

1. Extend the abdominal incision as high as possible and excise the xiphoid process (Fig. 14, A).

2. Elevate the left lobe of the liver with Weinberg or Harrington retractors.

3. Divide the gastrohepatic omentum high, near the esophagus and above the left gastric artery.

4. Retract the esophagus to the left with a Penrose drain (Fig. 14, B).

5. Palpate and visualize the aorta lying between the crura of the diaphragm.

6. Apply a long straight arterial clamp vertically to occlude the aorta (Fig. 14, C). Dissect around the aorta with long curved right-angle clamps and, if time permits, pass an umbilical tape about the aorta. Lift the aorta with the umbilical tape, holding the esophagus and stomach to the left.

7. Release the clamp for one or two minutes every fifteen minutes unless serious bleeding results. Release the clamp permanently when control of the aorta has been obtained above the aneurysm and below the renal arteries.

Transthoracic supradiaphragmatic control of aorta

1. Make an anterolateral submammary incision in the sixth or seventh interspace. One or two ribs may be divided anteriorly or posteriorly if necessary to provide sufficient exposure (Fig. 15, A). Tilt the operating table so that the left side of the chest is anterior.

2. Insert the rib spreader, retract the lung upward, and identify the pulsating aorta. For immediate control of bleeding, press the aorta against the vertebras.

3. Retract the diaphragm downward, open the pleural reflection over the aorta, and dissect about it.

4. Apply the Crafoord clamp or another suitable clamp to the aorta (Fig. 15, B).

5. Begin the abdominal operation, and obtain control of the abdominal aorta below the renal arteries as soon as possible.

6. Release the aortic clamp for one or two minutes each fifteen minutes, and

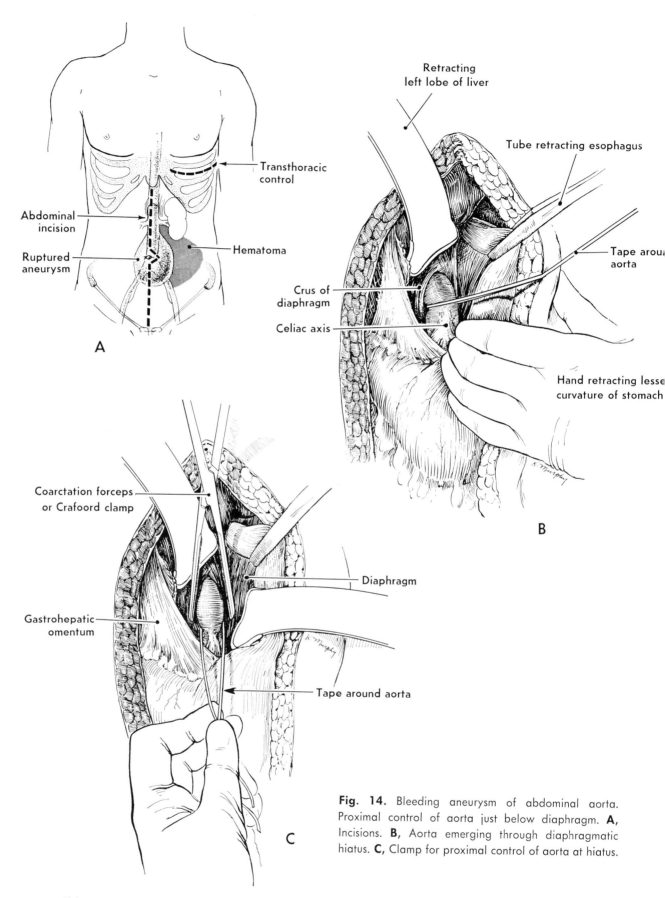

Transthoracic
control

Abdominal
incision

Ruptured
aneurysm

Hematoma

A

Retracting
left lobe of liver

Tube retracting esophagus

Tape arou
aorta

Crus of
diaphragm

Celiac axis

Hand retracting lesse
curvature of stomach

B

Coarctation forceps
or Crafoord clamp

Gastrohepatic
omentum

Diaphragm

Tape around aorta

C

Fig. 14. Bleeding aneurysm of abdominal aorta.
Proximal control of aorta just below diaphragm. **A,**
Incisions. **B,** Aorta emerging through diaphragmatic
hiatus. **C,** Clamp for proximal control of aorta at hiatus.

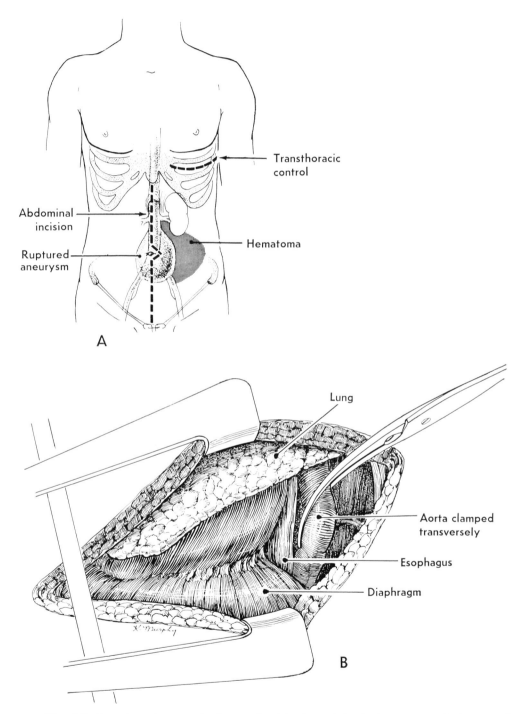

Fig. 15. Transthoracic control of aorta for bleeding abdominal aneurysm. **A,** Intercostal incision, supine view. **B,** Anterolateral view of aorta and adjacent structures through sixth or seventh rib intercostal incision. Operating table tilted to right.

release it altogether when the abdominal aorta has been clamped above the aneurysm and below the renal arteries.

Resection of bleeding aneurysms

The technique of resection of a bleeding aneurysm resembles the elective operation, except that the presence of a hematoma requires technical modifications, mainly intrasaccular anastomosis and reconstruction, because the hematoma obscures the usual landmarks.

1. A midline incision is made speedily. Divide the ligament of Treitz immediately. The hematoma usually will obscure all other landmarks. Retract the duodenum and small bowel mesentery to the right. Incise the peritoneum over the neck of the sac. To obtain proximal control of the aorta below the renal arteries, first identify the left renal vein crossing the aorta behind the ligament of Treitz. The inferior mesenteric vein will probably be encountered and divided as it crosses the aorta at this location. With proximal control in the chest, dissection is less impeded than it would be were the assistant manually compressing the aorta in the abdomen. The thumb and forefinger or a large curved clamp is used to dissect about the aorta in the free angle just below the renal arteries and between the aorta and the spinal column. Cross clamp the aorta vertically below the renal arteries and restore flow to the kidneys and liver by releasing any clamps that have been placed proximally on the aorta (Fig. 16, C).

2. Isolate and clamp the iliac arteries at any convenient site. Beware of ureters concealed by extensive hematoma.

3. The planes of dissection around the aneurysm are unclear. Therefore, open the aneurysm wide and remove clots (Fig. 16, D). This will give room to dissect in and around the sac. Identify and ligate the inferior mesenteric artery anteriorly and to the left inside the sac of the aneurysm.

4. Lumbar arteries may continue to bleed into the sac. These are easily sutured inside the sac (Fig. 16, F).

5. Trim the cuff of the sac (Fig. 16, E) and perform the anastomosis up in the neck of the sac close to the vertical aortic clamp (Fig. 16, G and H).

6. Peel out all intima and debris, leaving the fibrous sac. Do not resect the sac. Merely trim it and use it to suture over the prosthesis. (See Fig. 16, I and J).

7. Tube grafts are used when the iliac arteries are not involved and the distal end of the sac is suitable for anastomosis, as illustrated in Fig. 13, A and B. Otherwise, the customary bifurcation prosthesis is inserted.

8. Perform the distal anastomosis by the same method, using wide, deep, secure bites with sturdy 3-0 or 4-0 suture.

9. Suture the sac over the prosthesis (Fig. 16, I and J).

Postoperative care

The most serious complication is oliguria. Prolonged hypotension, multiple transfusions, temporary cross clamping of the aorta above the renal arteries, and pre-existing renal disease may all contribute to renal failure. Hourly observation of the urine volume and of the hematocrit is advisable during the immediate postoperative period. The central venous pressure is the best guide for blood and fluid replacement. Several liters of balanced electrolyte solution and blood should be supplied as needed, keeping central venous pressure less than 10 cm.

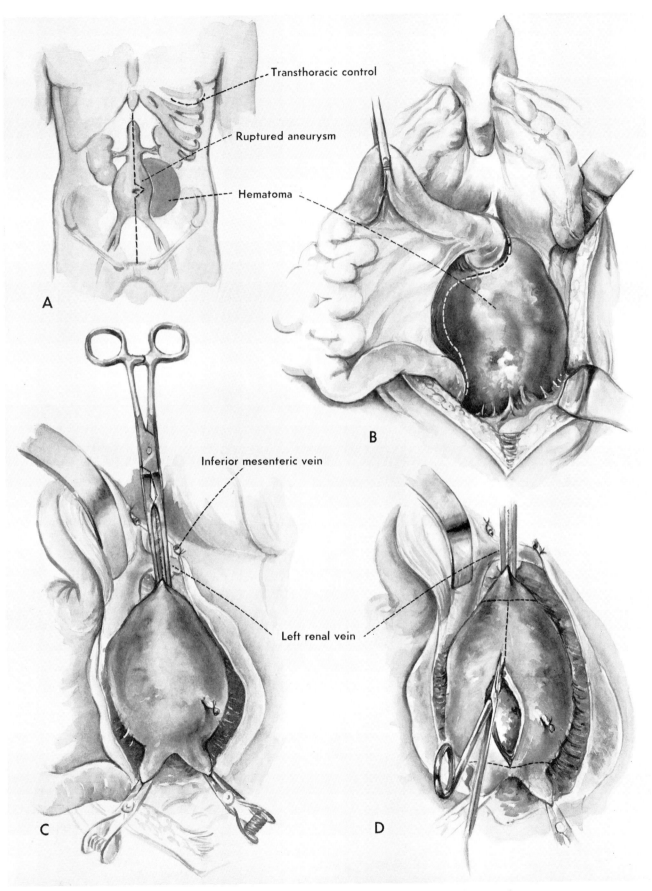

Fig. 16. Resection of bleeding aneurysm. **A,** Incision. **B,** Peritoneal incision over hematoma.
C, Proximal control of aorta below renal arteries. **D,** Open aneurysmal sac.

Continued.

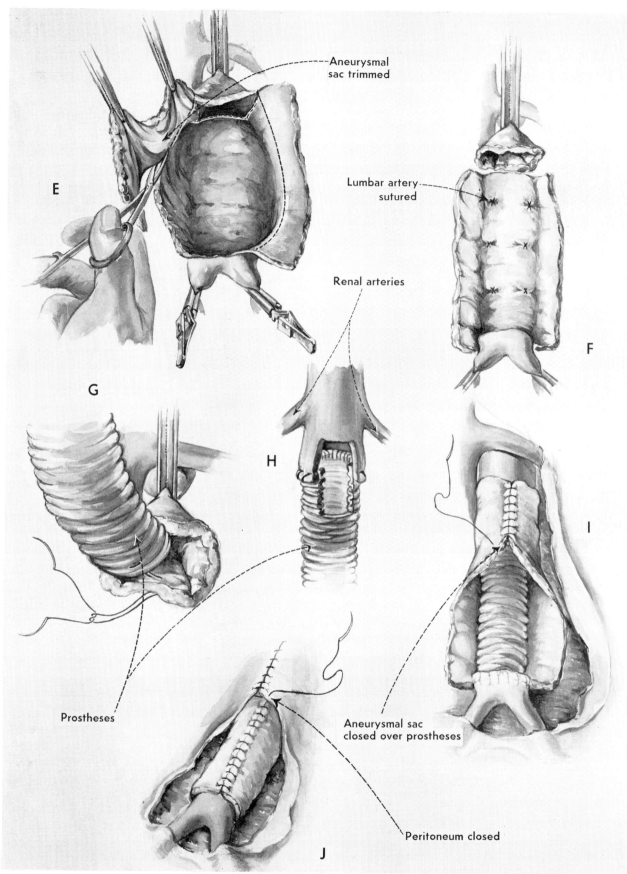

Labels within figure:
- Aneurysmal sac trimmed
- Lumbar artery sutured
- Renal arteries
- Prostheses
- Aneurysmal sac closed over prostheses
- Peritoneum closed
- E
- F
- G
- H
- I
- J

Fig. 16, cont'd. Resection of bleeding aneurysm. **E,** Trim excess aneurysm sac. **F,** Proximal cuff of aorta ready for anastomosis. **G,** Proximal aortic anastomosis. **H,** Cut-away view of anastomosis to show prosthesis up inside aortic cuff. **I,** Aneurysmal sac sutured over prosthesis. **J,** Peritoneum and left mesocolon sutured over prosthesis and sac.

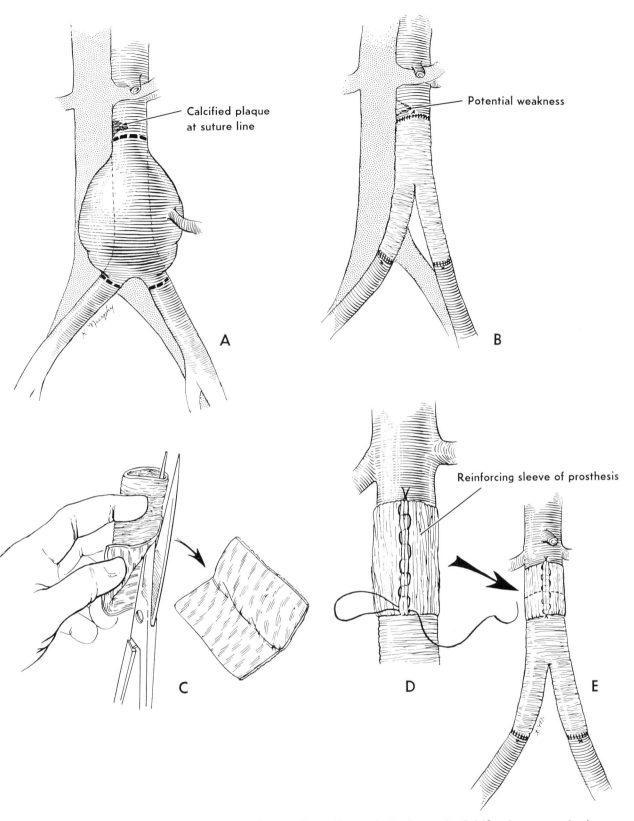

Fig. 17. Reinforcement of suture line with prosthetic sleeve. **A,** Calcific plaques proximal to aneurysm. **B,** Potential weakness after removal of calcific plaque. **C,** Cut-open prosthetic tube to make sheet or strip. **D,** Suture strip around anastomosis. **E,** Completed operation.

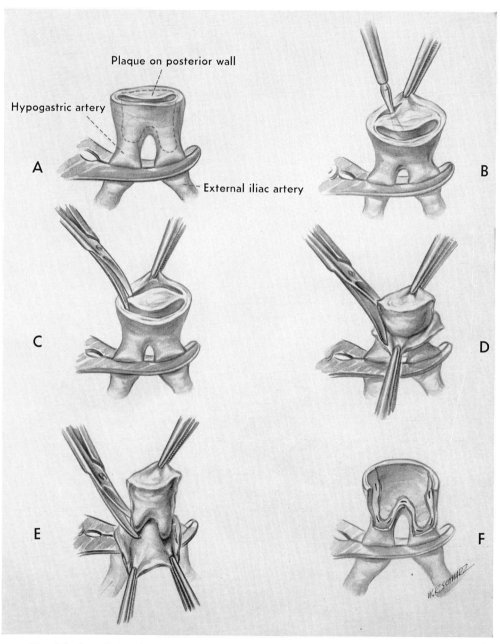

Labels in figure:
Plaque on posterior wall
Hypogastric artery
External iliac artery
A
B
C
D
E
F

Fig. 18, A to **F.** Local endarterectomy of iliac artery bifurcation. **A,** Plaque extends distally. **B,** Develop cleavage plane between plaque and media. **C,** Cut attachment of plaque to normal intima. **D** and **E,** Evert artery if necessary to visualize plaque and its distal extensions. **F,** Cutaway view to show mattress sutures reattaching distal intimal edge.

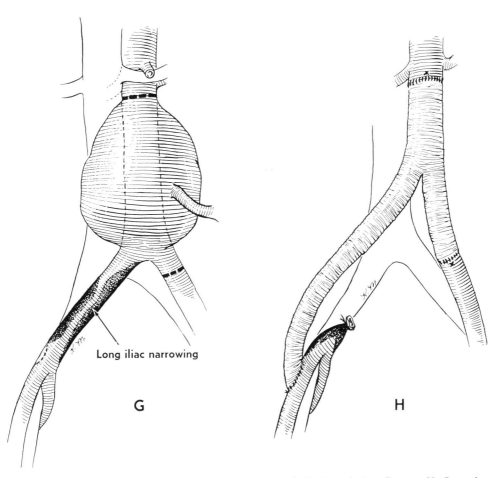

Long iliac narrowing

G

H

Fig. 18, cont'd. G, Combination of aneurysm and distal occlusive disease. **H,** Resection and bypass for extensive atherosclerosis of iliac artery distal to aneurysm.

and maintaining adequate urinary output. Other postoperative measures are identical with those for elective resection. Mannitol is also indicated for diagnosis and treatment of oliguria.

COMBINATIONS OF ANEURYSMS OF ABDOMINAL AORTA AND OCCLUSIVE DISEASE

Endarterectomy of proximal aorta and reinforcement of suture line

Aneurysm, occlusive disease, and calcific disease of the arterial walls are fairly common combinations and may require modifications of technique. The usual location of the calcific plaque is on the posterior wall of the proximal aorta or along the posterior walls of the iliac arteries. Calcific plaques frequently cannot be removed or sutured without weakening the aortic wall or the suture line. If possible, resection through such plaques should be avoided. Higher resection (Fig. 17, A and B) is preferable to reinforcement of the suture line.

If the arterial wall near the suture line has been weakened by calcific plaques and higher resection is not feasible, it is wise to reinforce the area with a sleeve of the unused prosthetic material. To do this, cut open the remaining cylinder of the prosthesis (Fig. 17, C), pass it under the anastomosis, and suture it snugly with a continuous everting mattress suture (Fig. 17, D). Trim off any extra prosthesis, leaving a 2 mm. cuff (Fig. 17, E). The prosthesis must be porous so that the surrounding fibrous tissue will infiltrate the pores and seal and reinforce the suture lines.

Endarterectomy of iliac arteries

Occasionally the iliac arteries must be transected through atherosclerotic plaques (Fig. 18, A). The atherosclerotic plaques are usually on the posterior wall and may extend far down into the internal and external iliac vessels. After endarterectomy the end of the prosthetic tube is anastomosed to the end of the artery.

The intimal plaque is detached from the media by blunt dissection with a small periosteal elevator (Freer). The plane of cleavage between the intima and media is usually obvious (Fig. 18, B).

Cut the edge of the plaque from the normal intima with a small scissors (Fig. 18, C). Evert the artery if necessary to permit more accurate dissection (Fig. 18, D and E). The long thin extension on the posterior arterial wall need not be totally excised and may be transected, beveled, and attached by suture.

Suture the remaining intima to the media of the artery (Fig. 18, F). Arterial silk sutures, 4-0 or 5-0, with needles at both ends are useful for this procedure. Pass the needles from within outward, pushing the intima toward the media and tying the suture outside the artery.

Comment: *Extensive iliac endarterectomy is unnecessary. If the calcific plaque on the posterior wall of the iliac artery is extensive, endarterectomy may be unsafe. In such instances, close the common iliac artery proximally and join the iliac limb of the prosthesis to the soft anterior surface of the artery at a more distal point.*

The bypass procedure (Fig. 18, H) avoids extensive endarterectomy and avoids sacrifice of the hypogastric artery. As a rule, the proximal end of the iliac artery would be oversewn rather than simply ligated, as shown in the drawings.

62

Chapter 4

Aortoiliac occlusive disease

Signs and symptoms

The surgeon who undertakes vascular procedures must realize that the basic pathological process of arteriosclerosis is diffuse. When occlusion is segmental, surgical replacement or bypass procedures are applicable. Many elderly persons have extensive occlusive disease, particularly in the lower extremities, but live out their lives without developing gangrene because collateral circulation is adequate to maintain viability of the limbs. Patients without symptoms or with nonprogressive symptoms, particularly those in whom intermittent claudication is the sole symptom, may develop collateral circulation and do not require surgery unless symptoms become severe or progressive.

Atherosclerotic disease affecting the legs is usually most pronounced and is most likely to be segmental at the aortic bifurcation or nearby iliac artery, in the upper femoral artery near the origin of the profunda branch, in the superficial femoral artery as it passes through the adductor canal, and in the distal popliteal artery at the branching of the anterior tibial or posterior tibial arteries.

Symptoms of occlusive disease depend on the pattern, on the degree of narrowing or occlusion, and on the adequacy of collateral circulation. When blood flow is insufficient during exercise, fatigue or pain results, and this intermittent claudication is usually the first and perhaps the only symptom. Occlusion in the iliac artery produces claudication in the hip or thigh. If the bifurcation of the aorta is involved (Leriche's syndrome), the patient complains of claudication in both hips and thighs. Occlusion in the superficial femoral artery usually results in claudication in the calf. If occlusions are multiple, there may be insufficient blood flow at all times. Atrophy of skin and muscle develops, and ischemic neuritis causes pain even when the limb is at rest. Nonhealing ulcers develop after trivial trauma or injections. Sometimes occlusion involves the most important collateral vessels as well as the major artery. A frequent example of this is occlusive disease in the superficial femoral artery, with narrowing at the orifice of the profunda femoris branch.

In the general spectrum of occlusive arterial vascular disease amenable to surgical correction, however, aortoiliac occlusion is the area in which surgical attack is most likely to be successful.

Frequently the patients are relatively young (that is, under 60 years of age), and their atherosclerosis is localized to the terminal aorta and the common iliac vessels. On exploration, the vessel is found to be plugged with atheromatous debris of a soft rubbery consistency that is rather easily removed. There is very little secondary calcification, and intimectomy is sufficient to relieve the obstruction.

Contraindications to elective surgery

We do not operate on patients with minimal disease whose condition may improve with development of collateral circulation. Poor-risk patients or patients with a short life expectancy from other diseases should not be operated upon. Patients with recent coronary occlusion, angina pectoris, or poor cardiac reserve in general are not surgical candidates unless the reasons for surgery are exceedingly compelling. Declamping shock in such patients after operations on the aorta has, in our experience, been more severe and cardiac arrest more likely. When declamping the aorta, rapid transfusion and a Trendelenberg position are employed to secure the maximum venous return to the heart at this critical time.

The most noteworthy failures in arterial reconstructive surgery in the lower limb occur in those patients in whom the popliteal artery and its branches are completely occluded at the time of operation. At times this information cannot be obtained preoperatively, or information obtained from preoperative angiography may prove unreliable. Operative angiography of the popliteal artery and lower leg is helpful in such cases.

Summary

At the present time treatment of occlusive disease by reconstruction below the popliteal level is rarely possible, and reconstruction proximally does little good when the distal outflow tract is too narrow to accept and distribute the flow from the graft. The problem of an inadequate outflow tract is not nearly so frequent in occlusive disease of the aortic bifurcation and/or the common iliac arteries. When femoral reconstruction is done, the prognosis is relatively good if the distal vascular tree has little or no atherosclerotic involvement and fair if at least one distal branch (usually the posterior tibial) remains open.

We have a conservative attitude toward patients with partial or complete aortic occlusion when they have obvious widespread atherosclerosis. The extent of this disease is estimated by taking into account the patient's age, any history of previous vascular accidents, and a thorough physical examination directed toward vascular disease. Most of these patients have claudication and in some instances will improve spontaneously or with the help of sympathectomy. Patients with ulceration, gangrene, intermittent numbness, and severe pain on rest are in danger of gangrene and must have angiograms and arterial reconstruction by bypass or endarterectomy whenever feasible. Extensive reconstructive procedures (that is, those extending from the aorta to the popliteal artery) may be advantageously staged.

Localized aortoiliac obstruction is readily relieved by endarterectomy, which is the procedure of choice. Older patients with extensive aortoiliac or iliofemoral disease or with mild and nonprogressive disease are probably best offered arterial reconstructions or grafts on a very selective basis according to the principles outlined previously.

AORTOILIAC ENDARTERECTOMY

Introduction

The purpose of endarterectomy is to remove intraluminal atheromatous obstructions and to restore arterial flow to the extremities through the artery. In the terminal aorta and proximal iliac artery, "atheromatous debris," a soft putty- or rubbery-like material, can be removed in many instances by establishing a subintimal cleavage plane. The media and adventitia are effective conduits for blood after endarterectomy.

Open endarterectomy is the simplest and most effective surgical procedure for localized occlusive disease in the terminal aorta and in the common iliac arteries. The occluding atheromatous material almost always is found in both iliac arteries. Occlusive disease that extends down the iliac arteries past the hypogastric arteries may be better treated by the bypass technique than by endarterectomy.

The usual indication is disabling intermittent claudication. In addition to the usual general systemic contraindications in poor-risk patients and patients with cancer or other terminal disease, endarterectomy should not be attempted when there is calcification of the arteriosclerotic plaques or of the media of the artery. It is also usually unwise to pursue endarterectomy far into the iliac vessels.

Preoperative care

Preoperative arteriograms reveal the site and degree of obstruction. The terminal aorta and iliac arteries are visualized by percutaneous retrograde arteriography via a femoral artery if a femoral pulse is palpable or by translumbar aortic injection. Preoperative digitalization and bowel sterilization are recommended.

Procedure

Exploration and evaluation

1. Place the patient in the supine position. Prepare and drape the entire abdomen, thighs, and legs.

2. Make a long midline incision from the xiphoid to the pubis. As in other surgical procedures involving the aorta and the iliac arteries, wide exposure is essential. Expose and explore the aorta and the iliac arteries by incisions of the peritoneum, mobilization and retraction of the small bowel, retraction of the sigmoid colon, and division of the ligament of Treitz, as illustrated (Fig. 11) and described previously.

Comment: *Careful palpation of the aorta and iliac arteries will reveal the extent of disease. The occlusions are usually worse than anticipated from preoperative evaluation of angiograms. Widespread endarterectomy is usually unwise. The bifurcation prostheses should be sterile and immediately available in the event aortoiliac or aortofemoral bypass operation is preferable. A long, thin atherosclerotic plaque usually occupies the posterior wall of the iliac artery. This need not be followed distally but may be cut across as detailed later in this chapter.*

Proximal and distal control

1. Pass umbilical tapes about the aorta proximal to the occlusive process.

2. Pass umbilical tapes about the external iliac and hypogastric arteries distal to all palpable atherosclerotic plaques.

3. Select appropriate clamps to apply at the proximal and distal limits of the operation. Complete circumferential exposure of the aorta is unnecessary.

4. Dissect along the left side of the aorta and apply a bulldog clamp to the inferior mesenteric artery. This vessel may be divided if occlusive disease is high and if retraction of the sigmoid mesocolon is necessary for satisfactory exposure of the lumbar arteries.

5. Dissect behind the aorta, isolate and identify the paired lumbar vessels, and occlude them with bulldog clamps or with large *temporary* silk ligatures secured by a single knot.

Arteriotomies

1. Place the aortic clamp across the aorta superiorly. Before closing the clamp, inject 30 mg. of heparin rapidly into the aorta just below the clamp and then immediately tighten the clamp. If occlusion time is over one hour, another supplementary dose of 20 to 30 mg. of heparin should be given intravenously. Apply distal clamps to iliac arteries. These are not shown in Fig. 19 in order to simplify the drawings.

Comment: *If aortic occlusion time exceeds ninety minutes, the atherosclerotic process was too extensive for endarterectomy and a bypass procedure would have been preferable.*

2. Incise the aorta vertically in the midline and extend the incision downward into the iliac artery on the side with the most extensive occlusion (Fig. 19, A).

3. Incise the other iliac artery (Fig. 19, A).

Comment: *The two incisions described should not join. An incision at the aortic bifurcation in the shape of an inverted Y is most undesirable. The two incisions are not joined so that a clamp may be applied between them on the proximal iliac artery, and the long incision extending into the aorta may then be closed to restore flow to one leg during completion of the operation on the opposite iliac artery. The aortic incision should not extend too high, usually stopping within 3 cm. of the renal artery. Plaques and atheromas above this level can be removed from below. When disease does extend to the level of the renal arteries, additional exposure will be necessary. In such an instance, the left renal vein must be dissected free and lifted from the anterior surface of the aorta. The origins of both renal arteries and the superior mesenteric artery must be exposed and temporarily occluded to prevent embolization of atherosclerotic debris loosened during the blind proximal endarterectomy.*

If it is discovered that endarterectomy must continue down to the groin, an incision should be made over the common femoral artery. Even though staged procedures are to be performed, it is desirable that the first operation restore flow as far distal as the profunda femoris. This vessel is never involved in the arteriosclerotic process except at its origin from the common femoral artery. Restoration of pulsatile blood flow into the profunda femoris is sufficient to preserve the leg.

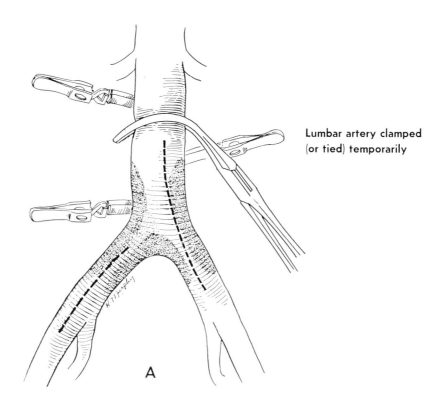

Lumbar artery clamped
(or tied) temporarily

A

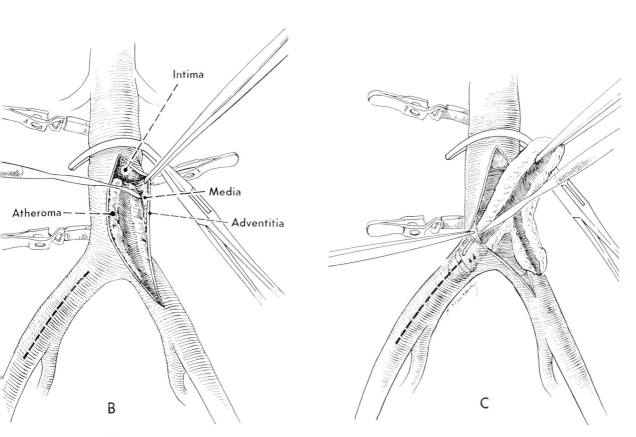

Intima

Media

Atheroma

Adventitia

B

C

Fig. 19. Aortoiliac endarterectomy. **A,** Incisions. **B,** Plane between plaque and media of aorta. **C,** Free up plaque from other iliac artery from above.

Continued.

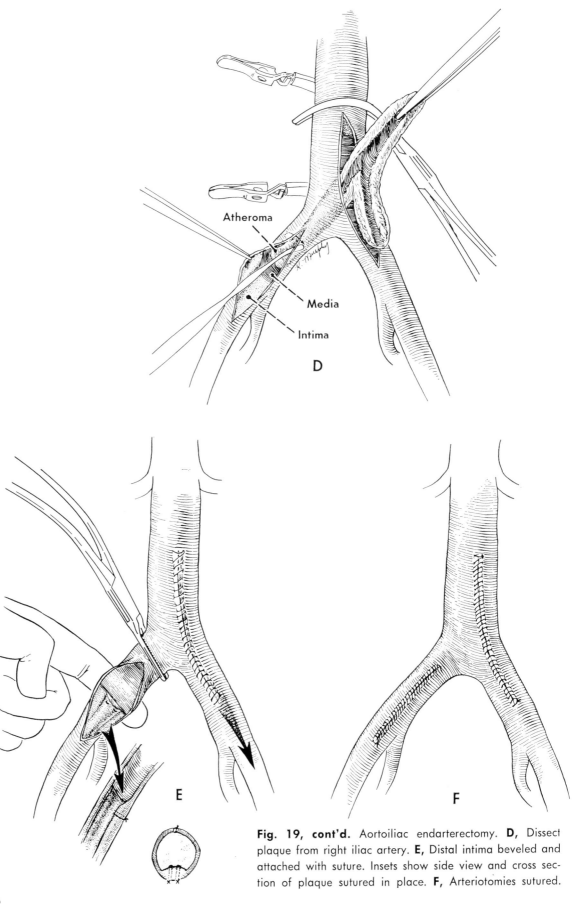

Atheroma

Media

Intima

D

E

F

Fig. 19, cont'd. Aortoiliac endarterectomy. **D,** Dissect plaque from right iliac artery. **E,** Distal intima beveled and attached with suture. Insets show side view and cross section of plaque sutured in place. **F,** Arteriotomies sutured.

Endarterectomy between the distal iliac artery and the bifurcation of the common femoral artery is done with a wire loop or a Wylie or a Leveen endarterectomy instrument passed between the femoral and iliac arteriotomies. It is tedious and unnecessary to open the full length of these arteries for open endarterectomy.

Endarterectomy

1. If occlusion is extensive and a groin incision has been made, endarterectomize the common femoral and iliac arteries by passing the endarterectomy loop upward from a longitudinal arteriotomy in the common femoral artery. At this point remove only easily accessible atheromatous material from the superficial femoral artery and concentrate on restoring blood flow to the bifurcation of the common femoral artery and the profunda.

2. Through the incision in the aorta, dissect out the mass of atheromatous material extending down into the iliac artery (Fig. 19, B). In dissecting the mass, place traction on the inside atheroma, not on the arterial wall. The subintimal plane of cleavage is recognized by the appearance of the circular fibers of the muscularis. A Freer elevator is a useful dissector for this procedure. Frequently the mass can be dissected from both iliac arteries and the aorta in one piece (Fig. 19, C and D). The area between the two incisions is gradually freed by working first from below and then from above (Fig. 19, D).

3. Visualize the distal end of the plaque, and cut the plaque from the normal intima with a scissors.

Restoration of blood flow to first leg

1. Irrigate the interior of the aorta with saline or heparin-saline solution.

2. Using an over-and-over suture, close the longer arteriotomy in the aorta and one iliac artery first, beginning at the aortic end and continuing to within 1 cm. of the distal end of the incision.

3. Clamp the opposite iliac artery proximally.

4. Release the proximal aortic clamp for a few seconds to flush out sludge and clots that may have accumulated proximally.

5. Close any distal arteriotomy in the common femoral artery, and fill the vessel with heparin-saline solution.

6. Release the distal iliac clamp on that side momentarily to backflush any clots. Quickly reapply the clamp.

7. Quickly finish the suture line. Release the distal clamp to fill the artery with blood and force out air before the last suture is tied.

8. Release the proximal aortic clamp slowly.

Comment: *When a thin atherosclerotic plaque continues down the posterior aspect of the iliac artery (Fig. 19, E), bevel the distal plaque and prevent further dissection by suturing the remaining intima and plaque to the arterial wall with several interrupted mattress sutures.*

Suture of iliac arteriotomy

Suture in the same fashion as the longer arteriotomy. Check back bleeding prior to completion of the closure, and force out air before completion of the suture line as described. Slowly release the proximal clamp. (Fig. 19, F.)

Closure

The peritoneum is loosely approximated over the arteries. As a rule, no drainage is necessary. The abdominal incision is closed. A mushroom catheter tube gastrostomy prevents postoperative distention.

Postoperative care

1. Anticoagulant treatment after aortoiliac endarterectomy is elective. However, this course should probably be followed if the endarterectomy has been extensive, particularly if it has extended into the femoral regions. We begin heparinization before closing the abdomen so that all pulses can be checked at this time. If endarterectomy has been limited to the aortic bifurcation, anticoagulation is probably unnecessary. The dose is conservative and should not exceed 25 mg. to 50 mg. every four to six hours.

2. Femoral and/or pedal pulses are observed hourly for the first forty-eight hours. Immediate reoperation is essential if the pulses disappear.

Comment: *Prolonged occlusion time should be avoided by choosing the correct operation. Endarterectomy should not be attempted when the procedure would involve extensive dissection. In such cases a bypass procedure should be elected. Disruption of the aortic suture lines is prevented by avoiding a Y-shaped incision. Also, in suturing the aortic arteriotomy, at least 1 mm. of aortic wall should be included in the bites. Double layers of sutures are ineffective if the adventitia is not utilized in closure and are unnecessary when it is. When weakness of the aortic wall appears to be a distinct problem, the aorta may be reinforced by a sleeve of prosthesis. High endarterectomy that is close to the renal vessels should not be attempted without proximal control of the aorta by a suitable crossclamp. Digital compression of the aorta is not safe, because when this method is used, the hand and fingers are in the operator's field during the surgical procedure.*

AORTOILIAC BYPASS OPERATION
Introduction

When aortoiliac occlusions are extensive, a bypass operation is used to restore pulsatile flow into the iliac or the femoral arteries. Extensive endarterectomy is not so safe or satisfactory as the bypass procedure. Before a bypass operation, patency of the outflow at the profunda femoris and at the popliteal arteries should be demonstrated by angiography. If one femoral vessel is open, retrograde aortography is the safest method to demonstrate the extent of occlusive disease. Poor outflow at the hypogastric artery or at the profunda femoris must be recognized, since the condition may require local endarterectomy.

The diagrams in Fig. 20 show the types of bypass procedures for more extensive occlusions. The end of the bifurcation graft may be anastomosed to either the common iliac or the external iliac artery. In some instances the most distal anastomosis will be in the popliteal region (Fig. 20, *A*). When such an operation is done, the profunda femoris must be perfused by another proximal connection in the femoral or the iliac artery.

Note that the aorta is not resected. Resection is unnecessary and troublesome.

70

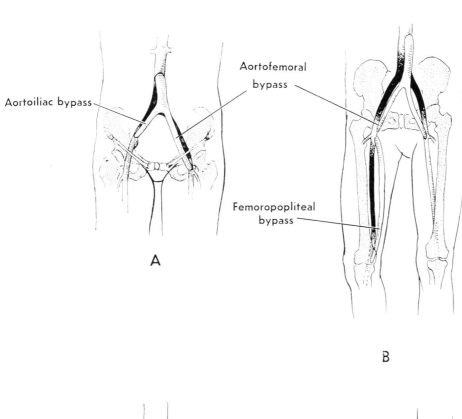

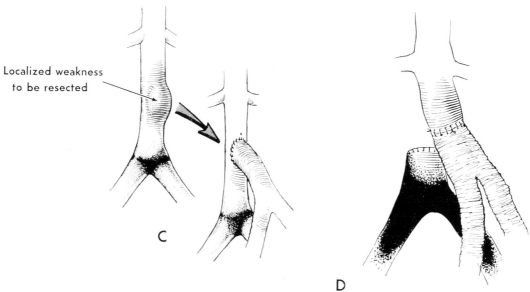

Fig. 20. Types of bypass for aortoiliac occlusion.

The proximal end of the bifurcation bypass prosthesis is attached to the front of the aorta at any convenient site below the renal arteries or to the end of the divided aorta (Fig. 20, D). An occluded aorta may present proximal localized thinning and early formation of aneurysm anteriorly (Fig. 20, C). In such cases the thin portion of the aortic wall is trimmed away and the defect is covered by the proximal end of the bypass prosthesis.

Severe occlusive disease is so commonly bilateral that bypass grafts from the aorta to one side are not shown.

Preparation

Preparation of the patient is the same as for other major surgery on the abdominal aorta. The large intestine should be sterilized preoperatively.

Procedure

Exposure and exploration

1. Place the patient in the supine position. Prepare and drape the entire abdomen, groins, and legs to below the knee.

2. Make a long midline abdominal incision from the xiphoid to the pubis. Expose and explore the aorta (see Chapter 3) by incising the peritoneum to the left of the small bowel, dividing the ligament of Treitz, and mobilizing the duodenum to the right of the aorta. Select the proximal aortic site for attachment of the bypass.

Palpate the iliac arteries. Compare the findings with the preoperative angiograms. Select the sites of the distal anastomoses. Incise the peritoneum over the iliac arteries at the proposed sites of the iliac arteriotomies and examine the patency of the vessels at these points.

Comment: *Since resection is not intended and the lumbar arteries need not be isolated, the peritoneal incisions for exposure of the aorta and iliac arteries are necessary only for exploration and for choosing the sites for anastomoses. In the average patient the small bowel and the ascending colon may be retracted to the right. In obese patients these must be lifted from the abdomen and enclosed in a plastic wrap or a Lahey bag. Incisions for this procedure are detailed in Fig. 11.*

Proximal control of aorta

1. Divide and ligate the inferior mesenteric artery to permit retraction of the sigmoid mesocolon to the left. Avoid the inferior mesenteric vein.

2. Dissect around the aorta, clearing approximately 1 cm. of vessel below the renal arteries and above the occlusive disease. Pass an umbilical tape about the aorta.

3. Free the remaining aorta by dissecting anteriorly from the bifurcation up to the previously placed tape. The lumbar arteries need not be visualized since they are controlled by the Crafoord clamp.

4. Rapidly inject 30 mg. of heparin in 30 ml. of saline solution into the aorta below the tape. Quickly apply the proximal aortic crossclamp at the level of the umbilical tape. The 60-degree Glover clamp usually lies with the handle comfortably out of the way (Fig. 21, A). A vertically applied clamp may fit better.

72

5. Apply the Crafoord clamp, pinching the distal aorta vertically (Fig. 21, A) as shown in the side view (Fig. 21, B). The tip of the S-curved clamp is posterior, close to the upper clamp, and temporarily occludes the lumbar arteries.

Comment: *Satisfactory control of the aorta for the bypass operation is obtained with only enough dissection for the proximal transverse clamp and the distal Crafoord clamp or DeBakey aneurysm clamp that controls the lumbar arteries without individual dissection and identification. Endarterectomy of the aorta above and below the site of the anastomosis may be necessary, and the surgeon may find that this must be done before the distal clamp can be safely applied.*

Early formation of aneurysm can accompany occlusive disease. If the operator observes weakening and bulging of the anterior aortic wall proximal to the occlusive disease, the area should be excised. Even though the resultant aperture is long and wide, the proximal end of the prosthesis can be tailored to fit it. Rapid outflow through the prosthesis prevents further weakening of the aortic wall proximal to the obstruction.

Aortic anastomosis

1. Incise the aorta longitudinally. Flush out any atheromatous debris at the site of the original incision. A decision whether to divide the aorta and insert the bypass by end-to-end anastomosis or to lengthen the aortic incision and make the proximal anastomosis of the bypass to the front of the aorta as illustrated in Fig. 21 must be made. For the end-to-side anastomosis, lengthen the incision to about one and one-half times the diameter of the aorta. If the aorta is small, trim its edges to leave an elliptical aperture. (See Fig. 21, A.)

2. Select a bifurcation prosthesis of the same size as the aorta. Measure the prosthesis so that the bifurcation will be no lower than the diseased aortic bifurcation. Cut the superior margin of the prosthesis (Fig. 21, B).

3. Begin the anastomosis with a mattress suture of 4-0 Dacron at the inferior end of the arteriotomy, using a double-armed suture (Fig. 21, B).

4. Suture one side of the anastomosis with a continuous over-and-over stitch, passing the needle from the prosthesis side to the aortic side (Fig. 21, C).

5. End the first side at the superior end of the aortotomy, with the needle emerging from the aorta (Fig. 21, C). Occasionally it may be necessary to lengthen the aortotomy superiorly or trim the tip of the prosthesis.

6. Suture the opposite side of the prosthesis to the aorta in an identical fashion. End the suture line with the needle emerging from the aorta, and tie the sutures together at the superior end of the anastomosis (Fig. 21, D).

Comment: *The best outflow through the prosthesis will be obtained by constructing apertures and anastomoses that conform to the shape of the normal arterial bifurcation. The longitudinal arteriotomy may not gap sufficiently and therefore some of the aortic wall must be removed to secure an adequate opening. Anastomosis should be begun at the inferior end of the prosthesis. The tip of the obliquely cut prosthesis is drawn up taut, and the corrugations are smoothed out as it is sewn to the aorta superiorly. This ensures that the completed anastomosis will branch obliquely from the aorta when it is filled with blood under pressure.*

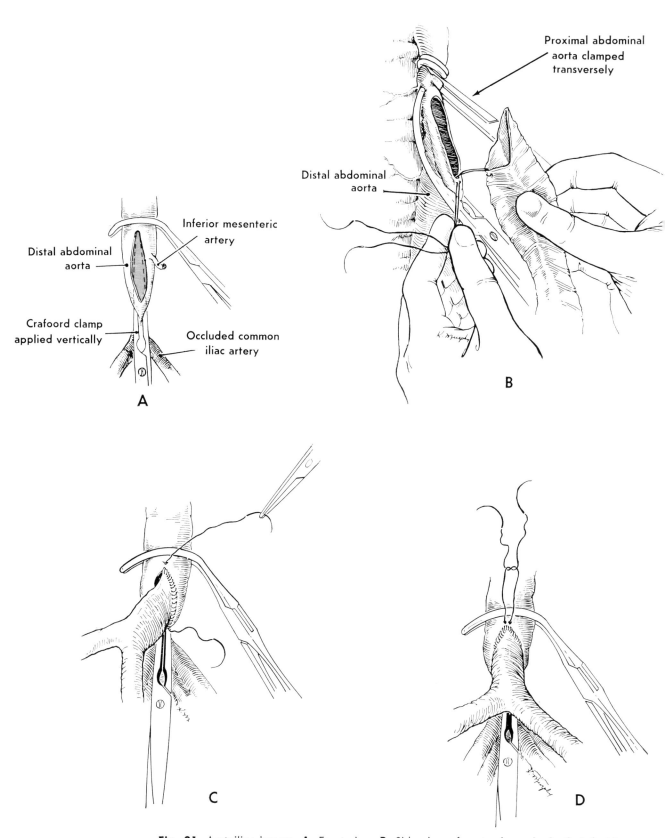

Fig. 21. Aortoiliac bypass. **A,** Front view. **B,** Side view of aorta shown in **A. C,** Left side of anastomosis completed. **D,** Completed anastomosis.

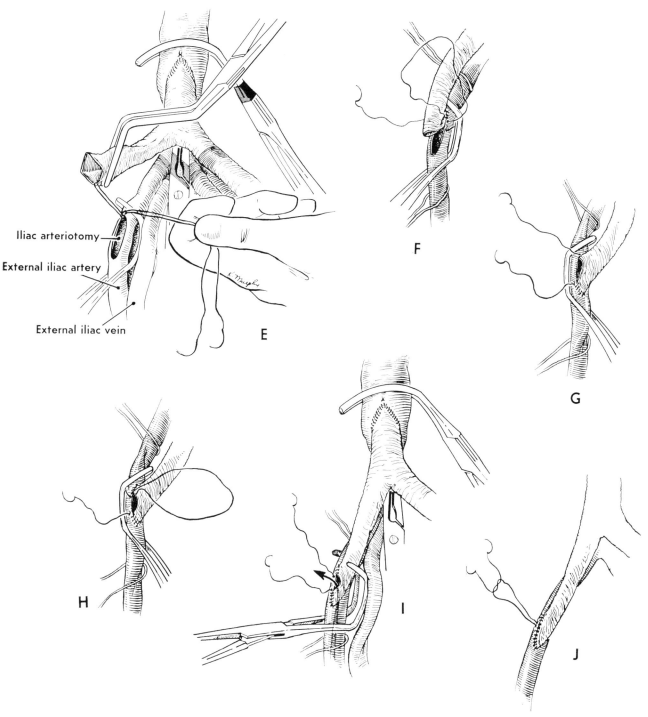

Iliac arteriotomy

External iliac artery

External iliac vein

E

F

G

H

I

J

Fig. 21, cont'd. Aortoiliac bypass. **E,** Start end-to-side anastomosis of prosthesis and iliac artery. **F,** Medial row of sutures. **G,** Continue medial suture around tip of prosthesis and rotate clamp to gain access to lateral side. **H,** Begin lateral row of sutures at oblique proximal angle. **I,** Check back bleeding. **J,** Completed anastomosis.

7. Preclot the graft and flush out the proximal aorta by releasing the proximal clamp momentarily to fill the prosthesis and its porous wall with blood under pressure. Quickly reapply the clamp and empty the prosthesis.

Comment: *This maneuver removes sludge and clots that may have accumulated proximal to the clamp. When prostheses with extremely small mesh are used, preclotting may be omitted. However, small-mesh prostheses are generally undesirable. If one iliac artery is still patent, flush out the aorta and iliac artery and then clamp the prosthesis and release the aortic clamp to restore flow to the corresponding leg.*

Iliac artery anastomosis

1. Draw the limbs of the prosthesis beneath the peritoneum on the right and beneath the peritoneum and the sigmoid colon on the left. Take care not to twist the limbs of the graft.

2. Apply a sidewise clamp to the iliac artery as it is elevated by two encircling tapes.

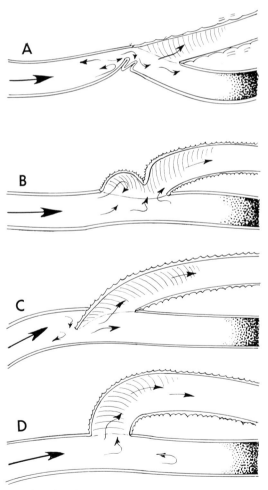

Fig. 22. Common errors in adjusting and completing an anastomosis. **A,** Excessive tension. **B,** Insufficient tension. **C,** Careless anastomosis. **D,** Right-angle exit not sufficiently oblique.

Comment: *A single sidewise clamp on the iliac artery at the site of anastomosis is preferable to bulldog clamps, since the handle can be used to steady the artery and the prosthesis and to turn the artery from side to side during the anastomosis. Choose a clamp of appropriate shape and apply it so that the handle is out of the way. The DeBakey tangential occlusion clamp or the Cooley, Beck, or small Satinsky clamp may be employed.*

3. Make a longitudinal arteriotomy in the iliac artery. Trim the edges to produce an oval opening or place stay sutures to hold the edges apart.

Comment: *It is unnecessary to trim the edges unless the artery is small.*

4. Draw the prosthesis downward, determine the correct length, and cut the end obliquely. Hold the prosthesis in position for anastomosis with an arterial clamp applied vertically about 1 cm. from the cut end (Fig. 21, E).

5. Hold the clamp so that the artery and the prosthesis are in the correct position for anastomosis. Begin the anastomosis with a mattress suture at the proximal end (Fig. 21, E). Sew over and over from the prosthesis to the artery.

6. Rotate the clamp on the artery and on the prosthesis to continue the suture around the tip of the prostheses and the distal end of the arteriotomy (Fig. 21, G). Stretch the tip distally and, if necessary, lengthen the arteriotomy distally to ensure an oblique attachment of the prosthesis to the artery.

7. Begin suture of the proximal end of the lateral side of the anastomosis with the remaining end of the first mattress suture (Fig. 21, H).

8. Release the iliac clamp momentarily to check the back bleeding and reapply the clamp (Fig. 21, I). Tapes maintain control during release of the clamp.

9. Reapply the clamp and rapidly complete the anastomosis (Fig. 21, J).

Comment: *Correct fit of the graft is essential. Some technical causes of narrowing and failure in end-to-side anastomosis are shown in Fig. 22. If exposure is poor, complete both sides of the anastomosis proximally at the acute angle and sew the distal tip last.*

Restoration of flow to first leg

1. Start a pint of blood running rapidly. Release the iliac clamp to permit back bleeding as high as the bifurcation.

2. Apply an occluding clamp to the completed side at the bifurcation of the prosthesis.

3. Release the aortic clamps briefly to flush clots and debris from the open limb of the graft.

4. Reapply the proximal aortic clamp momentarily.

5. Release the clamp from the completed side and reapply it to the open side at the bifurcation.

6. Release the proximal aortic clamp slowly, restoring flow to the leg through the completed anastomosis. Slow down the blood transfusion when bleeding stops and flow is restored to the first leg.

Second iliac anastomosis

1. Pass two umbilical tapes about the iliac artery at the site of anastomosis.
2. Select an appropriate sidewise clamp.
3. Inject 10 mg. of heparin in 10 ml. of saline solution distally.

4. Make a longitudinal arteriotomy and observe for back bleeding. Apply the sidewise clamp. Trim the sides of the arteriotomy and/or insert guide sutures on either side to hold the edges apart.

5. Proceed with fitting and anastomosis of the graft as described for the first side.

6. Remove the iliac clamp briefly before completion of the anastomosis to check back bleeding. Open the bifurcation clamp to flush out any clots and fill the graft with blood. Quickly close the proximal clamp, complete the anastomosis, and release the distal iliac clamp. Slowly release the proximal clamp.

7. Lumbar sympathectomy through the abdominal incision should be performed before closure (Fig. 25).

8. The iliac limbs of the bypass prosthesis are drawn beneath the peritoneum over the common iliac arteries so that closure over the distal anastomoses is simplified. Draw the mesocolon and mesentery of the small bowel together over the aorta anteriorly, covering the proximal portion of the prosthesis.

AORTOFEMORAL BYPASS
Importance of deep femoral artery

Prolongation of aortic grafts into the leg may be necessary to assure satisfactory outflow when the external iliac artery is narrowed. However, atherosclerosis of the external iliac artery commonly extends distally into the common femoral artery, and most of the patients also have associated narrowing or occlusions of the superficial femoral artery.

The deep femoral artery (profunda femoris) is the most important collateral artery in the leg, and in any operation on the arteries of the leg, normal pulsatile flow through the profunda femoris must be assured. Some of the various maneuvers performed on the profunda are illustrated in Fig. 24.

The profunda femoris is so important that restoration of pulsatile flow in it may save a leg even though the superficial femoral and popliteal outflow are both narrowed and inoperable. Aortofemoral bypass revascularization of the profunda femoris may not be ideal but may be all that is feasible. The outflow and collateral circulation via the profunda femoris is large. In many patients the femoropopliteal outflow is too poor for femoral endarterectomy or femoral bypass procedures. Other patients are poor risks, and the combined operation from the abdominal aorta to the popliteal arteries is too formidable even in two stages. In patients in whom the superficial femoral artery is also occluded, the surgeon must be absolutely certain that the profunda outflow is satisfactory.

When serving as collateral circulation, the profunda femoris may dilate tremendously. Its abundant large muscular branches are a superb "runoff," and in some patients pedal pulses return after aortoprofunda bypass even though the superficial femoral artery is occluded.

The orifice or the proximal centimeter of the profunda femoris is frequently narrowed by atherosclerotic plaques, particularly in those patients who need the profunda outflow most (that is, those with aortoiliac atherosclerosis extending down into the femoral artery). This is usually overlooked in the routine anteroposterior arteriograms because the shadow of the common femoral artery overlies the origin of the profunda femoris from the posterior side of the common femoral artery. The distal portion of the profunda femoris is usually free of atherosclerosis.

Procedure

The aortic portion of the operation has already been illustrated (Fig. 21, *A* to *D*) and described.

Exposure of common and deep femoral arteries

1. Make a vertical incision over the common femoral artery, and avoid dissection near the more medially placed lymphatic vessels and the femoral vein (Fig. 23, *A*).

2. Dissect out and isolate with umbilical tapes the profunda femoris, the common femoral, and the superficial femoral arteries. Palpate the vessels, and note localized plaques that may require endarterectomy. The arteriotomy will be made over the orifice of the profunda so that it can be inspected. This is frequently narrowed by plaques which must be removed to ensure adequate outflow.

Comment: *Inspection of the orifice of the profunda femoris should be part of all revascularization operations if the superficial femoral artery is occluded. In such cases the probability of narrowing of the profunda is so great, and the need for an adequate outflow from the profunda is crucial. The arteriogram does not visualize the origin of the profunda, where the narrowing may occur.*

3. Make a tunnel alongside and medial to the iliac artery by blunt dissection carried upward under the inguinal ligament and retroperitoneally to the common iliac artery or the aorta (Fig. 23, *B*).

4. Draw the prosthesis through this tunnel without kinks or twists. Adjust the length and apply an arterial clamp about 1 cm. from the proposed anastomosis. Trim the end of the prosthesis, leaving some excess.

Comment: *The correct length of the prosthesis must be carefully adjusted later, since too much tension or insufficient tension will disturb the blood flow at the anastomotic site (Fig. 22).*

Arteriotomy and inspection of profunda femoris artery

1. Make a longitudinal arteriotomy in the common femoral artery. Do not extend the arteriotomy distally past the orifice of the profunda femoris. It may be necessary to extend the incision into the profunda (Fig. 24, *A*).

Comment: *Dilation of the orifice of the profunda femoris (Fig. 24, C) is sometimes necessary because the fascial hiatus limits the dilation of the artery. Since the distal portion of the profunda is invisible behind the fascia, the common bile duct dilator (Fig. 24, C) is useful to explore, calibrate, and dilate the artery.*

Anastomosis

1. Rapidly inject 10 mg. of heparin into the deep and common femoral arteries, and apply an appropriate arterial occluding clamp (Fig. 24, *D*). Separate angled clamps are convenient to clamp the three arteries individually.

2. Begin the anastomosis with a double-armed suture, placed as a mattress at the acute angle between the graft and the arteriotomy (Fig. 24, *E*). Sew with an over-and-over stitch down each side of the arteriotomy, lengthening it if

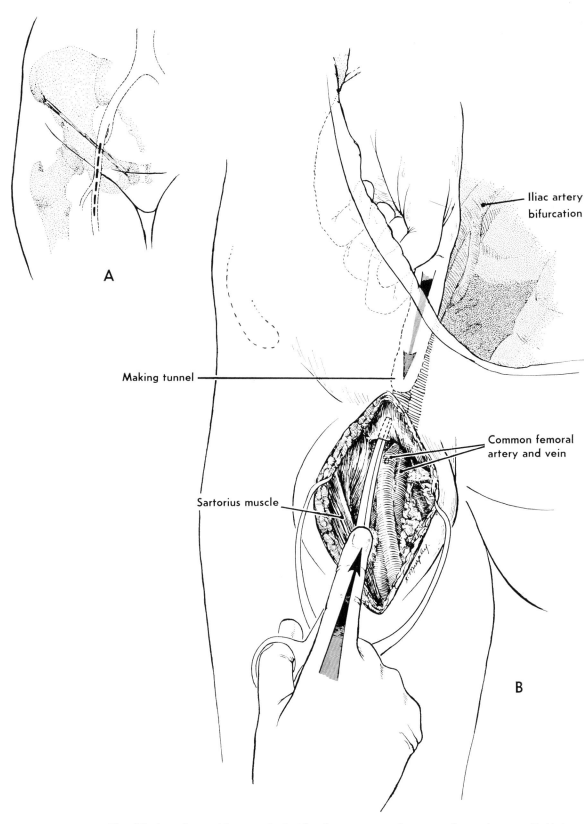

A

B

Iliac artery
bifurcation

Making tunnel

Common femoral
artery and vein

Sartorius muscle

Fig. 23. Aortofemoral bypass. **A,** Incision for exposure of common femoral artery. **B,** Make
a tunnel beneath inguinal ligament. (See also Fig. 24.)

80

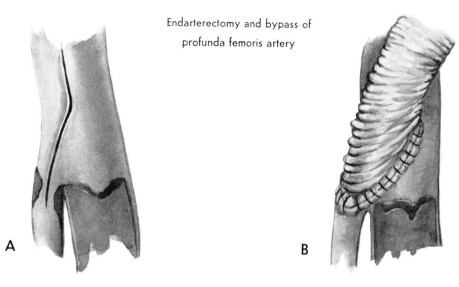

Endarterectomy and bypass of
profunda femoris artery

A

B

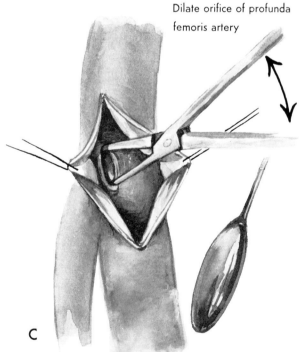

Dilate orifice of profunda
femoris artery

C

Fig. 24. Aortofemoral bypass. **A,** Arteriotomy extended onto deep femoral artery when orifice of profunda femoris is narrow. **B,** Enlargement of orifice by tip of prosthesis. **C,** Dilation of orifice.

Continued.

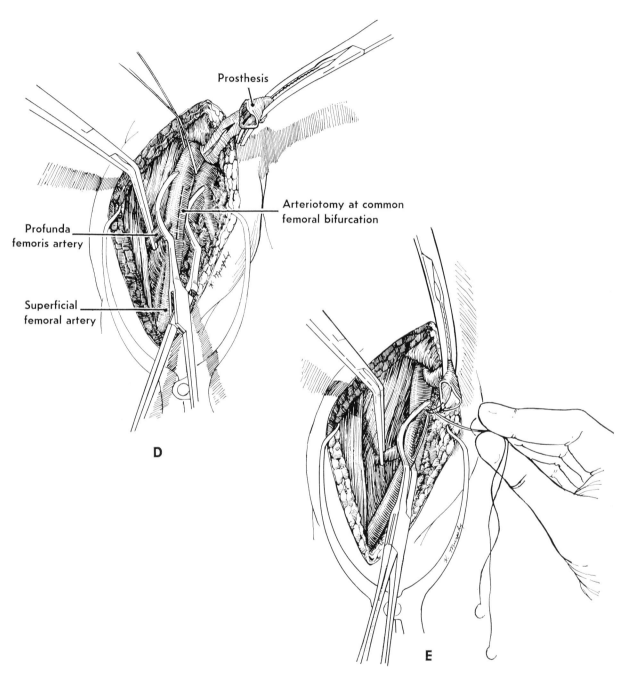

Prosthesis

Arteriotomy at common
femoral bifurcation

Profunda
femoris artery

Superficial
femoral artery

D

E

Fig. 24, cont'd. Aortofemoral bypass. **D,** Exposure of common femoral artery for aortofemoral bypass prosthesis. **E,** Begin anastomosis of prosthesis to front of common femoral
artery.

necessary. This procedure is similar to the anastomosis of the iliac bypass (Fig. 21, *E-J*).

3. Check back bleeding from the distal femoral artery. Flush clots from the prosthesis by releasing the proximal clamp before completing the anastomosis.

4. Finish the last portion of the anastomosis, and tie the sutures after releasing the distal clamp to extrude air from the femoral artery.

5. Restore flow to the leg by removing the proximal clamp slowly.

6. Soft tissues should be closed meticulously about the prosthesis to prevent collections of blood, lymph, or serum that can easily become infected.

Comment: *Delayed disruption and false aneurysms are more common in these anastomoses than elsewhere, probably due to motion of the prosthesis with flexion and the more common serum and lymph collections that prevent adherence and incorporation of the prosthesis and suture line in healthy tissue. Arterial silk loses its tensile strength after prolonged implantation, and Dacron, Tevdec, polyethylene, or polypropylene sutures are necessary for these as for other host artery–prosthesis anastomoses.*

Postoperative care

Anticoagulants are not used postoperatively. If the graft has been placed across the flexion crease of the groin, prolonged sitting positions should be avoided for a period of ten days.

Other maneuvers and variations

The arteriotomy for aortofemoral or aortoprofunda bypass described in detail earlier should be extended onto the profunda femoris as illustrated in Fig. 24, *A*, if inspection through the common femoral arteriotomy reveals a plaque causing narrowing of the orifice of the profunda.

The orifice of the profunda femoris can be widened whenever needed by inserting the tip of the aortofemoral prosthesis (Fig. 24, *B*). When aortoiliac endarterectomy must be extended into the femoral and profunda arteries, patch angioplasty is the best closure since it widens the profunda and wide secure stitches can be used for closure without narrowing the arterial lumen.

Local endarterectomy (that is, removal of the plaque) is performed in the profunda femoris only when the plaque is localized to the proximal centimeter and is thick or ulcerated. When an atherosclerotic plaque in a small artery has a smooth normal intima or extends a considerable distance, it is preferable to widen the lumen by patch angioplasty rather than by removal of the plaque.

Extended exposure of the profunda femoris is readily accomplished by incision of the fascia overlying it. Tributaries of the femoral vein cross in front of it and may be troublesome. The profunda gives off many branches posteriorly. To temporarily occlude these, use either loosely applied removable silver clips or a loop of 2-0 suture. Bulldog clamps are too bulky for this location.

BILATERAL ABDOMINAL SYMPATHECTOMY

Bilateral abdominal lumbar sympathectomy should be used routinely as an adjunct to either endarterectomy or bypass operations for aortoiliac occlusive disease. The lumbar sympathetic ganglia are removed from about the second or third lumbar segment to the pelvic brim. It is difficult to get as high on the chain of ganglia as during lumbar sympathectomy through a lateral retroperitoneal approach. However, the lumbar sympathetic chains are easily accessible at the time the aorta is exposed and may be removed either before or after the primary procedure.

Procedure

Technique—right side

1. Dissect the fat and lymphatic tissue from the right side of the inferior vena cava. Retract this tissue and the spermatic or ovarian vessels laterally.

2. Roll the inferior vena cava medially with a sponge stick, and palpate the anterior aspects of the fourth and fifth lumbar vertebras to locate the sympathetic chain. The chain is unique and may be identified by the small nodular ganglia.

3. Roll the nerve against the vertebral bodies. Lift the chain with a nerve

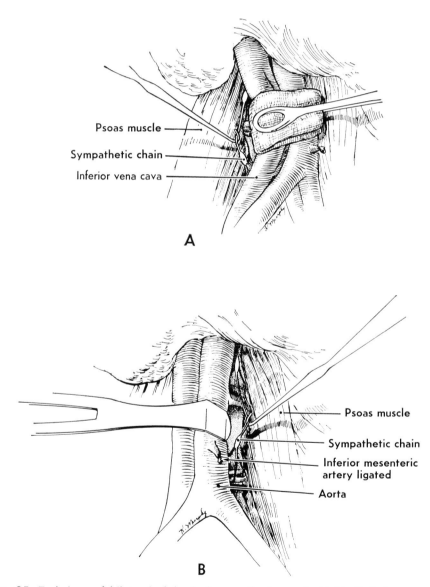

Fig. 25. Technique of bilateral abdominal sympathectomy. **A,** Right. **B,** Left.

hook, and dissect it from the groove between the psoas muscle and the vertebral bodies. Inferiorly carry the dissection to the right iliac vein. Divide the rami only, leaving the chain intact. The lumbar veins ordinarily are posterior to the sympathetic chain. However, care must be taken to visualize and to avoid injury of these vessels (Fig. 25, A).

4. The kidney is not displaced forward with the anterior approach. Follow the sympathetic chain upward, posteriorly, and somewhat deeper, until the right renal pedicle limits further dissection. Use a narrow Deaver retractor to expose the upper possible limit of dissection. Dissection may be extended slightly by using one's finger or a small "peanut" sponge to dissect a little farther up the sympathetic chain. Clip the upper end of the sympathetic chain with several silver clips and divide it.

Technique—left side

Sympathectomy on the left may be more difficult than on the right, particularly if there is much inflammatory or fibrotic reaction about the terminal aorta.

If exposure is difficult by the following method, the sigmoid colon may be reflected superiorly and medially and the sympathetic chain approached retroperitoneally after a posterior peritoneal incision is made.

1. Divide the inferior mesenteric artery, and retract the descending colon and its mesentery to the left. Retract the lymphatic and fatty tissues and gonadal vessels laterally. The sympathetic chain lies in the groove between the psoas muscle and the vertebral bodies and is located by palpation as a firm nodular cord.

2. Lift the sympathetic chain with a nerve hook. Dissect inferiorly, and apply silver clips at the pelvic brim. Divide the terminal rami of the lumbar sympathetic chain here, seize the chain with a hemostat, and dissect upward as described for the right side, dividing the rami of the sympathetic chain in the process. Apply silver clips to the superior limit of the dissection and divide the chain to remove it.

SURGICAL MANAGEMENT OF COMPLICATIONS OF PROSTHESES
Introduction

The technical precautions which avoid or reduce complications have been described in detail in each section and are not repeated here.

The following discussion is intended to reemphasize general principles and direct the reader to original articles for details not already included.

Rerouting arterial grafts—femorofemoral, axillofemoral, and iliofemoral via obturator foramen bypass procedures

Arterial grafts may be rerouted in patients in whom a prosthesis becomes infected or thrombosed. The new prosthesis need not be placed in or even near the normal course of the bypassed artery. Indeed, when a prosthesis is infected, a new one must not approach the contaminated area and must be inserted via new incisions. An example is the bypass via the obturator foramen from the iliac to the superficial femoral or popliteal artery to avoid an infected subinguinal incision.

Rerouting of grafts may also be necessary in poor-risk patients unsuitable for laparotomy who have acute ischemia due to thrombosis of the iliac artery. Blood flow may be restored to the ischemic leg by attaching the prosthesis to an opposite patent femoral artery (Fig. 26) or to the axillary artery on the same side. The prostheses are drawn through subcutaneous tunnels. The operations have been performed under local anesthesia when the use of general anesthesia involved too great a risk.

The femorofemoral crossover graft (Fig. 26) was first reported by Vetto.* The profunda femoris on the ischemic side is almost always open, and local endarterectomy of the common femoral artery and proximal portion of the profunda furnishes a site for the distal attachment of the femorofemoral graft. The subcutaneous tunnel over the pubis is made by blunt dissection connecting the two groin incisions. The ends of the 8 mm. prosthesis are attached to the sides of the two femoral arteries. The acute angle of the takeoff of the graft is theoretically undesirable but cannot be avoided. Some of these femorofemoral crossover prostheses have remained open as long as three years despite the unnatural turbulence. Details of the anastomoses follow the techniques previously described in detail.

The axillofemoral bypass graft was first described by Blaisdell and Hall† in three patients, two of whom had infected abdominal grafts that had to be removed. The third patient had cardiac arrest and could not tolerate general anesthesia. Although the length of the graft decreases the flow, it has saved lives and limbs. We have had no personal experience with this procedure.

Infected prostheses

When infection involves the anastomosis of a prosthesis and artery, disruption is inevitable. The false aneurysm, or pulsating hematoma, is a catastrophe that requires ligations of the artery and ultimately removal of the infected graft. Blood flow to the limb distal to the ligation is rarely sufficient to permit delay for elective revascularization. The new emergency bypass prosthesis must be placed through uncontaminated incisions and routed far from the infected field. The femorofemoral, axillofemoral, and iliofemoral via obturator foramen bypass procedures were described in the previous discussion.

Sometimes infection about a prosthesis does not extend to the anastomosis and for a time the prosthesis conducts blood. If this is recognized in time, early opening of the incision before gross suppuration develops and extends may permit debridement and meticulous secondary closure. This should be preceded and followed by massive antibiotic dosage and immobilization of the limb or bed rest to reduce lymph flow. The meticulous closure must obliterate dead space. Drains are seldom necessary.

Thrombosed-occluded prostheses

The technical aspects and inflow and outflow factors affecting graft patency have already been illustrated (Fig. 22) and discussed. However, these general principles need reemphasis.

---

*Vetto, R. M.: The treatment of unilateral iliac artery obstruction with a transabdominal, subcutaneous femorofemoral graft, Surgery **52**:342, 1962.
†Blaisdell, F. W., and Hall, A. D.: Axillary femoral artery bypass for lower extremity ischemia, Surgery **54**:563, 1963.

86

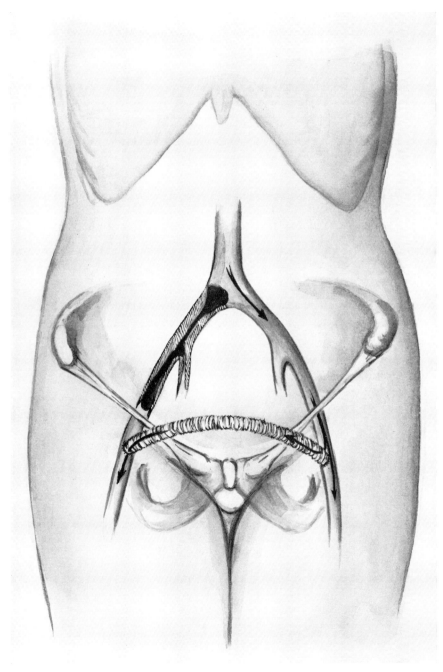

Fig. 26. Femoral crossover bypass.

1. Early occlusion of a prosthesis is always due to some small technical error that is correctible by immediate reoperation, reexploration, and revision of the anastomoses or graft unless, of course, the inflow or outflow was misjudged. If the occlusion was truly operable, the limb or operation is still salvageable by immediate reoperation.
2. Pulsatile flow into the profunda femoris can be restored by one of the maneuvers or rerouting procedures and will save many limbs even though the superficial femoral artery and its outflow are blocked or narrowed and inoperable.
3. Intraabdominal grafts that occlude need not be removed since the new grafts can be rerouted. Femoral grafts, however, must usually be excised.
4. Endarterectomy of a prosthesis is futile. The factors that led to the first occlusion must be corrected, and this almost always requires a new graft with better flow through.

Aortoenteric fistula

Aortoenteric fistulas are almost unknown since the need for separation of bowel from the prosthesis by sufficient living soft tissue was recognized. The two hazardous sites are the third part of the duodenum, which may cross the proximal portion of the prosthesis or anastomosis, and the cecum, which may overlie an iliac prosthesis or anastomosis. The mobilization of the third part of the duodenum so that it does not cross the prosthesis and the use of the sac of the aneurysm, mesocolon, or omentum to cover the prosthesis have been described previously. These procedures are essential in the prevention of aortoenteric fistula.

Chapter 5

Occlusive disease in the lower extremity

Introduction

Arteriosclerotic occlusive disease below the level of the common femoral artery is one of the most challenging problems in vascular reconstructive surgery and perhaps the one that is, to date, most elusive of solution. Many of the patients have extensive arteriosclerotic disease at the level of the popliteal artery and below and are inoperable unless there is a suitable outflow tract below the popliteal level. Evaluation of outflow requires good arteriograms and experience in their interpretation. At least one main branch of the popliteal artery must be open. Given, however, a suitable outflow tract at the popliteal level, a number of methods have been used to conduct blood from the common femoral artery to the popliteal level. Unlike atherosclerotic occlusion in the aorto-iliac region, which is frequently localized and suitable for endarterectomy, occlusive disease in the femoropopliteal region is usually more diffuse.

Endarterectomy is the ideal procedure to restore flow in short segments of large arteries occluded by atheromatous deposits in the intima and may also reopen muscular branches of the artery. Endarterectomy is difficult and sometimes hazardous in arteries with medial calcification. Endarterectomy of small vessels such as the distal portion of the popliteal artery is less successful. Endarterectomy of the femoral arteries is usually accomplished by passing loops between the arteriotomies and is therefore blind. Long open endarterectomies closed with an onlay graft of saphenous vein are very tedious. Combinations of onlay and bypass with the saphenous vein are under trial. The bypass procedures are preferred for long occlusions.

Bypass grafts of prosthetic material, even when distal outflow is adequate, frequently occlude, particularly where they pass the flexion crease of the knee. A more successful alternative is bypass with an autogenous saphenous vein, either removed and reversed or used in situ with the valves destroyed or reversed. Experiments with arteriovenous fistula and with arterialization of the venous system are of less clinical importance at present.

89

Of all these various methods, the most promising and most widely applicable is the use of autogenous veins as grafts for arterial bypass. Veins continue to function under the relatively unfavorable hydrodynamic condition of poor distal outflow that would ensure the failure of a prosthetic arterial replacement. The use of vein grafts also extends the range of bypassing to the distal popliteal artery.

In operations on the lower extremity, the importance of the profunda femoris artery cannot be overemphasized. At any time that the common femoral artery is exposed and opened, the orifice of the profunda femoris should be inspected and be cleared of any constricting arteriosclerotic plaque. In many patients the profunda has proved capable of nourishing the entire lower extremity. In these, as well as in other patients with borderline arterial circulation, lumbar sympathectomy should be employed routinely.

EXPLORATION OF POPLITEAL ARTERY

The common diseases involving the popliteal artery are atherosclerotic occlusive disease, popliteal aneurysm, and embolism. The medial approach as illustrated in this discussion is most advantageous for occlusive disease, embolism, and injuries. The midline posterior approach is applicable to excision and grafting procedures for aneurysm and for injuries. Important advantages of the medial approach are as follows:

1. Incisions can easily be extended upward and downward as the operative findings may dictate.

2. The popliteal artery is more accessible by the medial approach, particularly in its proximal and distal portions.

3. The artery is easily drawn forward toward the skin when the knee is flexed.

4. The tibial nerve and the popliteal veins are more easily avoided.

5. The patient is in the supine position so that the surgeon may work simultaneously in the groin and in the abdomen without repositioning.

The popliteal artery may be considered in three divisions. The proximal or upper portion begins at the adductor hiatus, the midportion lies between the heads of the gastrocnemius muscle at about the level of the knee joint, and the distal portion lies behind the upper parts of the tibia and fibula. The upper part of the popliteal artery is commonly affected by occlusive disease extending distally from the adductor canal (Hunter's canal). Plaques are commonly seen at the branching of the distal popliteal artery.

Procedure

Exploration of proximal portion of popliteal artery

1. Place the patient in the supine position with the thigh slightly abducted and externally rotated and the knee flexed and supported. The surgeon stands at the opposite side of the table.

2. Begin the incision medial and anterior to the saphenous vein in the lower part of the thigh and extend it downward to the lower border of the patella (Fig. 27, A). The saphenous nerve may cross the incision and can be divided or retracted gently. The saphenous vein should be preserved in case manipulation of the popliteal vein predisposes to thrombosis or it is needed as a vein graft.

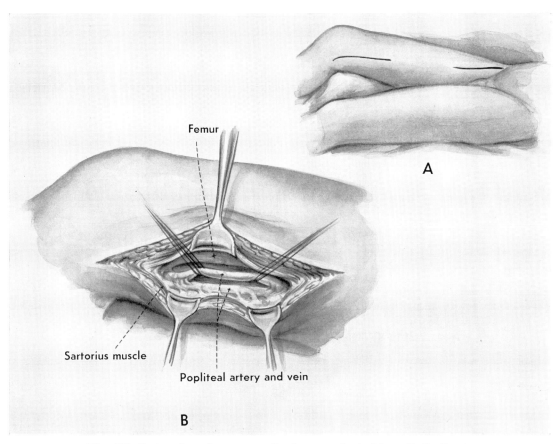

Femur

Sartorius muscle

Popliteal artery and vein

A

B

Fig. 27. Exploration of upper popliteal artery. **A,** Incisions. **B,** Popliteal exposure.

3. Open the deep fascia anterior to the sartorius muscle and retract the muscle posteriorly.

4. Identify the posterior edge of the vastus medialis muscle with blunt dissection and retract it anteriorly. Divide the adductor tendon to mobilize the artery (Fig. 27, B).

5. Identify the popliteal artery, which is the most superficial cordlike structure palpable through the exposure. Divide the overlying fascia and the sheath of the artery.

6. Mobilize a considerable length of the artery so that it can be easily drawn up into the incision with an umbilical tape.

Comment: *The tibial nerve and the popliteal vein lie posteriorly and well away from the proximal portion of the artery. The nerve need not be dissected out or otherwise disturbed. The vein is not usually troublesome posteriorly and laterally, but frequently the popliteal or superficial femoral vein is double and one of the channels may lie anterior and medial to the artery.*

Exploration of midportion of popliteal artery

The medial approach is useful if occlusive disease involves the upper portion of the popliteal artery, since an arteriotomy may be made in the more normal middle section for attachment of a vein or Dacron prosthetic bypass. Arteriotomy

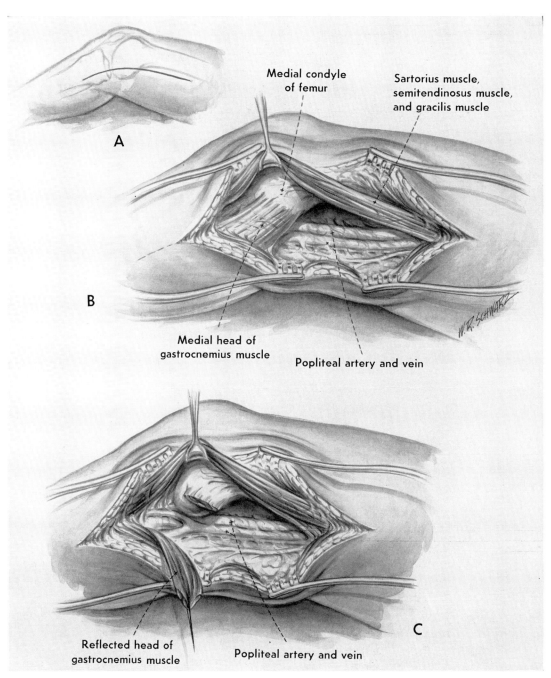

Medial condyle
of femur

Sartorius muscle,
semitendinosus muscle,
and gracilis muscle

A

B

W. R. SCHWARZ

Medial head of
gastrocnemius muscle

Popliteal artery and vein

C

Reflected head of
gastrocnemius muscle

Popliteal artery and vein

Fig. 28. Exploration of midportion of popliteal artery. **A,** Incision. **B,** Retraction of ham-
strings to expose upper popliteal artery and origin of gastrocnemius muscle. **C,** Division of
medial head of gastrocnemius muscle to reveal midportion of popliteal artery.

92

of the midportion of the popliteal artery is also preferred for embolectomy by the retrograde flush method.

The midportion of the popliteal artery is approached by mobilizing the hamstring muscles and tendons and retracting them posteriorly. The exposure is extended by dividing the medial head of the gastrocnemius muscle where it attaches to the medial condyle of the femur (Fig. 28, B and C).

1. Extend the skin incision employed for the proximal popliteal artery distally, anterior to the saphenous vein and nerve, and as far distal as the medial tibial condyle (Fig. 28, A).

2. Incise the deep fascia along the anterior edge of the sartorius and the hamstring muscles. Occasionally it is preferable to incise along the posterior edge of these muscles and to retract them anteriorly (Fig. 28, B).

3. Identify the medial head of the gastrocnemius muscle and divide it close to its ligamentous origin. Leave 1 or 2 cm. of the tendinous attachment to facilitate suture later and to avoid opening the knee joint (Fig. 28, C).

4. Turn the distal divided end of the gastrocnemius downward and medially. Note and spare the motor nerve and arterial branches that enter the muscle at a somewhat lower level.

5. Incise the sheath of the popliteal artery. It may be necessary to divide venous tributaries that cross the artery. The popliteal vein is not troublesome, except distally. The tibial nerve is posterior and well out of the way.

6. Flexion of the knee relaxes the artery so that it is readily drawn close to the skin level.

Exploration of distal portion of popliteal artery

Distal exposure is suitable for occlusive disease proximal to this level, arterial injuries (particularly the "quick-draw" pistol wound), arteriotomy for popliteal embolectomy, etc. Arteriotomies in the distal portion of the popliteal artery should be closed with vein patch to avoid narrowing. The technique of patch angioplasty is illustrated in Fig. 57.

1. Place the patient in the supine position with the leg externally rotated, the thigh abducted, and the knee moderately flexed.

2. Make an incision 8 to 10 cm. long along the posteromedial border of the tibia, below the medial condyle, and extending upward to the knee joint (Fig. 29, A).

3. Incise the deep fascia overlying the gastrocnemius muscle along the posterior edge of the tibia (Fig. 29, B).

4. Retract the medial head of the gastrocnemius muscle posteriorly away from the tibia, and expose the origin of the soleus muscle from the posterior aspect of the tibia. Elevate the thigh on a folded sheet or towel in order to flex the knee slightly and allow the calf muscles to drop downward.

5. Divide the tendons of insertion of the sartorius and other medial hamstring muscles that are attached to the medial condyle of the tibia.

6. Identify the popliteal vein along the medial edge of the soleus muscle. Dissect this and retract it with a small vein retractor to uncover the popliteal artery (Fig. 29, C).

7. Identify the origin of the anterior tibial artery on the opposite side of the popliteal artery. The point of origin is almost perpendicular to the popliteal

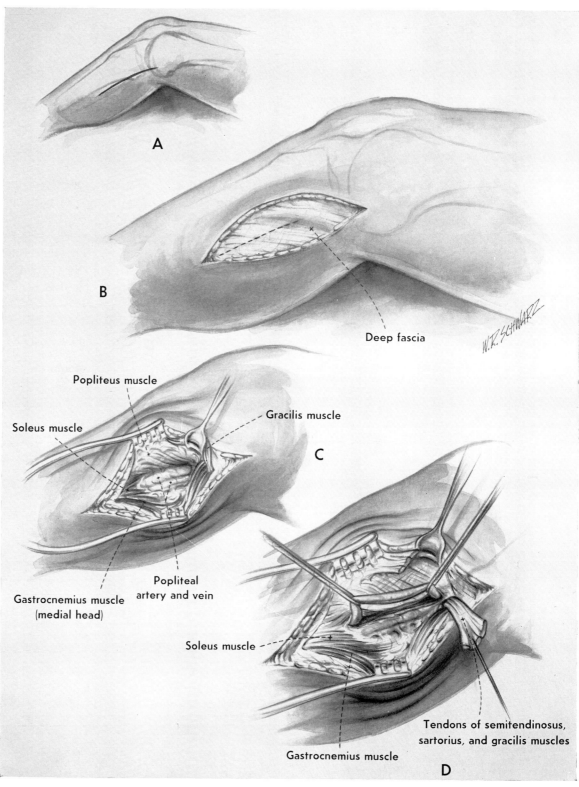

A

B

Deep fascia

W.R.SCHWARZ

Popliteus muscle

Soleus muscle

Gracilis muscle

C

Gastrocnemius muscle
(medial head)

Popliteal
artery and vein

Soleus muscle

Tendons of semitendinosus,
sartorius, and gracilis muscles

Gastrocnemius muscle

D

Fig. 29. Exploration of distal portion of popliteal artery. **A,** Incision. **B,** Incision in deep fascia at posterior border of tibia. **C,** Distal popliteal artery uncovered by retraction of muscles. **D,** Distal popliteal artery dissected free and drawn up toward skin. The knee is bent.

artery. After a very short course, the anterior tibial artery penetrates a hiatus in the interosseous membrane between the tibia and fibula.

Comment: *In an occasional patient the anterior tibial artery originates at a higher level. Another variation is the trifurcation, that is, simultaneous origin of the three outflow branches at one point. Normally, however, the popliteal artery continues another few centimeters before it terminates by division into the posterior tibial and the peroneal arteries.*

8. Expose the distal portion of the popliteal artery by dividing the attachments of the soleus muscle to the tibia for 2 to 5 cm.

9. Separate the popliteal veins from the artery at the site of the proposed arteriotomy. The popliteal vein at this low level is frequently double. Arteriotomy at the origin of the anterior tibial artery permits local endarterectomy of stenosing plaques at that level and assures perfusion of the anterior tibial artery by the flow from the graft.

10. With the knee flexed and the medial tendons divided, the artery is readily drawn forward into the incision (Fig. 29, *D*).

11. A tunnel can be made ready for the bypass, or an endarterectomy stripper can be readily passed upward.

FEMORAL ARTERY BYPASS
Introduction

Femoral bypass is a useful procedure to restore normal pulsatile flow and to heal ischemic lesions in the foot or leg that are caused by atherosclerotic occlusions in the superficial femoral artery. At least one of the branches of the popliteal artery must be patent. Intermittent claudication alone is not a sufficient indication for operation unless it is disabling.

Operability may be determined by preoperative angiography, which should show a patent popliteal artery. As mentioned, at least one of the arteries of the lower leg should be open. When in doubt, the popliteal artery should be explored as described earlier in this chapter or more precisely evaluated by operative angiography.

Candidates for bypass of the femoral artery should be chosen carefully. Patients with late changes (that is, muscle wasting in the calf, loss of hair, nail changes, and absent distal pulses) have obliterative disease that is too extensive for vascular reconstructive surgery. Other contraindications are of a general nature.

If proximal stenoses are present, these must be relieved by an appropriate earlier or simultaneous operation such as aortoiliac bypass or endarterectomy. Endarterectomy of the entire femoral artery has been employed by some surgeons for these severe conditions. We have used endarterectomy for localized occlusions and prefer bypass prostheses for more extensive occlusive disease.

Bypass with a long saphenous vein graft is less likely to be complicated by postoperative thrombosis than bypass with a Dacron prosthesis. Vein grafts are preferable for patients with borderline outflow. Prosthetic materials may be employed when bypassing to the proximal portion of the popliteal artery or when the saphenous vein is missing, diseased, or too small.

Preoperative care

Preoperative care should be thorough. Arteriograms must demonstrate patency of the major vessels proximal and distal to the proposed bypass. The risk to life in operations on the leg alone is small, but evaluation of cardiopulmonary and renal function is essential.

The skin should be prepared with antiseptic soap (pHisoHex or Septisol) for several days preoperatively.

Procedure

Place the patient in the supine position with the thigh slightly abducted and externally rotated and the knee flexed and supported laterally. Prepare and drape the entire groin, thigh, and leg to well below the knee.

Exploration of popliteal artery to assure operability

1. Incise the skin and deep fascia medial to the knee and posterior to the femoral condyle. Exploration of the popliteal artery is summarized here (Fig. 30, A and B) but is described in more detail on pp. 90-95.

2. Retract the sartorius muscle posteriorly, avoiding the saphenous nerve.

3. Divide the adductor tendon.

4. Enter the popliteal space anterior to the hamstring muscles.

5. Identify the popliteal artery, separate it from the vein, pass an umbilical tape about it, and palpate carefully to choose a site for anastomosis where the artery is soft and has an adequate lumen. Extend the incision and explore distally if this is necessary. If the findings and preoperative arteriogram are inconclusive, operative arteriography should be done (Chapter 2).

Comment: *Some apparently inoperable legs can be salvaged with distal implantation of vein grafts.*

Exposure of common femoral artery

1. Incise the skin and superficial fascia longitudinally over the femoral pulsation from about 2 cm. above the inguinal ligament inferiorly for a distance of about 10 cm. (Figs. 23, C, and 30, A).

2. Open the femoral arterial sheath directly over the artery and dissect upward and downward. Identify the profunda femoris and the superficial femoral branches of the common femoral artery.

3. Palpate the artery carefully. Plaques at the bifurcation of the common femoral artery are usually not demonstrated by the anteroposterior films made during arteriography. Therefore, the arteriotomy will be made over the bifurcation. Tapes are necessary about the common femoral, superficial femoral, and profunda femoris arteries. Arteriotomy over the bifurcation will allow inspection of the interior of the artery and examination of the orifice of the profunda. Plaques are frequently localized at the exit of the profunda and may be removed by local endarterectomy prior to anastomosis.

Femoral arteriotomy

1. Inject 30 mg. of heparin in 10 to 15 ml. of saline solution into the common femoral artery.

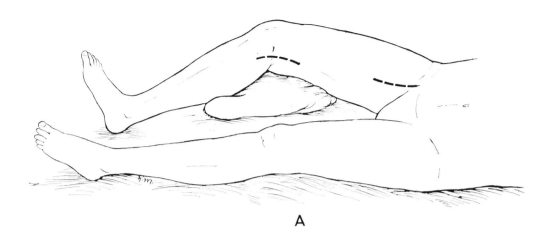

A

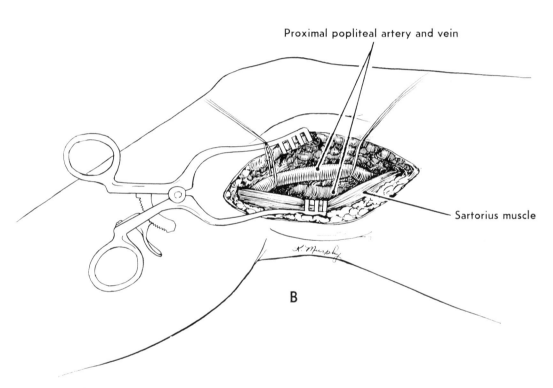

Proximal popliteal artery and vein

Sartorius muscle

B

Fig. 30. Femoropopliteal artery bypass. **A,** Position of patient and incisions. **B,** Exposure of proximal popliteal artery.

Continued.

2. Immediately apply occluding clamps. DeBakey angled clamps are convenient for controlling the common, superficial, and deep femoral vessels (Fig. 30, *C*).

3. Make a short longitudinal arteriotomy at about the junction of the profunda femoris and superficial femoral arteries. Begin the arteriotomy with a knife, and complete it with the Potts angled scissors. The arteriotomy is one and one-half to two times the diameter of the artery. If the ostium of the profunda is narrowed, a localized endarterectomy is performed at this time.

97

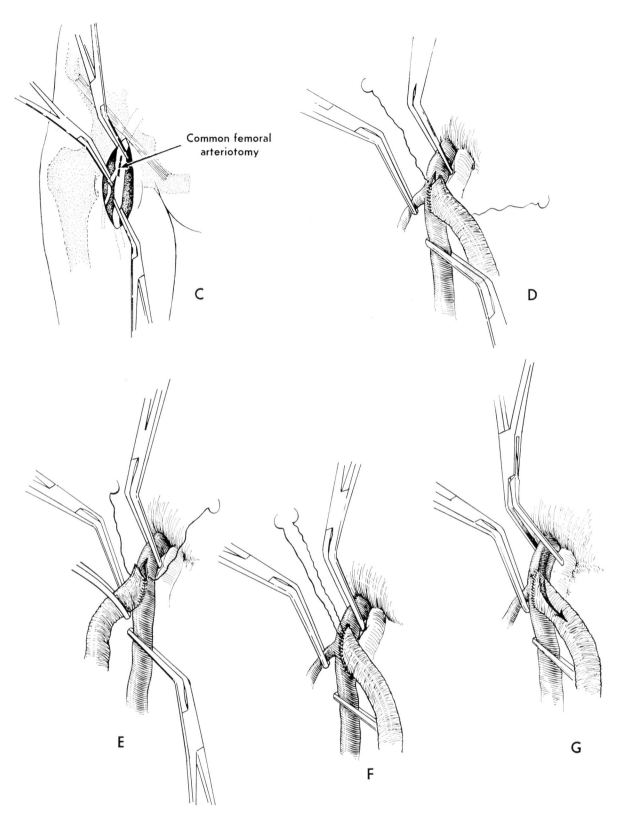

Fig. 30, cont'd. Femoropopliteal artery bypass. **C,** Exposure and control of femoral artery for proximal anastomosis. **D,** Lateral side of anastomosis. **E,** Medial side of anastomosis. **F,** Anastomosis completed. **G,** Flush artery and preclot prosthesis.

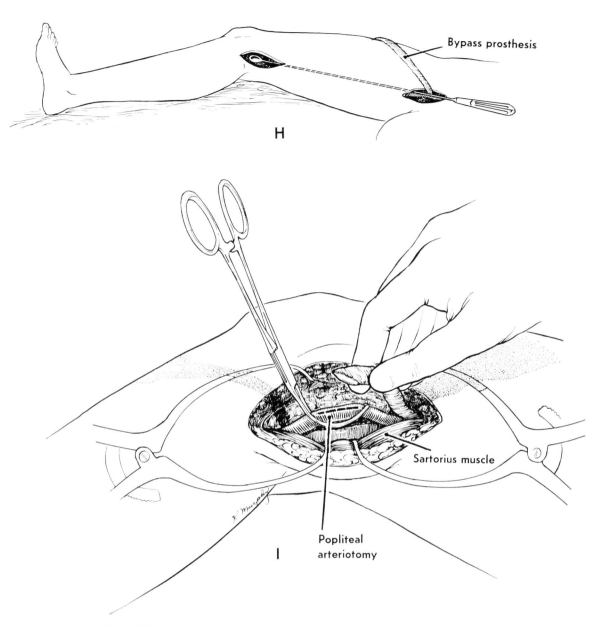

Bypass prosthesis

H

Sartorius muscle

Popliteal
arteriotomy

I

Fig. 30, cont'd. Femoropopliteal artery bypass. **H,** Subfascial tunnel. **I,** Exposure of proximal popliteal artery for anastomosis.

Proximal end-to-side anastomosis of prosthesis and artery

1. Select an 8 to 10 mm. Dacron arterial prosthesis. Smaller prostheses are likely to thrombose. The technique of end-to-side anastomosis is illustrated in Fig. 30, *D-F*. It is helpful to begin at the acute angle of the anastomosis—distally in this case. This permits proximal extension of the arteriotomy, accurate fitting at the tip of the graft, and the proper oblique attachment for nonturbulent flow through the anastomosis. Review Fig. 22 for common errors.

2. Cut the proximal end of the prosthesis obliquely, and hold it with an arterial clamp applied vertically.

99

3. Place a mattress suture of double-armed 4-0 arterial Dacron through the distal end (the oblique angle) of the prosthesis.

4. Suture a portion of the lateral edge of the prosthesis to the artery with a continuous over-and-over stitch, using one of the ends of the double-armed mattress suture (Fig. 30, D).

5. Suture the medial edge of the prosthesis and artery with the other end of the mattress suture (Fig. 30, E).

6. Stretch the tip of the prosthesis, lengthening the arteriotomy if necessary to fit the stretched tip, ensuring that the prosthesis will take off obliquely from the artery.

7. Continue one of the sutures around the upper end of the arteriotomy to meet the other suture (Fig. 30, F). End the suture line by tying the two ends securely (Fig. 30, G). Open the proximal clamp momentarily to flush and to preclot the graft (Fig. 30, G).

Preparation of tunnel for bypass prosthesis

1. Dissect free the medial edge of the sartorius muscle at the inferior end of the femoral incision.

2. Visualize the deep fascia. Thrust the DeBakey tunneling instrument between the sartorius and deep fascia along the course of the femoral canal (Fig. 30, H). Measure the approximate length of prosthesis required and cut the graft a little longer.

Popliteal arteriotomy

1. Flex the knee to relax the artery, and apply a curved DeBakey peripheral arterial clamp to the popliteal artery at the site of the proposed anastomosis (Fig. 30, I). Pull the artery outward toward the skin in a more accessible position.

2. Place a guide suture on either side of the intended arteriotomy to steady the artery. Make a stab wound with a No. 11 pointed scalpel blade, and enlarge the opening with the Potts angled scissors. The incision must be long enough to accommodate the oblique cut end of the graft.

Preclotting prosthesis and flushing proximal femoral artery

1. Release the proximal clamp on the common femoral artery, filling the graft under pressure (Fig. 30, G).

2. Reapply the clamp, and inject 10 mg. of heparin proximal to it. Empty the graft and artery of excess blood and clots, using a suction catheter if necessary.

3. Pass a sponge-holding forceps through the tunnel. Grasp the graft and draw it down so that it lies within the tunnel without twists or kinks. Stretch the graft to medium tension, apply an arterial forceps vertically, and trim the end of the prosthesis obliquely to adjust the length as necessary. Leave the prosthesis somewhat slack in the popliteal area.

4. Apply a mattress stitch of 4-0 arterial suture at the proximal end (that is, the acute angle) of the junction of the prosthesis and the popliteal artery. Tie this in place while the assistant holds the artery and prosthesis in approximation with the clamps.

5. Anastomose the lower end of the prosthesis to the popliteal artery in a manner identical to that for the upper anastomosis. The assistant holds the artery and prosthesis in approximation with the clamps and turns them to give access to the inferior edge of the anastomosis.

6. Momentarily release the popliteal clamp to test the back bleeding and then reapply it. Tapes around the artery give additional control and permit lifting the artery to reapply the clamp.

7. Before completing the popliteal anastomosis, release the femoral clamp to flush out any clots. Quickly reapply the femoral clamp and finish the anastomosis. Do not tie the suture until the air is forced out of the artery and prosthesis by the next maneuver.

8. Remove the popliteal clamp. If a separate clamp has been placed on the profunda femoris, remove it. Slowly remove the clamp on the common femoral artery.

9. Palpate pulses carefully and/or do a routine operative arteriogram to check the patency of the anastomosis.

10. Delay closure of the incisions for a few minutes to allow removal of any blood that may leak from the prosthesis shortly after blood flow is restored.

Closure of incision

1. No drains are necessary, and anticoagulation should not be used.

2. Close incisions carefully in layers, suturing soft tissue over the anastomosis and the graft.

3. Meticulous closure in the groin will prevent lymph and serum accumulations that lead to slow wound healing and infection. Do not allow dead space.

Postoperative care

The pressure of a tight bandage behind the knee is avoided. Keep the limb slightly elevated, and check the pedal pulses regularly. The pedal pulses may not be palpable immediately. If they are palpable but later disappear, reoperation is necessary at once.

Bed rest for seven to ten days is necessary until the incision has healed and soft tissue is adherent about the prosthesis. After that time, gradual flexion of the knee may be allowed. However, the knee must not be flexed past 90 degrees. Crossing the legs and all pressure behind the knee should be avoided.

Distal popliteal anastomosis for femoral bypass

Femoral bypass with distal popliteal anastomosis differs in several respects from the bypass to the proximal portion of the popliteal artery just described. Extremities with such extensive occlusion are more likely to be inoperable, although occasionally distal anastomosis, perhaps combined with endarterectomy at the division of the popliteal artery, can be accomplished. Vein grafts are preferable in this situation and, after further trial, the in situ utilization of the saphenous vein may become the best procedure.

Comment: *When vein grafts are used, the reversed vein lies in the tunnel or groove from which it was removed. The distal tunnel for the vein graft or for* *prostheses should not cause kinking of the graft when the knee is flexed. To prevent this, as well as to improve exposure of the distal anastomosis, we never hesitate to divide muscles or tendons.*

The first step is to explore the distal popliteal artery to determine operability (see pp. 90-95). If the condition is operable, a third incision is necessary to make the longer tunnel. This incision is made as follows:

1. Incise the skin of the lower third of the thigh for several inches along the medial border of the sartorius muscle.

2. If a prosthesis is used, make the distal tunnel along the popliteal neurovascular bundle and lateral to the medial hamstring group of muscles.

3. Dissect the tunnel along the neurovascular bundle behind the knee joint between the two heads of the gastrocnemius muscle. Divide the medial head of the gastrocnemius muscle if it appears to constrict or angle the graft.

4. From the distal popliteal incision dissect proximally with the fingertip behind the medial head of the gastrocnemius muscle along the artery to join the finger passing down from the proximal popliteal incision.

The prosthesis will have been previously preclotted and emptied and is now drawn through the tunnel to the correct length without twisting or kinking.

The distal anastomosis is less accessible than the proximal, but division of the tendons inserting on the medial aspect of the tibia gives ample room. Do not suture divided tendons if they will restrict or angulate the graft. The artery is drawn up into the incision with fine-toothed vascular clamps. The anastomosis begins with the first mattress stitch at the acute (proximal) angle as previously described.

Techniques of the arteriotomy, localized endarterectomy when necessary, and restoration of flow otherwise follow methods previously described in detail.

Vein graft for femoral bypass

Autogenous saphenous veins offer considerable advantages over fabric materials for reconstruction in the distal popliteal artery, across the popliteal crease, and into poor outflow tracts. Vein grafts are more likely to remain open when there is a marginal outflow. The best vein is the saphenous from the same leg. However, it may be diseased, too short, or too small. When it is short, it can be implanted lower on the superficial femoral artery. The proximal portion of the superficial femoral artery is then cleared by endarterectomy. Other maneuvers to utilize short veins are described below and illustrated in Fig. 31, *E-J*, and the technique of vein graft bypass in situ is described later in this chapter.

Procedure

1. Expose the popliteal artery by the medial approach (Fig. 31, *A*). Careful palpation and/or an operative arteriogram is necessary to confirm operability and the site of distal anastomosis. Do not divide the saphenous vein during the incision. Frequently this can be palpated at the time the incision is made or will be visualized soon after the incision is carried through the skin.

2. Carefully examine the saphenous vein in the distal portion of the incision (Fig. 31, *B*). If it was not found when the incision was made, it will usually lie

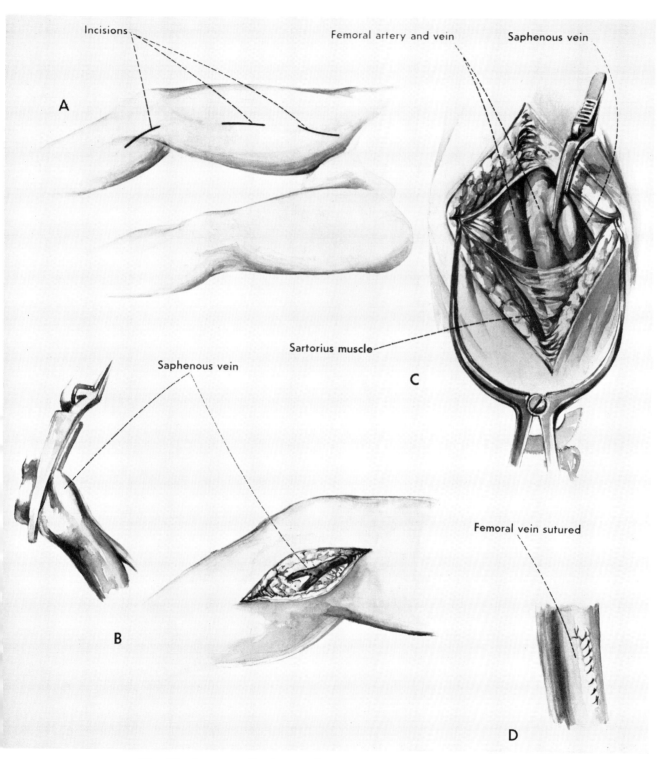

Fig. 31. Femoropopliteal artery bypass vein graft procurement. **A-D,** Incisions and exposure.

Continued.

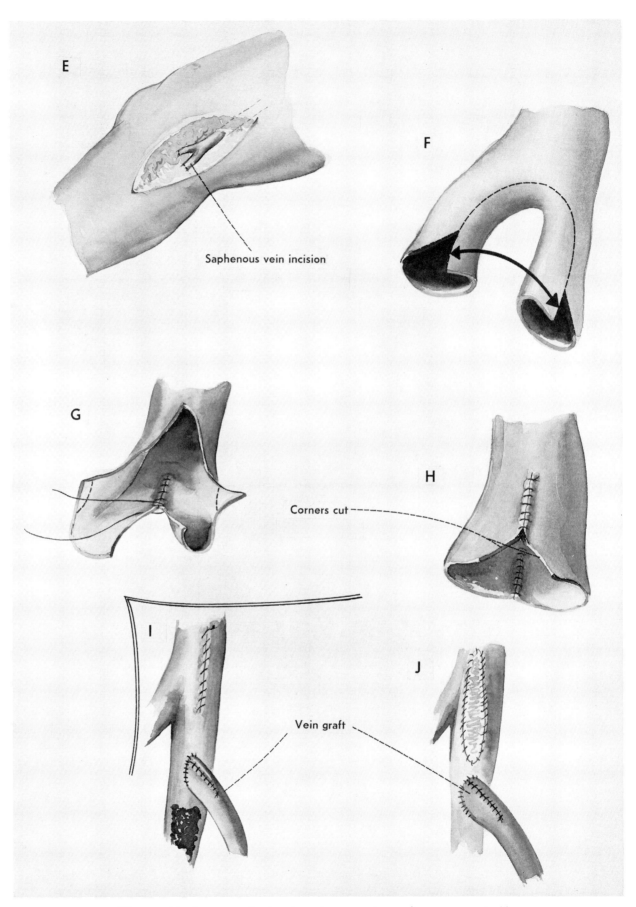

E

F

G

Saphenous vein incision

H

Corners cut

I

Vein graft

J

Fig. 31, cont'd. Femoropopliteal artery bypass vein graft procurement. Maneuvers to utilize short veins. **E-H,** Utilize tributaries to increase length of vein graft. **I** and **J,** Distal implantation of vein graft.

somewhat posterior to the incision. A small tributary may be followed to the saphenous vein. If in doubt, carefully reflect the posterior skin flap in the plane just deep to the superficial fascia. It is desirable for the distal portion of the saphenous vein to be at least 4 mm. in diameter.

3. Procure the saphenous vein graft beginning at the vertical groin incision used to expose the common femoral artery (Fig. 31, *C*). Ligate the saphenous vein flush with the common femoral vein to conserve length (Fig. 31, *D*). Trace the saphenous vein distally, making one or more shorter incisions to permit a rather meticulous dissection and removal.

Comment: *To utilize short veins, several maneuvers are helpful. The two distal tributaries can be divided as illustrated in Fig. 31, B, or they may be sutured together in order to gain length as shown in Fig. 31, E-H. Short grafts may also be implanted lower in the superficial femoral artery (Fig. 31, I and J) and the inflow to the graft restored by endarterectomy proximal to it. It is unnecessary and unwise to incise the skin the full length of the thigh.*

4. Remove the vein to a separate small table. Rinse it with heparinized saline solution. Tie all tributaries carefully. Tie the distal end of the vein over a beaded cannula, clamp the opposite end, and distend the vein with heparinized saline solution (Fig. 32, *A*). This reveals small tributaries and leaks and enlarges the lumen of the vein somewhat. Ligate and/or suture branches and tributaries (Fig. 32, *B*).

5. Remove the adventitia of the vein so that it will dilate further. Pull off the adventitia with fine thumb forceps (Fig. 32, *C*), or rub it off with moist gauze while the vein is distended with heparinized saline solution under pressure.

6. Prepare the proximal and distal arteriotomy sites. This is done by either the surgeon or his assistant while the vein graft is being prepared. *Reverse the vein before insertion.*

7. The technique of insertion of the vein graft (Fig. 33, *A* to *F*) is identical with that for the insertion of a Dacron prosthesis. If the vein graft is short, the proximal anastomosis may be made to the superficial femoral artery (Fig. 31, *I* and *J*) after a short proximal endarterectomy has been performed.

The saphenous vein is somewhat smaller and more delicate to suture than a Dacron prosthesis. It is helpful to use two guide sutures and to shape the end of the vein graft as shown in Fig. 2. When the vein is small, this guide suture should *not* be mattressed as shown in the drawing because this will cause some narrowing.

The proximal anastomosis is performed first (Fig. 33, *C* and *D*) and the vein allowed to distend and straighten under pressure before passing it through the tunnel (Fig. 33, *E* and *F*) and performing the distal anastomosis.

A vein graft can be reversed and replaced in the bed from which it came. No new tunnel is needed.

Comment: *When a saphenous vein is too small in diameter to serve as a tube, it can be utilized as an onlay graft (Fig. 33, H). Onlay grafts should be made over a 16-18 F. catheter stent to avoid excessive or irregular widening of the artery. Otherwise, local dilations and mural thromboses are prone to occur. In the popliteal region, the onlay can be continued as a bypass as described by Edwards. The onlay may be combined with endarterectomy of the open segment of artery.*

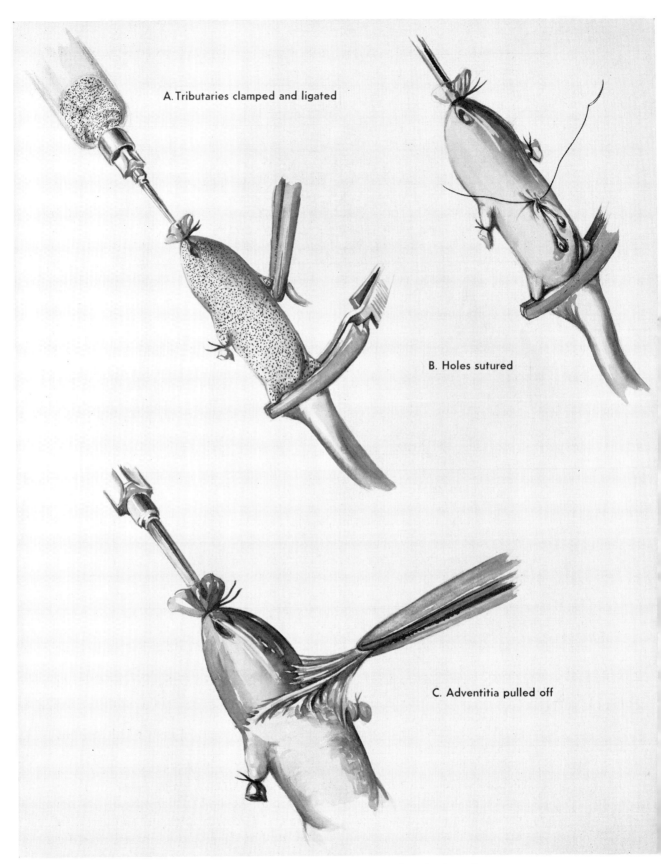

A. Tributaries clamped and ligated

B. Holes sutured

C. Adventitia pulled off

Fig. 32. Femoropopliteal artery bypass. Preparation of vein graft.

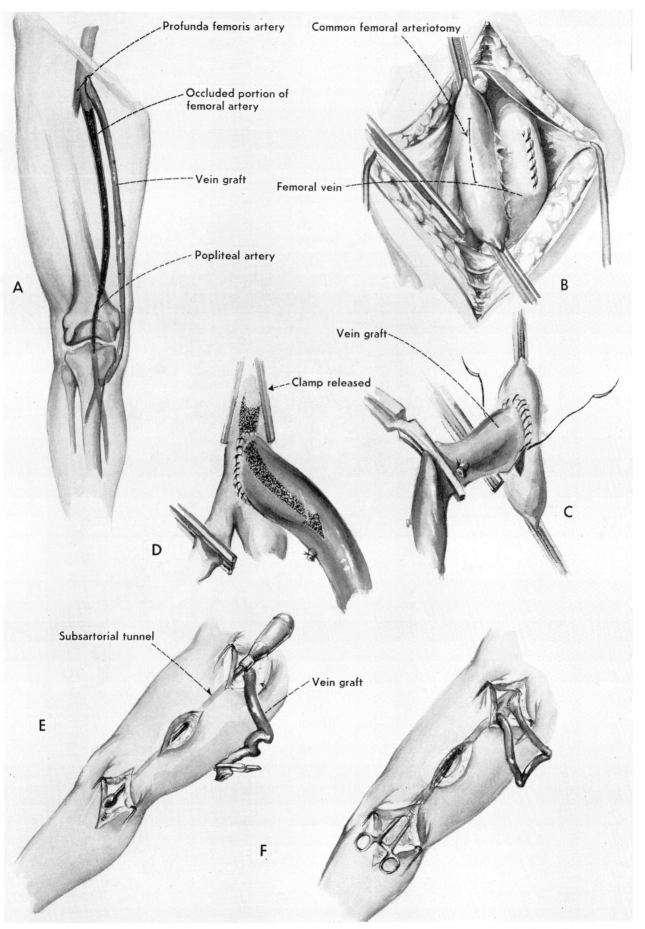

Profunda femoris artery

Occluded portion of femoral artery

Vein graft

Popliteal artery

A

Common femoral arteriotomy

Femoral vein

B

Vein graft

Clamp released

D

C

Subsartorial tunnel

Vein graft

E

F

Fig. 33. Vein graft for femoropopliteal artery bypass. **A-F,** Insertion of vein graft.

Continued.

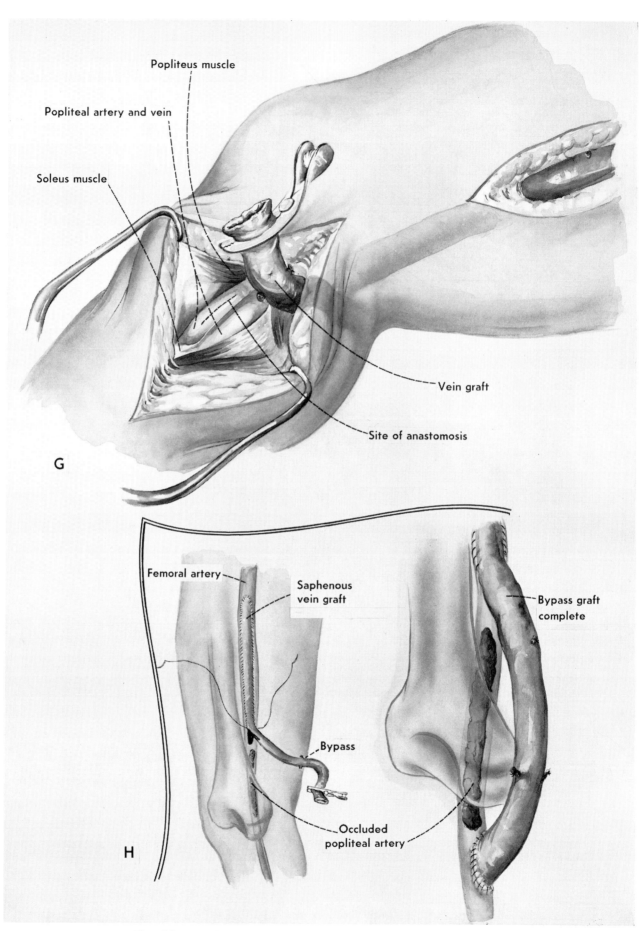

Popliteus muscle

Popliteal artery and vein

Soleus muscle

Vein graft

Site of anastomosis

G

Femoral artery

Saphenous vein graft

Bypass graft complete

Bypass

Occluded popliteal artery

H

Fig. 33, cont'd. Vein graft for femoropopliteal artery bypass. **G,** Distal anastomosis. **H,** Onlay graft with bypass extension.

In situ saphenous vein bypass

Indications are the same as for bypass with a reversed autogenous saphenous vein or a Dacron prosthesis. There may be certain advantages in not removing the saphenous vein. Incisions are shortened. The vein wall is not devascularized, and the intima remains viable in the early postoperative period. Since the vein is not reversed, its smaller end is anastomosed to the smaller portion of the bypassed artery. The valves of the saphenous vein obstruct the arterial flow until they are reversed. It is necessary also to locate significant tributaries by operative arteriography and to ligate them.

Procedure

1. Determine operability via the popliteal incision as previously described. Expose and note that the saphenous vein is of adequate size distally (that is, 4 mm. or more).

2. Expose the femoral artery and the proximal portion of the saphenous vein in the femoral triangle. Ligate and divide all accessible saphenous vein tributaries in the femoral triangle, particularly the accessory saphenous vein. Later it may be necessary to make another small incision over the saphenous vein in the midthigh to ligate other tributaries. Divide the saphenous vein flush with its junction at the common femoral vein.

3. Divide the vein distally. Reverse or destroy the valves in the saphenous vein by passing a flexible vein stripper with a torpedo-shaped tip 4 mm. in diameter from above downward. Pass the stripper from the femoral to the popliteal end of the saphenous vein several times without withdrawing it proximally. Follow the stripper with a Cannon or Wylie endarterectomy loop to make certain that the valves will not obstruct the reversed direction of blood flow.

4. Flush the vein with dilute heparinized saline solution and perform the proximal venoarterial anastomosis. When this is completed, a strong jet of arterial blood should emerge at the distal end of the vein. Administer heparin to the patient. Clamp the distal end of the saphenous vein, and adjust the length of the vein to the proposed site of bypass. Avoid angulation.

Comment: *It may be necessary to divide the adductor tendon and/or tunnel behind or divide the medial head of the gastrocnemius muscle to avoid angulation or excessive tension at the distal anastomosis.*

5. Perform the distal anastomosis by the techniques previously described. Flush and check back bleeding before the final sutures are placed. Observe and palpate pulses. Perform an operative arteriogram to note further tributaries in the thigh.

6. Close the popliteal and groin incisions while the films are being developed. If any tributaries have been missed, these may now be located and ligated. Small tributaries that later enlarge can be located and ligated under local anesthesia postoperatively.

FEMORAL ENDARTERECTOMY
Introduction

We seldom employ closed-loop endarterectomy of the superficial femoral artery. As in bypass grafting, an adequate outflow tract is necessary, and diffuse atherosclerotic disease involving the popliteal artery and its branches is a contra-

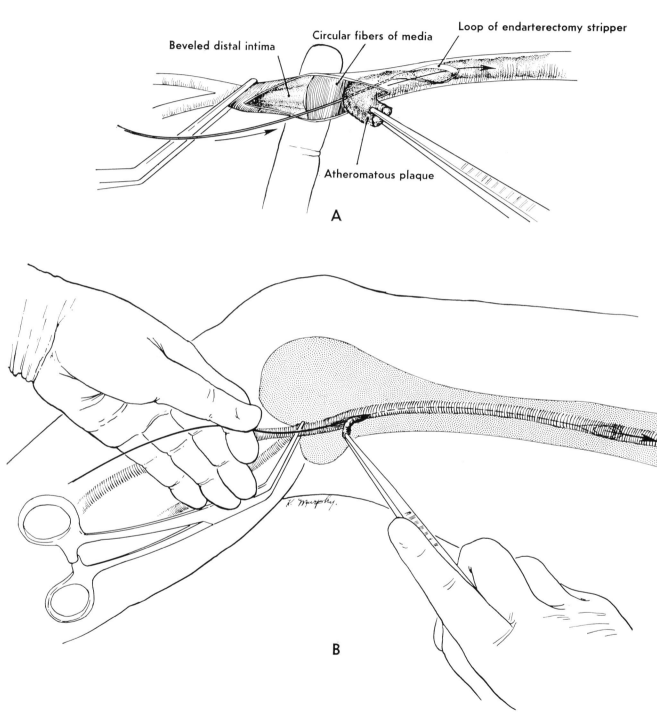

Beveled distal intima

Circular fibers of media

Loop of endarterectomy stripper

Atheromatous plaque

A

R. Murphy.

B

Fig. 34. Femoral endarterectomy. **A,** Begin endarterectomy by introducing stripper into popliteal artery. **B,** Pass stripper proximally.

110

indication. Vein bypass is superior to extensive endarterectomy. Open end-arterectomy of long segments of the femoral artery, closed by angioplasty with a long strip of vein, is under trial. Bypass prostheses should be available whenever endarterectomy is begun in case the femoral bypass precedure should become desirable.

Procedure

With endarterectomy loops

1. Prepare the skin for several days in advance. Place the patient in the supine position, with the thigh abducted and externally rotated and the knee flexed and supported. All levels of the popliteal artery are readily approached by the medial route (pp. 90-95).

2. Expose the common femoral artery in the groin. The proximal incision should expose the common femoral artery and permit endarterectomy at the branching of the profunda femoris and superficial femoral arteries. Identify the common femoral artery and its branches and isolate them with umbilical tapes.

3. Expose the popliteal artery as already described (pp. 90-95).

4. Inject 20 mg. of heparin into the popliteal artery distally and apply an angled arterial clamp. Give an additional 50 mg. of heparin intravenously.

5. Make a longitudinal arteriotomy at the distal end of the occlusion, extending it to the occluded area proximally and into relatively normal artery distally (Fig. 34, A).

Comment: *Transverse arteriotomies are now preferred.*

6. Separate the diseased intima and the thrombotic core from the media for a distance of several centimeters. The Freer elevator or a suitably shaped scissors is used, transecting the intima where it is suitably thin. The correct plane of cleavage is marked by the circular muscular fibers of the tunica media.

7. Distally, bevel the intima and suture it to the arterial wall with a double-armed mattress suture of 5-0 arterial suture. Pass the suture from within outward, tying it outside the artery.

8. Place the open loop of the stripping instrument over the end of the core, hold the end of the core for countertraction, and gently advance the stripper upward (Fig. 34, B).

Comment: *Distal introduction of the stripper ensures that it will not be too large for the artery as it is passed upward in the direction of increasing arterial diameter. Various types of closed-loop strippers are available. Loops may also be improvised from stiffer steel wire in the absence of instruments specifically designed for endarterectomy.*

9. Inject 20 mg. of heparin into the common femoral artery and place arterial clamps on the common femoral above the disease process and on the profunda femoris. Make a longitudinal arteriotomy at the bifurcation of the common femoral artery to allow visualization of disease at the ostium of the profunda branch.

10. Pass the stripper from below as far as the profunda femoris. Separate diseased intima from the media in the region of the bifurcation, and tease any plaque from the ostium of the profunda. Divide the intima above any thick plaques.

Comment: *Do not attempt blind endarterectomy at major arterial bifurca-*

tions. If the stripper becomes arrested, another skin incision and arteriotomy will be necessary or endarterectomy can be abandoned and a bypass prosthesis can be anastomosed to the upper and lower arteriotomies.

11. Withdraw the stripper through the popliteal incision and the core from above. Introduce a polyvinyl catheter the same size as the stripped segment of artery for its full length and irrigate with heparinized saline solution (0.1%). Back bleeding from collateral branches usually causes oozing.

Comment: *Remnants of attached intima are the cause of many failures. Those surgeons who advocate endarterectomy use many supplementary maneuvers. LaVeen passes size 01 tube gauze through the artery. A spring-handled nasal speculum prevents the gauze from dragging at the edge of the arteriotomy.*

12. Perform an operative arteriogram. Even small irregularities shown on the films are cause for concern, and such defects should be corrected by flushing, by drawing tube gauze through the artery, or by transverse arteriotomy at the site. The arteriogram is most readily performed through a whistle-tipped cardiovascular catheter held in the endarterectomized artery with a Javid clamp or umbilical tape.

The portable x-ray machine and the 14″ × 17″ grid-front cassette are the only pieces of radiographic equipment needed. The cassette is dropped into a sterile pillowcase. The entire leg has been prepared and draped as usual. The leg is lifted so that the film can be positioned accurately beneath it.

Irrigate the artery with heparinized saline solution to estimate the volume of contrast medium needed to fill the artery.

Inject a slightly larger volume of Conray 400, expose the film, release the distal clamp, irrigate again, and begin closure while the films are being developed.

Closure of distal and proximal arteriotomies

1. Close the distal arteriotomy first using a continuous 5-0 Dacron, Tevdec, polyethylene, or polypropylene arterial suture. The catheter stent is in place to prevent narrowing during the closure.

Comment: *If the popliteal artery is small, a patch of vein or prosthesis is sutured between the edges of any longitudinal arteriotomy to prevent narrowing. (See patch angioplasty, Fig. 57.)*

2. Partially close the proximal arteriotomy.

3. Withdraw the catheter stent that was used for irrigation, leaving the artery full of heparinized saline solution.

4. Cross clamp the superficial femoral artery, and momentarily release the clamp on the common femoral artery to flush out clots. Next release the clamp on the profunda femoris to check back bleeding.

5. Finish closure of the proximal arteriotomy, releasing the clamps on the popliteal, superficial femoral, and profunda femoris arteries before tying the suture. Lastly, slowly release the clamp on the common femoral artery.

Closure of popliteal and groin incisions

Close the popliteal incision, suturing all except the adductor tendon. Since anticoagulants will be used, a drain should be inserted, but this should not lie close to an arteriotomy. Close the fascia and skin. In closing the groin incision, be careful to eliminate all dead space.

Postoperative care

1. Avoid circumferential dressings.

2. Heparin, 30 mg. to 60 mg., should be given intravenously every four hours to prolong the clotting time. These frequent intravenous injections are made painlessly via a Teflon cannula inserted in a forearm vein for several days. The sterile obturator covers the hub of the cannula and is removed temporarily at the time of injection. Frequent intravenous injections of small doses of heparin maintains a more constant heparin effect.

3. Bed rest is advisable for a period of seven to ten days.

4. If the leg becomes ischemic, reoperate at once. Be prepared for operative angiography, retrograde flushing, bypass grafting, or patch angioplasty.

Chapter 6

Aneurysms of the popliteal artery

Operation for aneurysm of the popliteal artery is advisable even though the popliteal outflow is absent or poor. The diagnosis is usually made by palpation of the lesion. Arteriograms are needed to demonstrate outflow distal to the popliteal artery, size of the proximal and distal portions of the popliteal artery, and presence of collateral circulation. Lateral views show the artery and aneurysm best. Popliteal aneurysm is frequently found bilaterally.

The purpose of the operation is to remove the aneurysm and to restore normal blood flow to the leg. Any sizable or symptomatic aneurysm should be removed if the patient is a reasonable surgical risk and if there is no established distal gangrene. Aneurysms of the popliteal artery are exposed to the trauma of frequent flexion and often rupture or thrombose.

Distal occlusion by propagation of thrombosis or by the distal embolization of atheromatous debris often precipitates acute vascular insufficiency in unrecognized or neglected popliteal aneurysm. Reconstruction and limb salvage are difficult after these complications, and one-third to one-half of such compromised legs require amputation.

Choice of operation

The ideal operation is to excise the aneurysm and to restore vascular continuity with a prosthesis or with a vein graft. A Dacron prosthesis is used in larger vessels. A vein graft is best when the popliteal artery measures 4 to 6 mm. or when the outflow tract is narrow. When the outflow tract is completely blocked, the aneurysm is excised and sympathectomy is performed to improve collateral circulation. Collateral branches close to the aneurysm should be preserved. Oversewing the proximal popliteal artery permits excision close to collateral vessels.

If the outflow tract is poor, lumbar sympathectomy is a useful adjunct, and a vein graft lined with living intima is less likely to clot than is a prosthesis. A further advantage of vein grafts at the knee is their flexibility.

Since the usual cause of popliteal aneurysm is atherosclerosis, poor outflow through the arteries of the leg is not uncommon. Gangrene and ultimate amputation are often the outcome. Patients with acute thrombosis must be operated upon immediately. When the thrombosis extends distally, the popliteal artery may be cleared of thrombus by retrograde flushing from the ankle or with the Fogarty balloon catheter from above. Proximal occlusion, involving the superficial femoral artery in the adductor canal, may be managed by excising the aneurysm and bypassing with a Dacron prosthesis from the side of the patent proximal superficial femoral artery to the end of the distal popliteal artery.

Surgical approach

The posterior approach is sometimes preferred for aneurysms of the popliteal artery because the popliteal vein and the nerve trunks traversing the fossa are more accessible by this approach. They are frequently found to be adherent to a large sac. The proximal and distal portions of the popliteal artery are, however, deep, and the posterior incision is not easily extended. The medial approach described in the preceding chapter (pp. 90-95) is very satisfactory for a small aneurysm and must also be employed when a prosthesis is used to bypass from the proximal superficial femoral to the distal popliteal artery. The medial approach allows better access to the proximal and distal parts of the artery with highly placed aneurysms. The subsequent illustrations show the midline posterior approach. For the medial approach, see pp. 90-95.

Procedure

1. Place the patient in the lateral position, with the affected leg down and the opposite leg flexed (Fig. 35, A). Prepare and drape the entire thigh, leg, and foot.

2. Make a long midline posterior or S-shaped incision, placing the superior limb of the incision more medially (Fig. 35, B).

3. Open the popliteal fascia, avoiding the median popliteal (tibial) nerve which crosses from medial to slightly lateral superficial to the popliteal artery, giving off several branches on the way.

Proximal control

1. Retract the biceps femoris muscle laterally and the hamstring muscles medially (Fig. 35, C).

2. Identify the popliteal artery deep in the incision and slightly medially as it emerges from the adductor canal. The artery will usually be tortuous and dilated. Spare the superior geniculate artery and other collateral circulation.

3. Retract and spare the overlying popliteal vein when possible. The vein may be densely adherent to the aneurysmal sac. The median popliteal and the lateral popliteal (peroneal) nerves lie close together superiorly.

4. Pass umbilical tape around the artery preparatory to clamping.

Distal control

1. Retract the heads of the gastrocnemius muscle.

2. Free the popliteal vein from the artery distally. There may be two veins distally.

3. If necessary because of dense adhesions to the aneurysm, divide the popliteal vein (Fig. 35, D and E).

4. Pass umbilical tape about the artery preparatory to clamping.

Resection of aneurysm

1. Inject 20 mg. of heparin into the aneurysm, and quickly apply occluding clamps proximally and distally on the isolated portions of the popliteal artery (Fig. 35, *E*).

2. Free the nerves from the aneurysm, sparing the motor branches and the sural nerve.

3. Dissect close to the wall of the aneurysm, dividing and ligating any branches encountered.

4. Divide the popliteal artery proximal and distal to the aneurysm. Lift one end of the aneurysm, and dissect the posterior wall from the depth of the popliteal fossa. Leave part of the wall if it is dangerously adherent.

Reconstruction by end-to-end anastomosis

1. Select a suitable prosthesis at least 8 mm. in diameter. If the artery is smaller than 6 mm. or the outflow is poor, procure a saphenous vein graft (see Fig. 31 for technique of procurement and anastomosis of vein grafts).

2. The distal end of the popliteal artery may be trimmed obliquely to allow for anastomosis of a somewhat larger prosthesis.

Proximal anastomosis

1. Place mattress sutures of 4-0 arterial Dacron at each side of the prosthesis and tie in place (Fig. 35, *F*).

Comment: *Dacron maintains tensile strength during long implantation.*

2. Sew the front of the prosthesis to the artery with a continuous over-and-over stitch (Fig. 35, *G*).

3. Complete the front row by tying the continuous suture to one end of the other previously placed mattress suture (Fig. 35, *H*).

4. Rotate the arterial clamp so that the back row to be sewn is brought anteriorly. Use the other end of the already placed mattress suture to construct another continuous suture line to complete the anastomosis (Fig. 35, *I*).

Comment: *Vertically applied clamps and the end-to-end anastomosis as illustrated in Fig. 12, F-I, may be easier than rotation of the clamps.*

5. Preclot the prosthesis as follows. Pinch the distal end of the prosthesis closed, and open the proximal clamp briefly to fill the prosthesis with blood under pressure, and preclot it (Fig. 35, *J*).

6. Empty the prosthesis of blood and clots.

7. Cover the proximal anastomosis with gauze saturated with bacitracin solution.

Distal anastomosis

1. Pull the prosthesis down under tension, and cut it to the correct length with the leg straight (Fig. 35, *K*). Do not allow kinks or laxity.

2. Check back bleeding by momentary release of the distal clamp (Fig. 35, *L*).

3. Apply an arterial clamp to the distal prosthesis and hold the distal artery and prosthesis in approximation for anastomosis (Fig. 35, *M*). If rotation of the artery for access to the back row is difficult, reapply the clamps vertically and use the technique detailed previously for the iliac artery (Fig. 12).

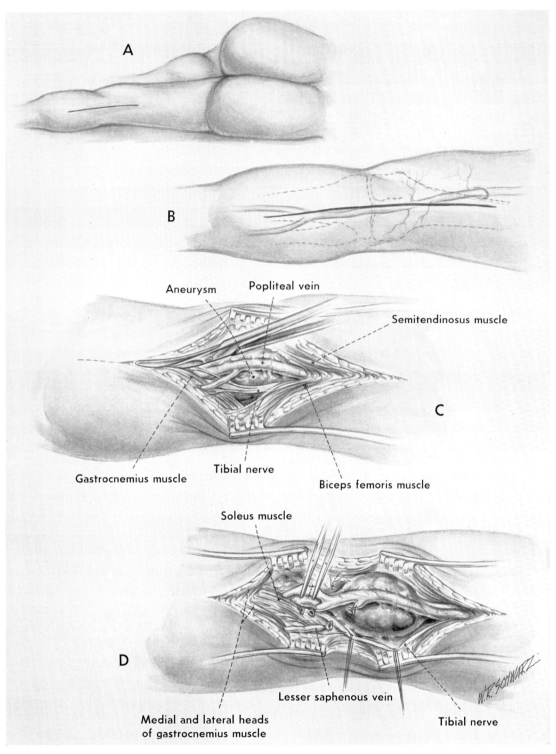

Fig. 35. Resection and graft of aneurysm of popliteal artery. **A,** Position. **B,** Incision. **C,** Exposure of aneurysm by retraction of muscles. **D,** Dissect vein and nerves from aneurysm.

Continued.

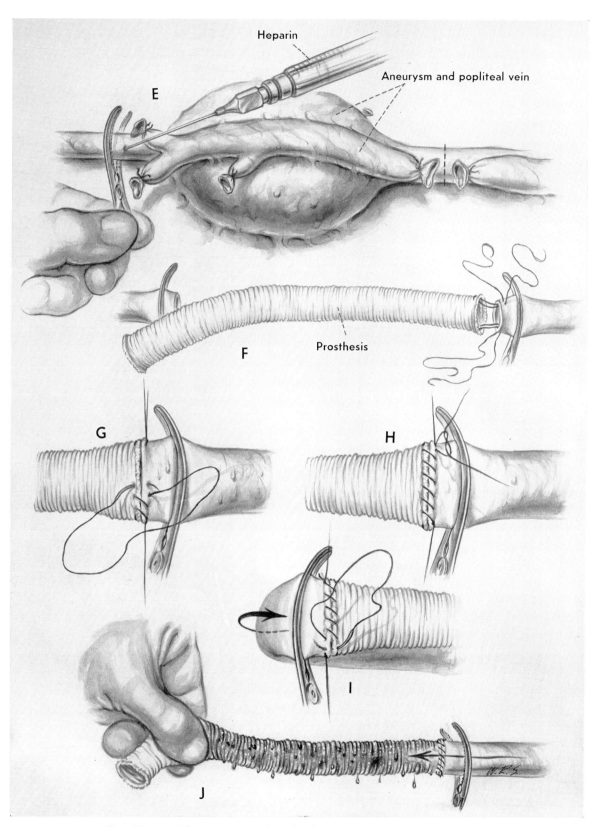

Fig. 35, cont'd. Resection and graft of aneurysm of popliteal artery. **E,** Regional heparinization before occlusion of artery. **F,** Begin proximal anastomosis. **G** and **H,** Anterior row of anastomosis. **I,** Posterior row of proximal anastomosis. **J,** Preclot prosthesis.

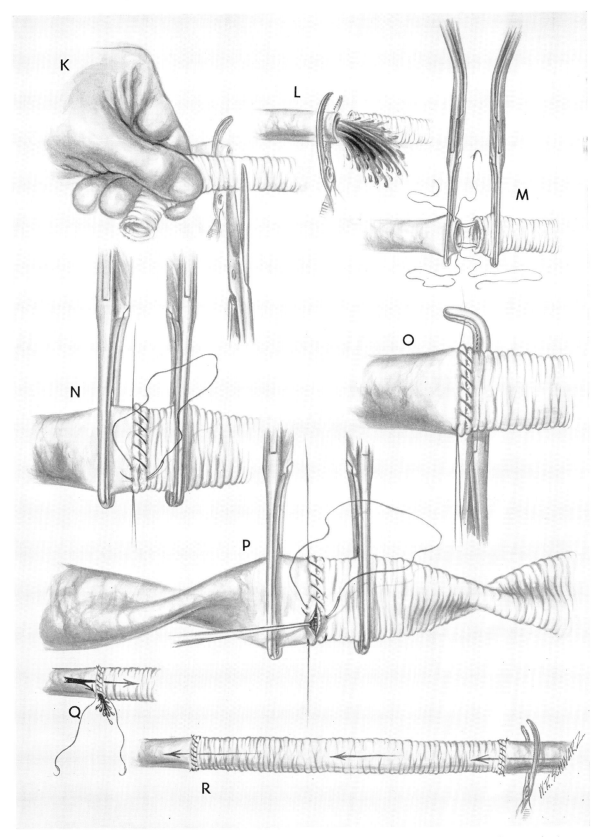

Fig. 35, cont'd. Resection and graft of aneurysm of popliteal artery. **K,** Cut prosthesis to correct length. **L,** Check back bleeding. **M,** Begin distal anastomosis. **N,** Front row. **O,** Rotate artery. **P,** Back row. **Q,** Back bleeding fills graft before last stitch is tied. **R,** Restore flow slowly.

4. Place a mattress suture at each side, and tie as the artery and prosthesis are held together by traction on the clamps.

5. Suture the front row of the anastomosis with a continuous over-and-over suture (Fig. 35, *N*). Tie one end to the opposite mattress suture.

6. Rotate the clamps 180 degrees so that the back row is anterior (Fig. 35, *O* and *P*), and complete the back row without tying the suture. If the anastomosis has been difficult or delayed, another proximal and distal flushing should be performed before the suture row is completed.

Restoration of flow

1. Release the distal clamp to fill the prosthesis and drive out air.
2. Tie the already placed arterial suture.
3. Remove the proximal clamp slowly.
4. Observe for satisfactory local and distal pulsation, and check color in the foot before closing the incision. Observe the graft as the knee is flexed. Divided tendons should be sutured with sturdy silk.

Postoperative care

1. Close the fascia carefully.
2. Drainage is not usually necessary.
3. Anticoagulants are contraindicated.
4. Observe and chart distal pulses hourly.
5. Start quadriceps exercises early.
6. Ambulate with crutches early, and allow weight bearing after ten days when the tendon repair is fairly secure.
7. Never flex the knee past 90 degrees unless a vein graft was used instead of the prosthesis.

Chapter 7

Embolic disease–acute arterial occlusion

Introduction

All emboli in major arteries should be removed, even if the limb is viable and the collateral circulation seems adequate. Embolectomy prevents proximal and distal propagation of the clot and prevents irreversible ischemic changes in the limb. No arbitrary time limit should be set, since limbs may be salvaged hours or even days after embolism by retrograde flushing or extraction of remote clots with balloon catheters. Major exceptions to this policy are moribund patients or patients with established gangrene. Surgery is performed under local or spinal anesthesia at low risk. When emboli arise in seriously diseased hearts, the mortality of both nonoperative and operative treatment is high.

Several new concepts need emphasis:

1. Maximum collateral circulation develops within a few hours and further improvement with vasodilators, sympathetic nerve blocks, etc. cannot save legs with major ischemia. Only operation restores normal blood flow.

2. Frequently legs remain viable and can be saved even after much delay. The clot propagates distally. However, distant clots can be extracted readily with balloon catheters. As long as the distal arterioles are still open, the leg is viable.

3. Multiple emboli, distal thrombosis or "tail thrombi," and fragmented or migratory emboli are more common than we realized and are the most frequent cause of postembolectomy "spasm." The routine use of operative arteriograms reveals the presence of these clots, and balloon catheters extract them.

Diagnosis of embolism is usually not difficult. The classic clinical picture of arterial embolism is a patient with some thrombogenic cardiopathy leading to formation of an embolus and sudden arterial occlusion. The pulses disappear distal to the site of occlusion, and the coincident onset of acute arterial insufficiency is manifested by ischemic pain, coldness, pallor, loss of sensation, and finally loss of motor function and obvious gangrene. As a rule, emboli lodge at the sites of major arterial bifurcations. These areas are also the commonest places for atherosclerotic narrowing of the blood vessels, and embolism or acute thrombosis may be superimposed upon this narrowing.

Special problems

Diagnostic problems arise when there are multiple emboli in the same extremity, when embolic occlusion is superimposed on arteriosclerosis, when embolic occlusion is incomplete, or when an embolic occlusion is present without an apparent source for the emboli. Late and repeated embolectomy, embolectomy of the visceral branches of the aorta, and embolism associated with long-term anticoagulation treatment pose special therapeutic problems. Some of these diagnostic and therapeutic problems and their solutions may be summarized as follows:

1. Embolism or acute thrombosis superimposed on arteriosclerotic narrowing may require either bypass or endarterectomy in association with thrombectomy.
2. Embolism originating in an aneurysm, or thrombosis of an aneurysm, should be treated by excision of the aneurysm.
3. Clot propagated distally should be removed by retrograde flushing or balloon catheters.
4. Restoration of circulation after prolonged ischemia may be followed by massive edema of the limb and this, in turn, requires fasciotomy.
5. Multiple emboli in the same extremity are frequently unrecognized. Operative arteriography or second incisions may be required to remove a more distal embolus in the same extremity if the balloon catheter cannot be passed.
6. Repeated embolism may require reoperation, sometimes on the same extremity.
7. Embolism during mitral valvulotomy continues to be a frequent problem. A careful record of pulses before operation with frequent observation and palpation after surgery will ensure prompt detection of emboli.

Balloon catheters (Fogarty)

The balloon catheter devised by Fogarty is a significant advance in vascular surgery and an indispensable instrument in embolectomy. Proximal emboli (that is, at the aortic or iliac bifurcation) and peripheral emboli at or below the knee can be extracted through a single arteriotomy in the femoral artery. Routine passage of the balloon catheter distally before an arteriotomy is closed frequently extracts distal fragments of clot and improves the results of the operation. The adequacy of back bleeding is difficult to judge, and profuse back bleeding may occur from proximal collateral channels even while the distal popliteal artery is still occluded.

The balloon catheter has other uses such as follows:

1. Extraction of clot from the iliac veins and vena cava (see femoral vein thrombectomy, Fig. 80)
2. Passage down the leg prior to the last iliac anastomosis after resection of the abdominal aorta

The balloon catheters are 80 cm. long, are available in sizes 4 F. to 7 F., and have delicate inflatable balloons at the tip. The catheter passes through the

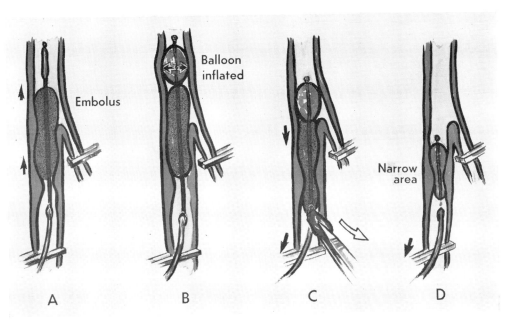

Fig. 36. Balloon catheters (Fogarty) for embolectomy. **A,** Catheter passes through clot. **B,** Balloon is inflated. **C,** Catheter is withdrawn, extruding clot. **D,** Delicate balloon deforms to pass narrow area.

clot readily without dislodging it (Fig. 36, *A*). After passage, the balloon is inflated (Fig. 36, *B*) with the correct volume of saline solution. The catheter is withdrawn, extracting the clot ahead of it (Fig. 36, *C*). The balloon is fragile and ruptures if it is overdistended. It glides by narrow places (Fig. 36, *D*) because when resistance is encountered, the fluid is displaced into the proximal part of the balloon.

Preoperative and postoperative medical and surgical teamwork

The site of the embolus must be localized by palpation, oscillometry, or arteriography. When pulses are absent in the opposite extremity, associated arteriosclerotic disease should be strongly suspected. A grid cassette and x-ray machine should be in the operating room for operative arteriography. Skin preparation and draping should include the whole extremity, so that retrograde flushing may be performed without interruption of the operative procedure to prepare and drape the extended surgical field. Bleeding, clotting, and prothrombin times should be obtained preoperatively, since anticoagulant therapy may be necessary in the postoperative period.

Failure to restore circulation may be caused by unrecognized distal embolism, and arteriograms or distal exploration may be needed if the limb is still in peril. Anticoagulants are indicated for prevention of recurrent mural thrombi or when the surgical procedure has included endarterectomy. Anticoagulants seldom lead to serious complications in groin incisions that are carefully closed—popliteal incisions should be drained and abdominal incisions should be avoided if immediate anticoagulant therapy is intended.

Medical-surgical teamwork is essential because all of the patients have

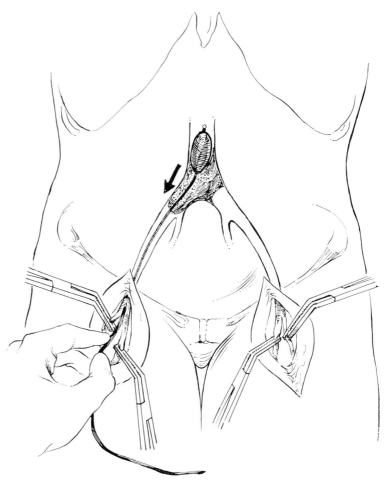

Fig. 37. Aortic embolectomy with balloon catheter introduced via femoral arteries. Details of groin incisions shown in Fig. 38.

serious associated medical problems. Although small emboli in distal popliteal or brachial arteries do not imperil the limb, there is no medical method to restore sufficient flow after major arterial occlusions. The medical treatment is concerned with four problems:

1. Treatment of the heart disease. The internist will avoid excessive use of digitalis or diuresis which may predispose to further thrombosis. A special problem is the occasional case of left ventricular failure precipitated by embolic obstruction of the abdominal aorta. Embolectomy may relieve the heart strain and may usually be accomplished under local anesthesia by introducing balloon catheters via the femoral arteries (Fig. 37).

2. Management of the ischemic limb. Extremities may survive without operation when small emboli plug only the distal brachial or popliteal arteries. In bedridden or poor-risk patients, these emboli need not be removed. The ischemic limb should be protected from injury or pressure and kept at room temperature in a slightly dependent position. Active cooling causes vasoconstriction of the skin and active warming increases

blood requirements, and both are harmful. In a slightly dependent position, the limb is usually more comfortable, the veins are full, and the color improves.

3. Vasodilation of the collateral arteries is desirable, but vasodilation elsewhere is useless or possibly even harmful to an ischemic limb. Vasodilator drugs or physiological stimuli to vasodilation such as warming the patient's body are not used. Sympathetic nerve block causes vasodilation in the affected extremity but will not save a limb when major ischemia is present. Sympathetic block may be helpful in patients with minor ischemia unless contraindicated by anticoagulant treatment.

4. Anticoagulants, beginning with heparin, should be used to prevent formation of more clots in the heart. Despite their use in high dosage, however, multiple or recurrent embolism occurs very frequently.

AORTIC BIFURCATION EMBOLECTOMY
Choice of procedure

The abdominal approach is seldom necessary now, but preparations must be made for both the abdominal and the femoral approach, since either route alone may not be satisfactory. The patient is placed in the supine position, and the entire abdomen, the groin areas, and the thighs are prepared to a point slightly below the knees. In most patients balloon catheters can be passed up normal common femoral and iliac arteries, and the embolus lodged at the bifurcation of the aorta can be removed by withdrawal of the catheter. This is the preferred approach because general anesthesia is unnecessary and heparin may be given postoperatively more safely. Laparotomy and arteriotomy at the bifurcation are described later.

Femoral approach—aortic embolectomy by retrograde catheterization of femoral arteries
Indications and preparation

Aortic or iliac bifurcation embolectomy via the femoral arteries may be done under local infiltration anesthesia and is preferable. In some patients laparotomy may become necessary. Therefore, the entire abdomen should be prepared and draped, and atropine should be included in the preanesthetic medication. Heparin may be given preoperatively, since the bleeding produced in the small incisions is not particularly troublesome. The balloon catheters (Fogarty) are preferred, although the open-ended polyvinyl cardiovascular catheters and suction are also described and are still useful.

Procedure
Retrograde aortic embolectomy with balloon catheters

1. Make a vertical incision over both common femoral arteries extending from Poupart's ligament superiorly downward for a distance of 6 to 7 cm. (Fig. 38, A). Open the fascia over the arteries. If there is no clot at the bifurcation of the femoral artery, distal control of the vessels may be obtained proximal to the profunda femoris (deep femoral) artery.

2. Dissect around the common femoral arteries, and pass umbilical tape around the artery above and below the proposed arteriotomies.

125

3. Slowly inject 20 mg. of heparin in 20 ml. of saline solution into the femoral artery. Lift the distal umbilical tapes and apply arterial clamps to both femoral arteries.

4. Make a 1 cm. vertical incision between the umbilical tapes on one femoral artery.

5. Pass the large (6 F.) balloon catheter proximally in the femoral artery until the tip is well above the navel.

6. Inflate the balloon with the *correct* amount of sterile saline solution and withdraw the catheter and the embolus. This is followed by forceful arterial bleeding.

7. Apply an arterial clamp above the femoral arteriotomy.

8. Release the distal clamp on the femoral artery. Back bleeding may be brisk from proximal collateral vessels, but we always pass the appropriate-sized balloon catheter distally in the femoral artery to remove distal fragments of clot in the popliteal artery.

9. Pass the 4 F. size balloon catheter distally as far as it will go gently, inflate the balloon with the correct amount of sterile saline solution, and withdraw the balloon. Unexpected distal small emboli are frequently removed.

Comment: *The surgeon holds the inflating syringe in one hand while withdrawing the inflated catheter with the other hand. If resistance is encountered at narrow areas, the balloon is deflated slightly.*

10. Pass the balloon catheter into the profunda femoris artery also, inflate the balloon, and withdraw the catheter.

11. Close the arteriotomy with 5-0 arterial suture.

12. Make an arteriotomy of the opposite femoral artery where fragments of embolus from the aortic bifurcation usually have been swept down to be arrested by the occluding clamp which was placed prior to the proximal passage of the balloon catheter into the aorta.

13. Proximal and distal passage of appropriate-sized balloon catheters guarantees that the iliac, femoral, popliteal, and profunda femoris arteries are all open. Repeat the procedure described for the opposite side.

Retrograde aortic embolectomy with suction catheters

1-4. The incision, exposure, femoral arteriotomy, etc., are the same as described in the first four steps for retrograde aortic embolectomy with balloon catheters.

5. Choose a catheter that fits rather snugly into the arterial lumen and has an oblique opening at the tip. A glass connector is used to connect the suction catheter to the remainder of the suction apparatus. Cut a hole in the side of the suction tubing close to the glass connector to control suction (Fig. 38, *B*). Pass the catheter upward toward the heart, and observe for bleeding through the glass connector. A glass T tube or Y tube may also be used as a connector and makes the hole in the tubing unnecessary.

6. Bleeding through the glass connecting tubing ceases when the catheter tip passes the hypogastric artery and touches the embolus. Advance the catheter until bleeding stops. At this point turn on the suction line and apply suction to the catheter by closing the hole or the side arm with the thumb. Withdraw the catheter slowly as suction holds the clot against its tip. As the clot is extracted,

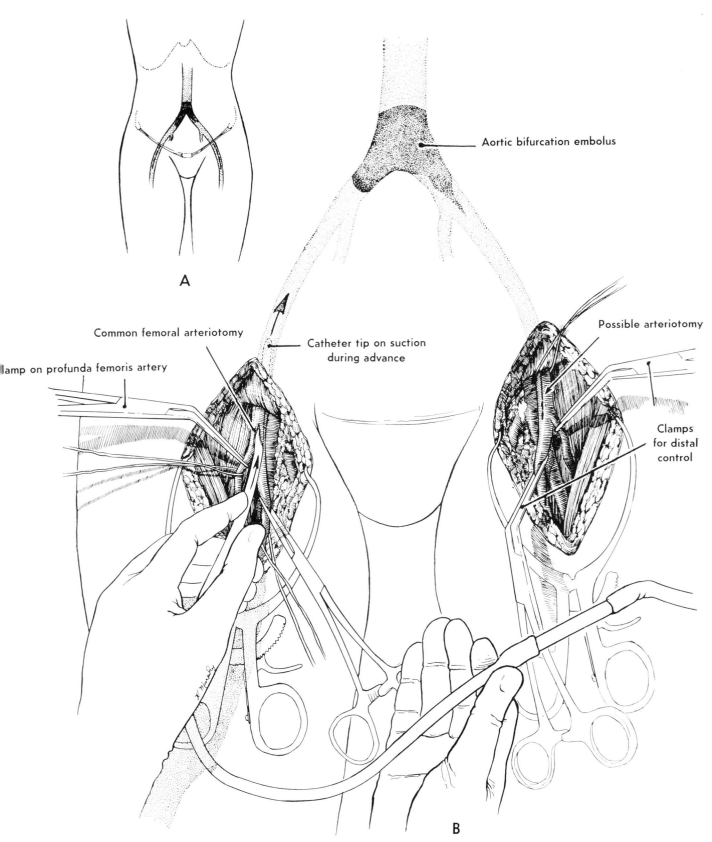

Aortic bifurcation embolus

Common femoral arteriotomy

Catheter tip on suction during advance

Clamp on profunda femoris artery

Possible arteriotomy

Clamps for distal control

A

B

Fig. 38. Aortic embolectomy by retrograde method. **A,** Incisions. **B,** Simultaneous control of both femoral arteries and retrograde catheterization.

127

clamp the femoral artery proximal to the arteriotomy. It may be necessary to pass the catheter several times.

7. Repeat the procedure on the other side. At this point, pieces of embolus may have been pushed over to the side that was originally cleared, and a second aspiration may be necessary to obtain an abundant, forceful, and pulsatile flow of blood from both sides.

Comment: *The combined abdominal and femoral approach may be necessary if catheters cannot be passed readily or if they do not clear the obstruction* (Fig. 38, *B*).

8. Check back bleeding from both the deep femoral and superficial femoral arteries by removing the distal occluding clamps. Rinse the blood clot away. Reapply the clamps, and suture the arteriotomy with 4-0 arterial suture as a continuous over-and-over suture. Close the femoral sheath and fascial layers carefully, avoiding dead space where oozing blood could accumulate during anticoagulant therapy.

Postoperative care

Anticoagulants may be used more safely with the femoral approach, since an occasional hematoma in the groin incision is easily noted and managed. Postoperative care includes medical management of associated heart disease.

Abdominal approach

Because the abdominal approach is used only after the femoral approach with retrograde catheters has failed, and because retrograde catheters fail mainly because of atherosclerotic narrowing, the embolectomy may have to be supplemented with endarterectomy. However, the classic abdominal aortic embolectomy is described.

Procedure

1. Make a long paramedian incision from the pubis to well above the umbilicus (Fig. 39, *A*). Expose the aortic bifurcation by packing off sigmoid colon to the left and small bowel to the right. For further details, see Chapter 3. Incise the peritoneum over the bifurcation, and observe the location of the embolus.

Comment: *The retroperitoneal approach to the bifurcation is also simple, but mobilization of the peritoneum over a large area results in more oozing in the heparinized patient.*

2. Incise the peritoneum over both iliac arteries distal to any apparent clot, and pass umbilical tapes about the arteries. Slowly inject 20 mg. of heparin into each iliac artery, and apply the arterial clamps. (See Fig. 39, *B*.)

3. Application of clamps to the iliac vessels ensures against distal propagation of the embolus. Now dissect around the aorta above the embolus, pass an umbilical tape to elevate the aorta, and select an aortic clamp of suitable size. Apply it to the aorta, but do not close it immediately. (See Fig. 39, *B*.)

4. Open the proximal portion of the iliac artery on the side where the embolus is largest. As the blood pressure extrudes the embolus, close the aortic clamp. (See Fig. 39, *C*.)

5. Open the iliac clamps one at a time to check for complete removal of the

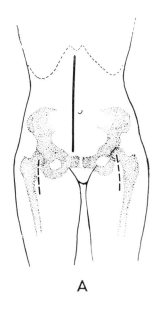

A

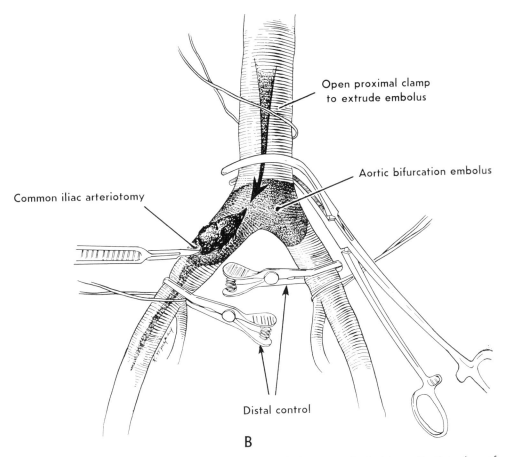

Open proximal clamp
to extrude embolus

Aortic bifurcation embolus

Common iliac arteriotomy

Distal control

B

Fig. 39. Transabdominal aortic bifurcation embolectomy. **A**, Incisions. **B**, Extrusion of embolus.

Continued.

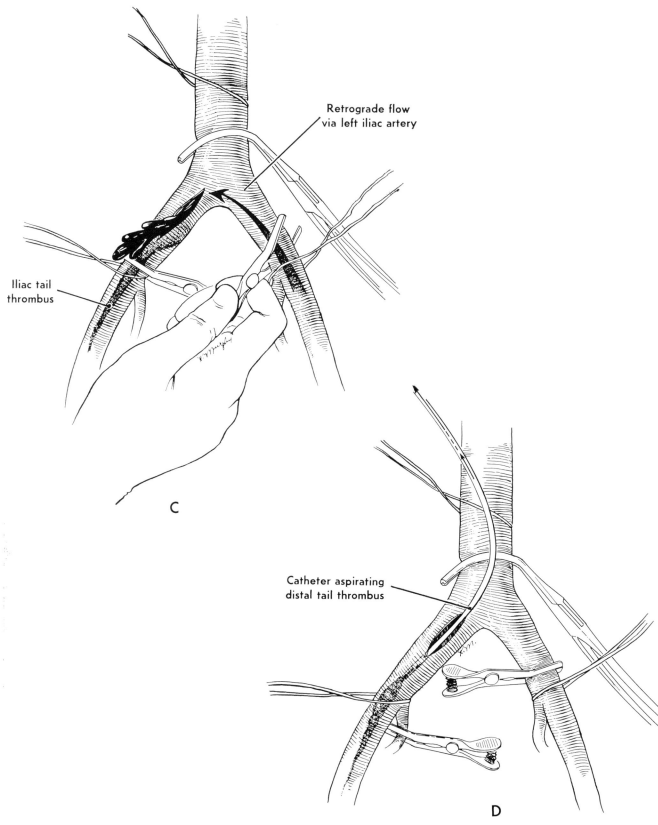

Retrograde flow
via left iliac artery

Iliac tail
thrombus

C

Catheter aspirating
distal tail thrombus

D

Fig. 39, cont'd. Transabdominal aortic bifurcation embolectomy. **C,** Check back bleeding from other iliac artery. **D,** Remove "tail thrombus" if present.

embolus (Fig. 39, C). A brisk gush of blood should result. If back bleeding is not abundant, a catheter attached to suction should be passed distally to remove any remaining thrombus (Fig. 39, D).

6. Close the arteriotomy with a continuous over-and-over suture of 3-0 or 4-0 arterial suture. Before the last few stitches are taken, release both the iliac clamps to fill the arteries with blood and to extrude any air within the artery. Finish the arteriotomy closure and tie the stitches.

7. Release the aortic clamp slowly and check pulses in the iliac vessels, the groins, and the popliteal fossae. If pulses are not present in the groin, the femoral arteries must be explored before the abdomen is closed. Secondary emboli must be removed at this time, and any arteriosclerotic occlusions present must be treated. Blood clot in or distal to the iliac arteries may be removed by femoral arteriotomy and retrograde suction with catheters as described earlier in this chapter. Popliteal or pedal pulses may be slow to return, particularly in patients with cardiac disease, prolonged occlusion, and spasm.

FEMORAL EMBOLECTOMY

Indications

The femoral artery must be explored for embolus when there is acute arterial insufficiency of the leg and pulses are absent below the bifurcation of the common femoral artery. Since the procedure may be done under local infiltration anesthesia, there are no contraindications except established gangrene.

Preparation

Preoperatively the entire leg and foot should be prepared and draped so that the popliteal and posterior tibial arteries are accessible for retrograde flushing and to facilitate operative arteriography if needed.

Procedure

1. Make a longitudinal incision over the course of the femoral artery (Fig. 40, A). Superiorly the incision extends to the inguinal ligament, and inferiorly it should be distal to the bifurcation of the common femoral artery. Diagnosis is confirmed by a visible embolus and by the absence of pulsation at the femoral bifurcation.

2. Dissect around the superficial femoral artery, and apply an arterial clamp distal to the embolus to prevent displacement and distal migration of the thrombus.

3. Dissect and pass an umbilical tape around the common femoral and profunda femoris arteries. Because of the very brief operation time, it is usually unnecessary to inject heparin.

4. Cross clamp the common femoral artery. Make a short vertical arteriotomy in the common femoral artery.

5. Release the distal clamp on the superficial femoral artery. Carefully pull the embolus out, being careful to withdraw it slowly so as not to lose any propagating tail thrombus in the superficial artery or the profunda femoris artery.

6. Pass the Fogarty balloon catheter (4 F.) distally as far as possible without force. Inflate the balloon gently, and withdraw the catheter to extract any distal fragments. Pass the Fogarty irrigating catheter and instill 30 ml. of dilute heparin

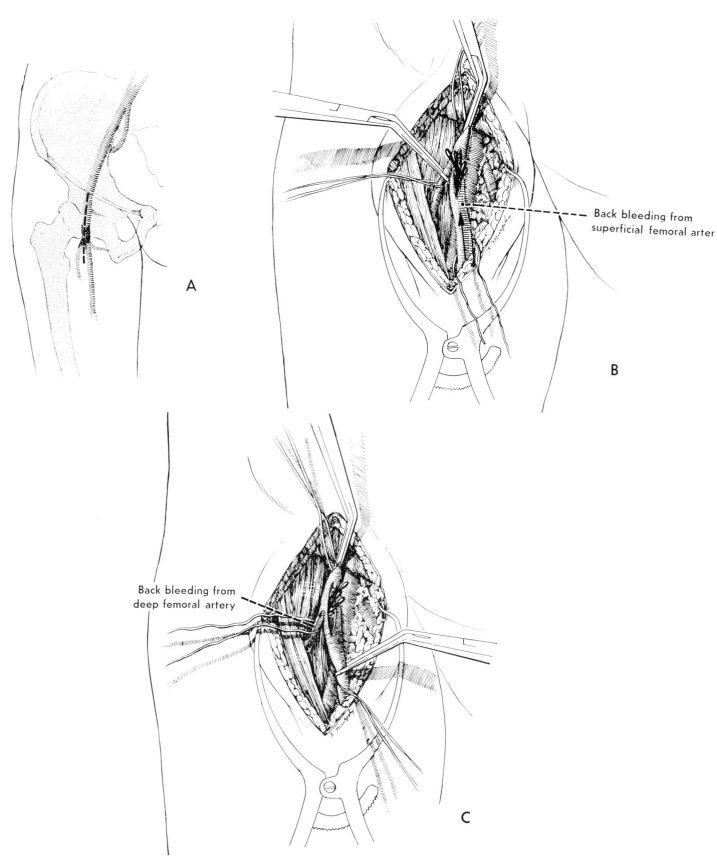

Fig. 40. Femoral embolectomy. **A,** Incision. **B,** Check back bleeding from superficial femoral artery. **C,** Check back bleeding from deep femoral artery (profunda femoris).

132

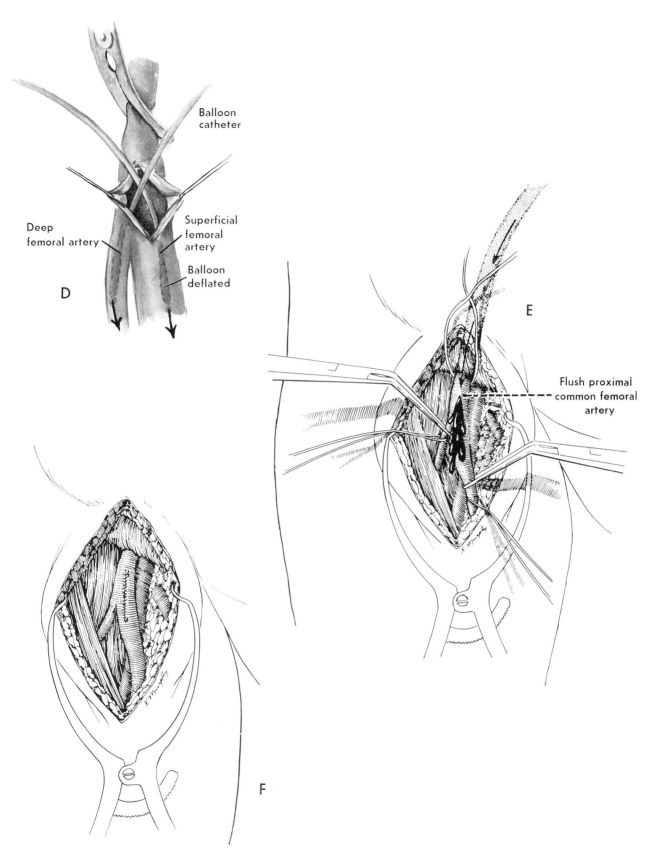

D

Balloon
catheter

Deep
femoral artery

Superficial
femoral
artery

Balloon
deflated

E

Flush proximal
common femoral
artery

F

Fig. 40, cont'd. Femoral embolectomy. **D,** Pass balloon catheters into superficial and deep femoral arteries. **E,** Flush proximal artery. **F,** Closure of arteriotomy.

as it is withdrawn. Clamp the superficial femoral artery. Further details about these balloon catheters are described on pp. 122 and 123.

7. Pass a small Fogarty balloon catheter into the profunda femoris artery and repeat the procedure just described.

Comment: *Poor back bleeding may signify the need for endarterectomy of the orifice of the profunda femoris or dilation of the orifice. Good back bleeding may be present even when distal fragments of clot are present, and the balloon catheters should be used in all cases to extract these distal fragments.*

8. Open the clamp on the common femoral artery. Proximal clot will be extruded. Reapply the clamp after forceful pulsatile flow is observed (Fig. 40, *E*).

9. Rinse away blood clots, and close the arteriotomy with an over-and-over stitch of 4-0 or 5-0 arterial suture (Fig. 40, *F*). Release the distal clamp momentarily before the last stitch is placed to allow back bleeding to extrude any air in the lumen.

10. Close the femoral sheath and subcutaneous fascia carefully to prevent collections of serum, blood, or lymph.

Comment: *Calcification of the media of the femoral artery may render it fragile and interfere with closure. A secure closure can be obtained by suturing adventitia only, as after endarterectomy. If necessary, the suture line may be reinforced with a sleeve of prosthesis (Fig. 17, C and D), or the diseased part of the arterial wall may be trimmed away and the defect closed with a patch of prosthesis (Fig. 57).*

Postoperative care

Anticoagulants may be used to prevent further thrombus formation in the heart. Careful closure of the incision obliterates dead space and helps to prevent hematoma when anticoagulants are necessary.

DELAYED EMBOLECTOMY—FASCIOTOMY
Indications

Operation is sometimes delayed due to poor facilities or the desperate condition of the patient, and delay may cause new complications. However, we have restored circulation and saved limbs even after a delay of many hours or days, and embolectomy or arterial repair must not be denied because of any arbitrary time limit. The distal thrombosis does not become inaccessible in the tiny arterioles until irreversible muscle damage has occurred. This is signified by the development of rigor of the muscle.

Heparin injections may be useful to prevent or limit distal propagation of the clot. However, these "tail thrombi" or other distal thrombi that are not continuous with the original embolus may occur. Balloon catheters have made it possible to remove these remote thrombi from the main channels without separate incisions.

When severe ischemia has persisted six to twelve hours, restoration of flow is followed by severe swelling, which may imperil the extremity. Edema is confined by closed fascial compartments and compresses the capillaries, resulting in muscle necrosis and gangrene. After delayed embolectomy, this dangerous edema is manifest by tightness and/or firmness of the calf of the leg without visible subcutaneous swelling or pedal edema.

134

Fasciotomy is frequently necessary if embolectomy has been delayed longer than six to twelve hours, particularly if the collateral circulation has been poor. However, prophylactic fasciotomy cannot be prescribed after any arbitrary time limit. The indications for fasciotomy are disappearance of pedal pulses that had been restored by embolectomy, recurrent pain, numbness, or pallor of the limb, and stiffness or tightness of the calf muscles.

Procedure—fasciotomy of leg

1. Make a long incision in the skin and fascia in the posteromedial aspect of the calf. The skin incision need not be so long as the incision in the fascia, which can be slit with the scissors proximal and distal to the skin incision.

2. Cut the fascia proximally and distally until pale muscle no longer bulges through the incision. Observe the return of color to the bulging muscle and to the foot. Note and mark the pedal pulses.

3. Incise the skin and fascia over the anterior tibial muscle compartment also.

Comment: *Whenever fasciotomy of the leg is indicated, both fascial compartments must be opened. Rarely, fasciotomy of the anterior compartment only is needed for the "anterior tibial syndrome."*

4. Close the skin partially at the ends of the incision unless closure causes tension.

5. Apply dressings, leaving the foot exposed for inspection and for palpation of the pulses. The edema rapidly subsides, soaking the dressings, which must be changed daily. Secondary closure of the skin in five days is usually feasible.

RETROGRADE ARTERIAL FLUSH

Retrograde flush procedures are seldom needed since the advent of the balloon catheters to remove other clots in the extremity. Balloon catheters, however, may be difficult to pass below the bifurcation of the popliteal artery. Retrograde arterial flush beginning at the ankle becomes necessary when the balloon catheter does not remove a thrombus which has extended distally from the popliteal artery and there is poor back bleeding after popliteal embolectomy. Persistent arterial insufficiency after embolectomy may also be due to multiple distal emboli.

If posterior tibial flushing is not successful, flush may be attempted via the dorsalis pedis artery.

Occasionally, squeezing the calf or wrapping it with a sterile snug Esmarch bandage from the toes proximally has extruded clots or assisted the flushing procedure. We have never regretted using these procedures. Flushing the posterior tibial artery will occasionally yield a branched clot. If perchance no clot is found, no harm has been done.

Procedure

Flush of posterior tibial artery

1. Make a vertical incision posterior to the medial tibial malleolus (Fig. 41, A).

2. Divide the thickened fascia of the laciniate ligament (flexor retinaculum). Identify the posterior tibial nerve or the medial and lateral plantar nerves, the

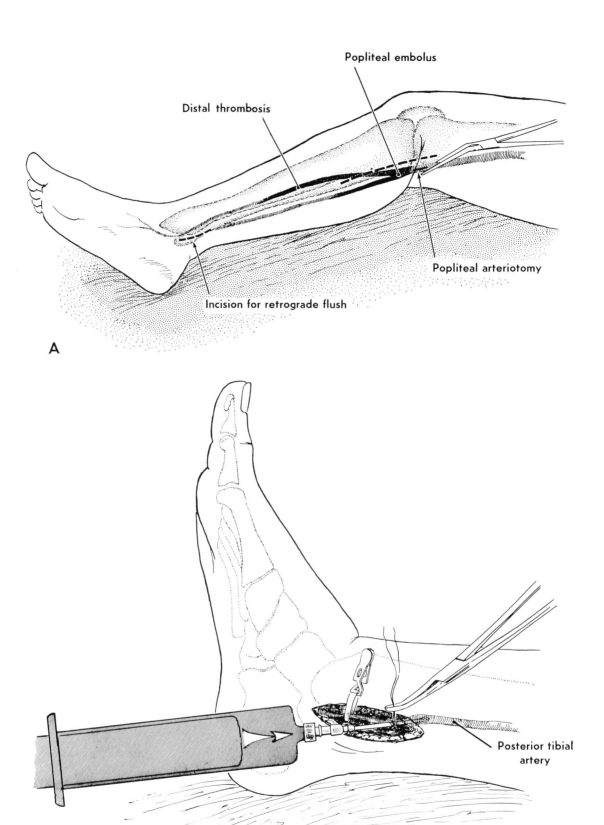

Fig. 41. Retrograde arterial flush at ankle. **A,** Incisions. **B,** Cannulation of posterior tibial artery at ankle.

136

posterior tibial artery, and the posterior tibial vein between the tendons of the flexor digitorum longus and the flexor hallucis longus.

3. Isolate the posterior tibial artery, and occlude it distally with a rubber-shod bulldog clamp. Incise the artery longitudinally proximal to the clamp (a very small incision will do), and insert a No. 13 to No. 15 thin-walled beaded cannula in the proximal direction. Secure the cannula with a temporary ligature. (See Fig. 41, B.)

4. Attach a 50 ml. large-bore syringe filled with warm heparinized saline solution. Empty the syringe rapidly and forcefully. Sometimes more than one irrigation may be necessary. Remaining clot will be extruded from the popliteal arteriotomy and should be followed by a profuse flow of clear saline solution.

5. Close the popliteal arteriotomy with a simple over-and-over suture of continuous 5-0 suture. If it appears that such a closure will constrict a small popliteal artery, use a small patch of vein or prosthesis so that constriction is avoided.

6. Remove the proximal popliteal clamp, and observe the pulsatile flow into the syringe at the ankle.

7. Remove the temporary ligature about the cannula at the ankle, remove the cannula, and close the arteriotomy in the posterior tibial artery with a few fine interrupted sutures of 6-0 or 7-0 silk placed in the adventitia only. Apply Gelfoam or oxidized cellulose and gentle pressure over the arteriotomy until leakage ceases. Close the incision.

Retrograde flush of dorsalis pedis artery

1. Expose the dorsalis pedis artery by a transverse incision on the dorsum of the foot, about 1 inch below the malleoli.

2. Divide the deep fascia (inferior extensor retinaculum or cruciate crural ligament).

3. Locate the artery between the tendons of the extensor hallucis longus and the extensor digitorum longus.

4. Isolate the artery, occlude it distally, and flush by the technique described for the posterior tibial artery.

Comment: *We have never regretted the incision at the ankle, even when retrograde flushing of one of the vessels was unsuccessful. Opening only one of the main arteries at the foot and calf may save the leg.*

Chapter 8

Arterial injuries

Introduction

Interruption of the major artery to an extremity causes gangrene in a high percentage of instances. All surgeons must be acquainted with the principles and techniques of treating arterial injuries because prompt reconstruction and restoration of arterial blood flow is essential. Complications in untreated patients are as follows:

1. Secondary hemorrhage
2. False aneurysm
3. Peripheral propagation of thrombosis
4. Distal embolism
5. Irreversible ischemic change in muscle and nerve

Even if a limb remains viable, usefulness is impaired because of arterial insufficiency, and fibrosis, contractures, claudication, or other signs of interference with blood flow and nutrition may appear.

Penetrating trauma

Arterial injury should be suspected when there is any penetrating trauma near a large artery, particularly in the neck, groin, axilla, or popliteal areas. Further indications of arterial injury are (1) pulsatile bleeding, (2) active bleeding, (3) distal arterial insufficiency, and (4) pulsating, extensive, or enlarging hematoma.

If a patient has a penetrating abdominal wound, major vascular injury should be suspected if shock does not respond to rapid transfusion of 1,500 ml. of blood. For wounds of extremities pressure dressings will stop the bleeding temporarily. Thoracic and abdominal hemorrhage may require operation to arrest bleeding before the shock can be treated.

Nonpenetrating trauma

Arterial insufficiency can follow nonpenetrating trauma from dislocations and fractures about the knee or elbow or from compression of arteries in the tight fascial compartments of crushed extremities. Compression-occlusion may also result from massive venous occlusion or from the interstitial edema that follows restoration of arterial circulation after prolonged ischemia from other causes. Following nonpenetrating injury, loss of pulses, coldness, pallor, progressive hypesthesia, anesthesia, and paralysis are danger signs and indicate urgently the need for accurate diagnosis and surgical exploration or other treatment.

Traumatic vasospasm may occur in patients with nonpenetrating arterial injury. If the arterial insufficiency is severe and is not relieved immediately and dramatically by sympathetic nerve block, the suspected artery should be explored immediately. Return of pulses following sympathetic block is reassuring, but increase in skin temperature and color alone merely signifies improvement in collateral flow and does not exclude arterial injury. The diagnosis of traumatic vasospasm must be verified and treated by operation. The condition is myogenic in origin and is independent of nervous control but responds to topical application of papaverine. Spasm, when present, is often accompanied by contusion and thrombosis, and resection of a section of damaged artery will be necessary.

Methods of repair

The method of repair varies with the type, severity, and location of the injury. Lateral repair of tangential injuries is seldom advisable. If debridement is unnecessary or very limited, closure of the laceration with a patch of vein or prosthetic material prevents narrowing at the closure. End-to-end anastomosis is performed when the ends can be approximated. If adequate debridement of the artery prevents anastomosis without extensive mobilization of the artery, a vein graft or prosthetic tube is preferable. Extensive mobilization tends to sacrifice collateral vessels and may put the anastomosis under undue tension.

Various arterial substitutes have been used, and arterial homografts enjoyed extensive use during the Korean War. However, the thrombosis rate in homografts is high. The patient's own living vein is preferable. The saphenous vein is sturdy and needs no external support. Vein grafts are always preferable in small arteries.

Of the various prosthetic materials available, the knitted Dacron (DeBakey) of moderate pore size is highly satisfactory. This and other prostheses are available in a wide range of sizes. However, prostheses less than 8 mm. in diameter should not be used. Prostheses are necessary in large arteries such as the iliac because vein grafts dilate and form aneurysms in these locations and all forms of external support have failed. Prostheses or vein grafts must be covered with living tissue.

Preoperative and postoperative care

Preoperative care should include antibiotics, tetanus and gas-gangrene prophylaxis, blood replacement, and immobilization of the injured extremity. Successful anastomosis results in prompt postoperative improvement. For reasons that are not clear, pedal pulses may not return for a period of six or eight hours. Theoretical reasons for this delay are (1) vasoconstriction persisting because of inadequate blood replacement, (2) reflex vasoconstriction from excessive tension on the anastomosis, (3) air embolism from residual air in the arteries, and (4) distal thrombosis or embolism. Sympathectomy or sympathetic blocks are not necessary postoperatively when arterial continuity has been restored and are useless when it has not been restored. The only treatment indicated if arterial insufficiency recurs is reoperation. Anticoagulants are not necessary and may prove dangerous. Vasoconstricting drugs, local heat, and excessive elevation of the extremity should be avoided. The limb should be immobilized for a period of ten to fourteen days.

Principles of surgical treatment

The essentials of surgical treatment in arterial injury may be briefly summarized as follows:

1. Early exploration and definitive treatment, preferably anatomical restoration
2. Adequate surgical exposure secured by a longitudinal incision along the course of the artery
3. Proximal and distal control of the artery and vein before incision into a hematoma or false aneurysm
4. Removal of distal clot by balloon catheters (pp. 122 and 123) or by the retrograde flush technique (pp. 135-137) if there is inadequate back bleeding from the distal arterial segment
5. Restoration of continuity of all major or critical arteries
6. Correct care of remainder of wound, including drainage when indicated, coverage of arterial anastomoses, and fixation of fractures
7. Early recognition of and fasciotomy for closed-space injuries or edema

REGIONAL CONSIDERATIONS
Neck, supraclavicular region, and upper thorax

Patients with injuries in the neck, supraclavicular region, and upper thorax have a high mortality rate, and many do not survive long enough to reach a hospital. Rapid control of hemorrhage is essential. Exposure of the subclavian artery requires resection of the clavicle. However, proximal control at the origin of the artery may become necessary. The origin of the subclavian artery and other great vessels is approached by splitting the upper sternum. Details of these exposures are found in the discussion of the upper extremity (Chapter 14).

Associated injury of the great veins may require ligation or repair of the subclavian or internal jugular veins. The superior vena cava should not be ligated. The innominate, subclavian, or jugular veins may be either repaired or ligated. Ligation of the great arteries in the superior mediastinum and neck should be avoided. Injuries of these vessels that do not kill instantly can usually be repaired. Gangrene of the arm may follow ligation of the second and third portions of the subclavian artery. Massive cerebral necrosis and death follow ligation of the innominate artery in 9% of patients. Morbidity after ligation of the common carotid artery is even higher, reaching 20% to 30%.

Aneurysm in the upper thorax and first portion of the subclavian artery can be approached safely only after adequate exposure to permit proximal control of the great vessels.

Thorax and abdomen

Most injuries of the heart and aorta are incompatible with survival. The same general principles of prompt exploration and control that apply to injuries in the neck and upper thorax also apply to injuries of the thorax and abdomen.

Surgical exposures are described elsewhere. Celiac, hepatic, and mesenteric arteries can also be repaired.

Iliac artery

With regard to the leg, the prognosis is about the same as for the common femoral artery in that gangrene will result in about 80% of patients if the circulation is interrupted. Management is often complicated by associated abdominal injuries. The distal portion of the iliac artery may be exposed in conjunction with the femoral artery by dividing the inguinal ligament. This should be done without hesitation to obtain proximal control and to stop hemorrhage. Ligation of the external iliac or common femoral vein may lead to massive edema. Therefore, these should also be repaired when possible. Restoration of continuity of the iliac artery is absolutely essential. When primary suture is not possible, a prosthetic tube must be inserted. Vein grafts are neither large enough nor strong enough to replace the iliac and larger arteries.

Femoral artery

Interruption of the common femoral artery results in gangrene in about 80% of patients. Associated atherosclerosis may be troublesome in older persons and may require more extensive exploration and replacement than indicated by the injury alone. The greater saphenous vein from the opposite leg can be used as a replacement, but prosthetic materials are satisfactory for replacement of the common femoral artery.

Injury to the superficial femoral artery produces gangrene in 45% to 55% of patients. The accompanying vein may be ligated with little risk of subsequent edema of the leg. The saphenous vein is the best replacement for the superficial femoral and popliteal arteries.

Brachial and axillary arteries

Gangrene is much less likely to occur after interruption of arteries in the upper extremities than in the lower extremities. Interruption of the brachial artery above the profunda brachii, however, results in gangrene in about 56% of patients, whereas gangrene results in only 25% when ligation is below the profunda. The brachial artery is easily exposed by a longitudinal incision along the medial side of the biceps muscle. Continuity should be restored whenever possible because of disability as well as the risk of gangrene.

Details of exposure of the brachial artery in the antecubital fossa and the upper arm are described in the discussion of the upper extremity. If the injury is above the midarm, adequate exposure will usually require division of the tendon of the pectoralis major muscle. The veins may be divided and ligated. Injured brachial arteries can usually be reanastomosed. When reconstruction requires a graft, brachii comites or the saphenous vein is the best replacement.

Noncritical arteries in lower leg and forearm

Penetrating injury or nonpenetrating injury may impair circulation in the lower leg or forearm. Arteries may be injured with or without associated fractures. Swelling within the tight fascial sheaths can cause arterial insufficiency by compression. A longitudinal incision on the volar aspect of the forearm is the best location for fasciotomy in this location. Below the knee, anterolateral and posteromedial incisions release pressure in the anterior and posterior compartments. Fasciotomy interrupts the vicious cycle in which impairment of capillary circulation leads to further edema. The objection that incision can interrupt collateral circulation through the skin is a theoretical one, and the skin and fascia, which tolerate ischemia better than muscle or nerve tissue, will survive and heal if deep circulation is restored. Without restoration of circulation to the muscle, fibrosis and contracture will ensue.

Occasionally, injury to a "noncritical" artery will result in arterial insufficiency because collateral circulation has been compromised, so that primary repair is indicated. The technique of anastomosing small arteries is given on pp. 151-156. This requires special instruments and sutures and meticulous technique for best results.

Popliteal artery

The popliteal artery is frequently injured by penetrating missiles or after distal femoral fractures. Posterior displacement of the distal fragment of a broken femur may compress or occlude the artery and injure the veins. Interruption of both the saphenous and popliteal veins can lead to massive edema that will require fasciotomy. This edema may not appear until arterial continuity has been restored. Surgical approaches to the popliteal artery are shown in Chapter 5. The artery is small, so end-to-end anastomosis must be precise. When debridement makes a graft necessary, a saphenous vein graft is preferred. The incidence of failure and gangrene after repair of the popliteal artery is higher than that for any other major vessel, being about 25% to 35% (Korean War statistics). Without primary repair, however, the leg amputation rate following popliteal injury is 78% (World War I and World War II statistics).

Associated venous injury

The accompanying veins are almost always injured in penetrating arterial wounds. Formerly it was believed that ligation of the veins would improve the circulation to the injured extremity and would reduce the incidence of gangrene when the artery was ligated. Ligation of veins may be necessary in debridement of gunshot wounds, but an occasional knife wound can be successfully repaired. No immediate harm will result from ligation of veins, but edema and stasis ulceration almost invariably follow interruption of the common femoral or external iliac veins. When all the veins of an extremity are thrombosed, massive edema may interrupt the arterial circulation by compression within the tight fascial compartments in the forearm or in the lower leg. If this happens, fasciotomy is necessary and repair of the veins and/or thrombectomy should be considered.

Vascular injury during elective surgical procedures
Inferior vena cava

The inferior vena cava may be injured during a number of procedures (for example, right nephrectomy, right lumbar sympathectomy, or right retroperitoneal lymph node dissection). Usually the source of bleeding is a small tear that results from traction on a small tributary. Bleeding is profuse but usually can be easily controlled by the local pressure of a small sponge on the fingertip—

large bulky packs may prove ineffective and always prevent visualization of the injury. Repair is simple after application of an Allis forceps or a sidewise partially occluding clamp such as the Satinsky and can be accomplished without further mobilization and without proximal and distal control of the vein.

Portal vein

The portal vein may be injured in pancreatoduodenal resections (Whipple operation). The vein may be invaded by cancer or may be adherent because of accompanying pancreatitis. Injury usually occurs as the operator uses his finger to dissect bluntly through the venous tunnel under the pancreas. To avoid injury to the vein, uncover it by dividing the pancreas to the left of the midline, and lift the proximal end of the divided pancreas anteriorly and to the right, approaching the portal vein and the superior mesenteric artery from the left side. Small branches may then be visualized and ligated as the vein is uncovered.

Left iliac vein and artery

The left iliac vein and artery may be injured during removal of a fifth lumbar herniated nucleus pulposus. If the anterior part of the annulus fibrosus is ruptured, the underlying vein may be torn. Hemorrhage is profuse and immediate. Laparotomy is necessary if packing the intervertebral space does not arrest the hemorrhage.

Left hepatic vein

The left hepatic vein may be injured during mobilization of the left lobe of the liver for abdominal vagectomy. This vein is more superficial than expected but is covered with a dense fibrous sheath that is readily distinguished from the areolar tissue between the left lobe and the diaphragm.

Hepatic artery

The hepatic artery may be resected with gastric cancer or during gastrectomy for duodenal ulcer. The right hepatic artery is occasionally ligated during cholecystectomy. In such instances, when the injury is recognized, the blood flow must be restored to the liver and the end of the splenic artery may be implanted into the side or anastomosed to the distal end of the hepatic artery. End-to-end anastomosis may be feasible.

Puncture wounds of arteries

Arterial puncture is usually innocuous. However, we have observed false aneurysms and arteriovenous fistulas following venipuncture near the femoral and brachial arteries and in the popliteal and brachial arteries secondary to puncture by Kirschner wires or Steinmann pins or arterial puncture for retrograde catheterization.

FALSE ANEURYSM AND ARTERIOVENOUS FISTULA

False aneurysms and arteriovenous fistulas are usually the result of penetrating injuries to blood vessels. When an artery is completely severed, the ends retract and contract and often the hemorrhage stops spontaneously. If, however, a vessel is partially severed, only the cut portion of the vessel is able to retract. The wound is held open, allowing rather profuse hemorrhage. If the soft tissue wound associated with the vascular wound is large, the hemorrhage is visible externally. When associated soft tissue wounds are small and there is no opportunity for external blood loss, blood may be trapped in muscle and fascial planes, with formation of a pulsating hematoma. The blood clot and the hematoma acquire a laminated organized exterior. The blood in the center of the hematoma remains fluid and is free to flow in and out of the tear in the arterial wall.

Organization of the wall of the hematoma produces a fibrous tissue sac lined with a glistening intima-like layer. Such false aneurysms assume shapes according to the contour of the surrounding anatomical structures. Accompanying veins and nerves are commonly incorporated into the walls of this false aneurysmal sac.

When the associated veins are injured in addition to the artery, blood escaping under high pressure from the arterial injury may follow the path of least resistance, enter into the vein, and form a fistulous tract. Such fistulas are prone to develop where the artery and vein are enclosed in a common sheath. Commonly, the false aneurysmal sac makes up a portion of the fistulous lesion. If two veins accompany the artery, all three vessels can become involved. The feeding artery proximal to the fistula usually becomes larger than normal, and the associated veins become enlarged and thickened.

Differential diagnosis

The following points help to differentiate false aneurysms from arteriovenous fistulas:

1. Arteriovenous fistula is usually accompanied by continuous rough vibratory thrill that is easily palpated. Auscultation reveals a rough, machinery-like murmur. False aneurysms have a murmur only during systole or perhaps not at all.
2. Large arteriovenous fistulas are accompanied by a rapid heart rate that slows when the fistulous tract is manually occluded (Branham's sign).
3. Dilatation of superficial veins is usual with arteriovenous fistula.

There are no systemic manifestations of a false aneurysm, but large arteriovenous fistulas cause cardiovascular manifestations. Branham's sign, a decrease in pulse rate with compression of the fistula, has already been mentioned. Early in the formation of arteriovenous fistulas there may be a decrease in both systolic and diastolic blood pressure, but after a time the systole pressure tends to recover. With the increase in blood volume and the increased work load on the heart, there may be gradual dilatation of the heart and later hypertrophy and cardiac failure.

Certain local changes may accompany arteriovenous fistulas. These are cool skin, trophic changes in the skin and appendages, edema, ulceration, cyanosis, pallor, and perhaps gangrene distal to the site of the fistula. The area near the fistula itself is usually warmer to the touch, and oscillometric readings are increased locally.

Although not always necessary, arteriography may be employed in differential diagnosis.

Surgical treatment

The goal of treatment is to eliminate the fistula and to restore normal arterial flow. Repair may be undertaken as soon as the patient's general condition permits and the associated soft tissue injuries are healed. Delay permits further dilatation of the aneurysmal sac and associated veins and other complications and disability. The expanding sac may erode bone and damage adjacent nerve trunks. In long-standing fistulas troublesome scarring, ectopic bone formation, and dilatation of all regional veins and their collateral vessels may develop.

Years ago quadruple ligation was the best treatment, and delay in operation was advised in order to allow development of collateral circulation. Quadruple ligation eliminated the fistula but was frequently followed by crippling arterial insufficiency. Therefore, this procedure is now used only for small, noncritical arteries.

Small fistulas in large vessels may occasionally be exposed and closed by transvenous repair. This method is subject to the limitations of primary lateral arteriorrhaphy already mentioned. Sometimes a false aneurysm may be closed laterally, or the fibrous wall may be used for the support of a vein graft. The Matas operation (intrasaccular suture and repair) has been unnecessary since the techniques of arterial replacement have been developed. Therefore, when an arterial prosthesis or vein graft is employed, it should be sutured to normal artery proximal and distal to the excised aneurysm.

EXPLORATION OF GUNSHOT WOUND OF FEMORAL ARTERY AND VEIN

Restoration of arterial continuity is essential for all wounds of major arteries. However, the most meticulous arterial suture may fail unless infection is forestalled by debridement and unless there is correct treatment of associated injuries such as fractures. These important matters have been discussed in various books and articles and are not discussed here.

Adequate exposure requires long incisions over the course of the artery. Details of the surgical approach to various parts of the femoral and popliteal arteries are described and illustrated in Chapters 3 to 6. In the drawings included in those chapters, as well as in the illustrations in this chapter, the drapes and skin towels are omitted in order to show clearly the anatomical landmarks.

In the appraisal of the amount of resection or type of treatment, it is usual to underestimate the extent of injury. One must look for minimal clues that may indicate damage. Concussion or spasm of injured arteries that does not respond to local applications of 2% papaverine requires resection of that portion of the artery. Such specimens usually show subintimal damage and thrombosis. Tangential repair of arteries or veins should be reserved for knife wounds. The partial or tangential lacerations that are the result of gunshot wounds require resection. In gunshot wounds the accompanying vein is usually injured. Its repair is seldom successful. Because of the high velocity of the bullet, arterial injury is usually more extensive than anticipated, and the usual error is to resect insufficient artery. If two of the three major veins of the thigh are injured or occluded, massive and dangerous edema may result in gangrene. Prophylactic fasciotomy of the calf is mandatory for such patients, and restoration of venous continuity with a graft from the opposite leg should be considered. If the accompanying vein has not been injured, it should be preserved. There is no evidence that ligation of the accompanying vein improves blood flow to the injured extremity.

The method used to restore arterial continuity depends in part on the length of the defect after the resection and on the location of the injury. Primary end-to-end anastomosis is seldom practicable for defects longer than 2 cm. without extensive dissection for mobilization of the artery proximal and distal and without sacrifice of collateral vessels. Saphenous vein grafts or prostheses are preferable for longer defects. Autogenous vein grafts are preferable in the superficial femoral or popliteal artery. Experience has shown that they do not need support by surrounding muscle or fascia. The saphenous vein is sturdy, will not dilate, and is suitable for replacement of the femoral or brachial arteries. The cephalic and brachial veins are thin walled. The saphenous vein graft is procured from the normal leg when the accompanying superficial femoral or popliteal vein is injured. Knitted prostheses of Dacron (DeBakey) are available in various diameters and lengths and should be used in large arteries such as the common femoral artery, because vein grafts in these locations will dilate despite external support with fascia, pericardium, etc. The techniques for use of such prostheses are described in the discussion of occlusive disease in the lower extremity.

It must be remembered that veins are not elastic and therefore the vein graft must not be too short. The veins are so thin walled that the edges, at the cut end, fold, wrinkle and collapse unless held by mattress sutures. Triangulating mattress sutures are essential. In this fashion the ends can be held open, manipulation with forceps can be avoided, and accurate placement of sutures is assured.

The most meticulous arterial suture may fail due to infection, improper fixation of associated fractures, or postischemic swelling in closed fascial compartments. Infection is usually the result of contamination and inadequate débridement. Adequate débridement of high-velocity missile wounds may result in sizable defects of soft tissue. Arterial anastomoses should be covered by living tissue, and muscle or skin flaps must be mobilized for this purpose. Dead space collects serum that can become infected, and this must not be permitted. Radical débridement of soft tissue is unnecessary for most civilian gunshot wounds. Drains may be placed in soft tissue and led out through a small separate and dependent drainage incision. They are not placed in contact with vascular anastomoses and are removed early.

Fasciotomy of the calf or forearm may be necessary to prevent compression of arteries and arterioles by edema within the tight fascial envelope. Fasciotomy is mandatory after popliteal artery injuries because of the associated venous outflow injury and obstruction. Fasciotomy should be done prophylactically in other instances when venous outflow is seriously impaired or when ischemia of the muscles of the calf has persisted over twelve hours. In such cases the muscle swells markedly when arterial continuity is restored. Swelling of muscle inside tight fascial compartments is evident only by firmness of the calf. Any evidence of arterial insufficiency of the foot in the presence of a firm calf is sufficient indication for fasciotomy. The surgeon will observe the edematous muscle bulge through the incision and be gratified at the return of distal pulses.

Procedure
Débridement of femoral artery and vein

1. Make a long incision over the course of the femoral artery (Fig. 42, A). Do not hesitate to divide the inguinal ligament if this is necessary to obtain proximal control of the bleeding.

146

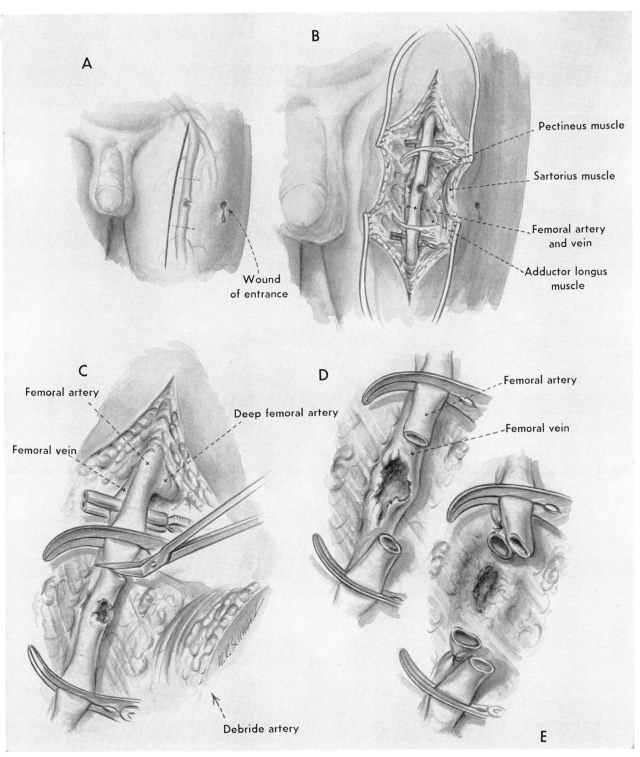

Labels in figure:
A

B

Pectineus muscle

Sartorius muscle

Femoral artery and vein

Adductor longus muscle

Wound of entrance

C

Femoral artery

Femoral vein

Deep femoral artery

Debride artery

D

Femoral artery

Femoral vein

E

Fig. 42. Vein graft for gunshot wound of femoral artery. **A** and **B,** Exploration of wound of femoral artery and vein. **C** and **D,** Débridement of femoral artery and vein. **E,** Vein ligated.

Continued.

2. Identify the femoral artery and the femoral vein, and obtain proximal control using serrefine arterial clamps before approaching the actual area of injury (Fig. 42, *B*). For occlusion of the veins, rubber-shod bulldog clamps are satisfactory and somewhat less traumatic. The superficial femoral vein usually has sizable posterior branches that must also be controlled. Approach the injury by dissecting progressively from normal tissues toward the area of hematoma. In the drawing the superficial femoral artery is almost completely divided and the vein has a through-and-through perforation.

3. Debride from 1 to 2 cm. of artery at each end of the wound (Fig. 42, *C*). Closely inspect the adventitia for tiny hematomas at the origins of small branches. The intima of the artery should be normal at the site of transection. Temporarily remove the distal clamp to observe back bleeding and to aspirate distal clots that may have formed during the period of occlusion. After the injured segment of artery has been resected, the remainder of the vessel retracts rather markedly.

4. Prepare the ends of the artery for anastomosis by trimming off any adventia that might protrude into the edges of the anastomosis (Fig. 42, *D*). In some instances arterial continuity may be restored by end-to-end anastomosis. In most gunshot wounds, however, adequate débridement leaves a considerable gap. Divided arteries retract, so that a gap of 6 to 7 cm. may result from resection of half that amount of artery. In this instance a 6 cm. vein graft was necessary. Measure the length of graft required without traction on the arterial clamps and take the vein graft a few centimeters longer than necessary.

5. Ligate the accompanying superficial femoral vein if repair is not feasible (Fig. 42, *E*).

Procurement of saphenous vein graft

1. Expose the saphenous vein in the upper thigh through a longitudinal incision (Fig. 42, *F*).

2. Uncover a sufficient length of vein. Ligate small tributaries prior to division of the vein. Employ sharp Potts arterial scissors to partially divide the vein distally (Fig. 42, *G*). Then place the first guide suture. Fig. 42, *I-M*, shows placement of other guide sutures before complete division of the vein.

3. Pass a double-armed 5-0 arterial suture through the vein distally, 0.5 mm. from the edge, for use as a horizontal everting mattress suture (Fig. 42, *H* and *I*). Hold both ends in a rubber-shod bulldog clamp. Continue division of the vein (Fig. 42, *J*).

4. Place the second suture one third of the distance around the circumference of the vein (Fig. 42, *K*).

5. Place a third horizontal everting mattress suture in the vein so that the three stitches form an equilateral triangle (Fig. 42, *L*).

6. Apply a toothed bulldog clamp proximally. Complete the division of the vein several centimeters longer than necessary (Fig. 42, *G*). *The vein must be reversed when it is inserted.*

Comment: *Divide the vein 1 to 2 cm. longer than necessary and place the triangulation sutures at the other end after completion of the first anastomosis. The judgment of the correct length for the vein graft is easier after the first anastomosis is completed, particularly if close to a joint.*

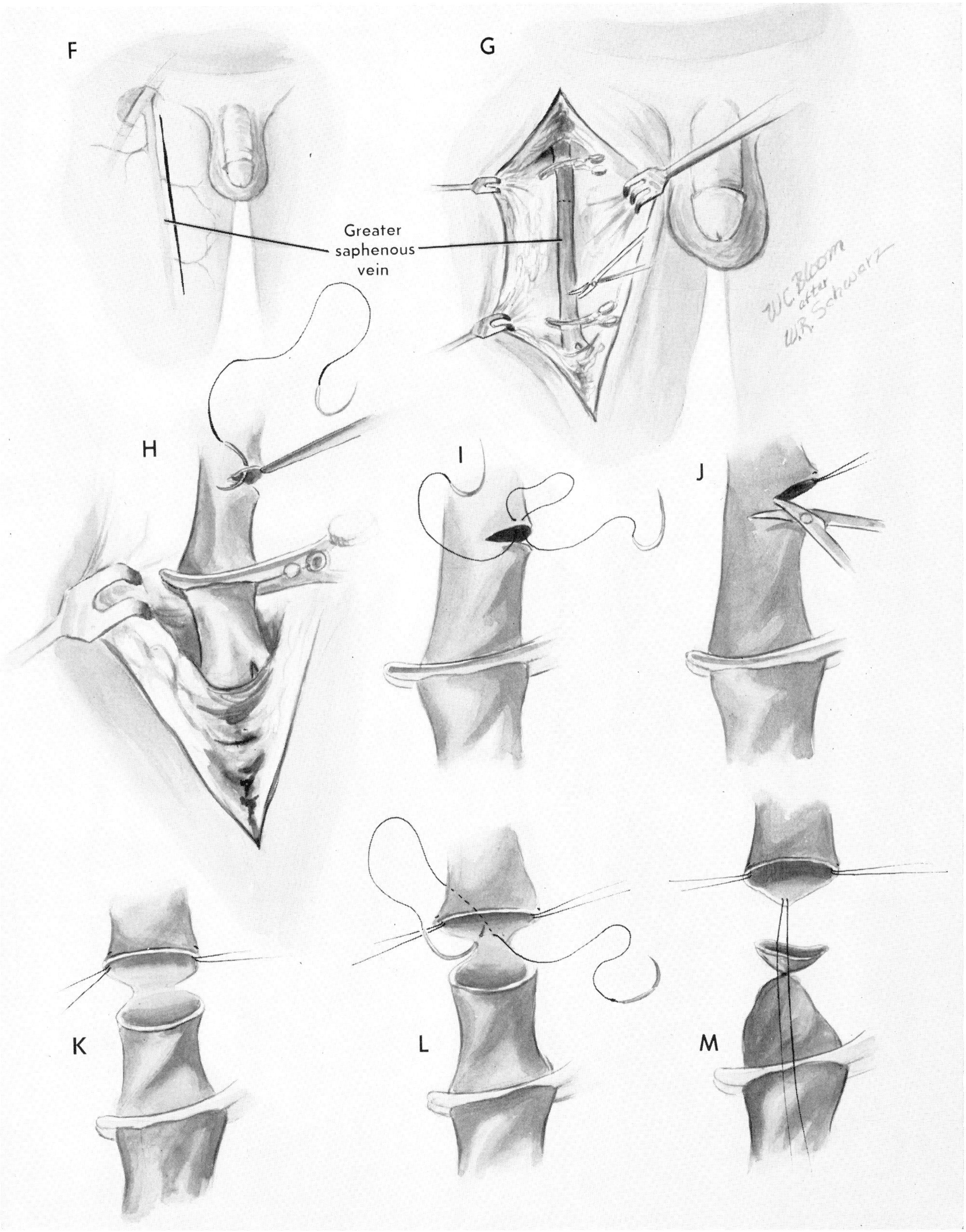
F
G
Greater
saphenous
vein
H
I
J
K
L
M

Fig. 42, cont'd. Vein graft for gunshot wound of femoral artery. Procurement of saphenous vein graft. **F,** Incision. **G,** Partial division of vein. **H** and **I,** First triangulation suture. **J,** Further division of vein graft. **K,** Second triangulation suture. **L** and **M,** Third triangulation suture.

Continued.

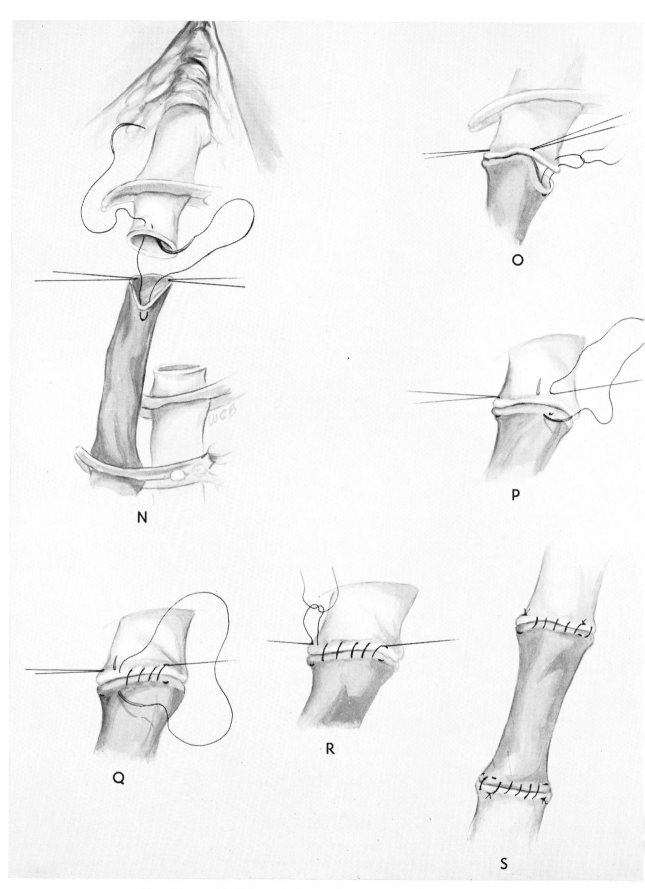

Fig. 42, cont'd. Vein graft for gunshot wound of femoral artery and vein. End-to-end anastomosis of vein graft and femoral artery. **N** and **O,** Triangulation sutures passed through artery and tied. **P** to **R,** Continuous suture of everted edges. **S,** Completed vein graft.

End-to-end anastomosis of vein graft and femoral artery

1. Insert, in the fashion illustrated, the previously placed guide sutures at the end of the vein into the prepared end of the artery as shown in Fig. 42, *N*. *Reverse the direction of the vein.*

2. Tie the mattress sutures without traction on the arterial clamps (Fig. 42, *O*). When the sutures are tied, the resulting eversion of the edges facilitates the remaining maneuvers.

3. Hold the suture line taut by placing traction laterally and medially on one of the limbs of the previously placed mattress suture. Sew the vein to the artery with small stitches about 0.5 mm. from the edge of the vessels, using an over-and-over continuous suture (Fig. 42, *P*).

4. Continue until the next mattress suture is reached (Fig. 42, *Q*).

5. End the continuous suture by tying it to one limb of adjacent mattress suture (Fig. 42, *R*). Release the proximal clamps to flush the proximal artery of the graft.

6. Reapply the bulldog clamp to the distal end of the vein graft to allow it to distend and lengthen under arterial pressure after release of the proximal arterial clamp.

7. Determine the correct length of the vein graft with the graft distended. If the graft is near a joint, judge the length with the joint extended and flexed.

8. Reapply the proximal arterial clamp, divide the vein graft partially, and place the first mattress suture for triangulation. Divide the graft more, and place the second and third triangulation sutures (as shown in Fig. 42, *H-M*).

9. Perform the distal anastomosis as described previously in steps 1-5 and illustrated in Fig. 42, *N-R*.

10. Before closing the last sutures, flush by momentarily releasing the proximal and distal clamps. Then tie the last suture. Remove the distal clamp till the graft fills with blood, and then slowly and intermittently release the proximal clamp. Bleeding from the needle holes or from the suture line will stop after five minutes. That the saphenous vein is slightly narrower than the artery should not be a cause of concern. Arteriograms in six or eight weeks will show that the vein has accommodated itself and is the same size as the artery.

11. Reconstruct the femoral sheath and soft tissues about the vein. Debridement of soft tissues need not be radical for wounds caused by low-velocity missiles. Associated injuries should be treated. The fascia of the thigh is closed loosely.

ANASTOMOSIS OF SMALL ARTERIES
Introduction

Restoration of continuity by direct vessel anastomosis should be performed in all traumatic interruptions of major arteries. When collateral circulation has been compromised, this principle must be extended to smaller vessels below the elbow and below the knee. Such vessels can be anastomosed with a fair rate of success by use of meticulous surgical technique. In emergency treatment of such injuries, use of hemostats to clamp severed vessels should be avoided. Wide operative exposure of the vessel at the site of injury is essential. If the injury is relatively old (that is, over twenty-four hours), extraction of the thrombus distal to the site of injury may prove difficult. However, this should be attempted, both by direct methods and by retrograde flushing.

The technique of anastomosis to be described employs fine 7-0 silk or monofilament suture on small atraumatic needles. The surgeon should make use of every aid to render his work precise, including adequate lighting and a magnifying binocular loupe. He should sit and arrange the field so that his elbows or forearms are supported. Microsurgery on very fine blood vessels using the binocular microscope has been described by Jacobson. This facilitates anastomosis of these small vessels. The Nakayama stapler is under trial in our laboratory.

Procedure

1. Debride the injured vessel. Occlude the vessel proximally and distally with rubbed-shod bulldog clamps. Wash blood clot from the ends of the vessels with warm saline solution or warm 0.1% heparin in saline solution. Two stay or guide sutures are now inserted with double-armed fine silk sutures at opposite ends of the vessel (Fig. 43, A).

Comment: *Following injury, small arteries may be highly spastic. Smooth muscle spasm may be overcome by topical applications of pledgets soaked with 2% papaverine. If this is ineffective or unavailable, the ends of the vessels must be mechanically dilated by very gently spreading the tips of a fine hemostat within the lumen of the vessel. At this stage, and before the anastomosis has begun, the distal portion of the vessel must be cleared of thrombus by using a wire loop or a small balloon catheter or by retrograde flushing.*

2. Have the assistant place traction on the tied guide sutures. Begin the anastomosis of the vessel with a simple over-and-over stitch, the surgeon sewing toward himself (Fig. 43, B).

3. When the end of the row is reached, tie the suture (Fig. 43, C).

4. Pass the three pieces of thread at one end to the assistant, and rotate the vessel 180 degrees (Fig. 43, D). Complete the remainder of the suture line with a simple over-and-over stitch (Fig. 43, E).

5. The suture line is completed in a manner similar to that used for the first row (Fig. 43, F).

Comment: *The operator should feel a pulsatile flow of blood when the anastomosis is complete and the bulldog clamps are released. If the vessel remains spastic, a sponge soaked in warm (not hot) saline solution may be employed in an attempt to relax muscle spasm and increase blood flow locally. It may be necessary to perform operative angiography in order to assure patency of the anastomosis and the distal vessels.*

In this and other chapters we have illustrated the use of double-armed sutures. It is obvious that the same procedures may be carried out with single-armed sutures. The double-armed suture allows the surgeon to sew in either direction from either end of the anastomosis. In addition, should one of the threads break—and this is not unusual when using very fine material—the spare suture and needle are available and the anastomosis can proceed without delay.

To avoid damage, vascular sutures should never be grasped or tagged with a hemostat unless it is rubber shod. Preferably, traction on these fine sutures

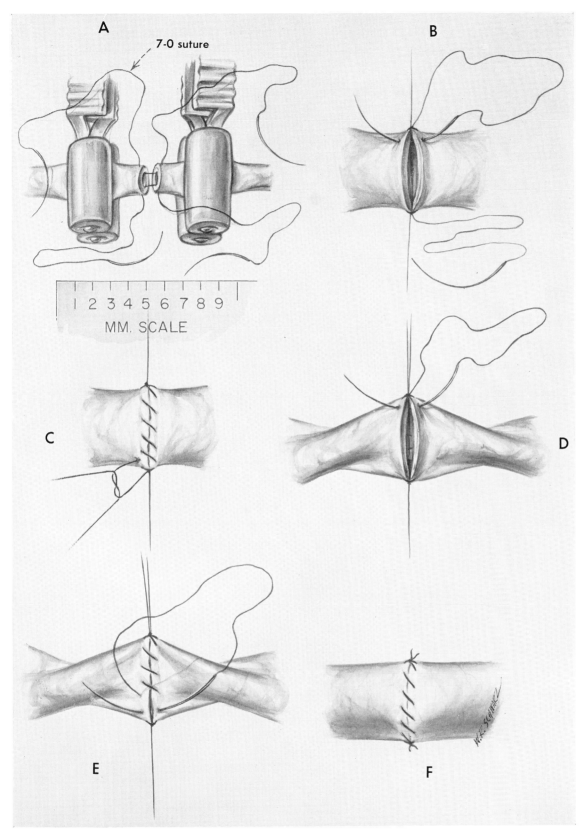

7-0 suture

1 2 3 4 5 6 7 8 9
MM. SCALE

Fig. 43. Anastomosis of small arteries. **A,** First sutures. **B** and **C,** Continuous suture of anterior row without excision or narrowing of lumen. **D** and **E,** Posterior row of continuous sutures. **F,** Completed anastomosis.

should be exerted directly through the gloved hand of the operator or his assistant without the intervention of an instrument.

ANASTOMOSIS OF SMALL VESSELS
WITH NAKAYAMA STAPLER

We have used the Nakayama vascular stapler* for rapid and accurate anastomosis of normal arteries or veins 2 mm. to 4 mm. in diameter. The vessels are anastomosed with two thin metal rings with prongs and holes which act as staples. Each of the two flat rings of stainless steel or tantalum has six tiny prongs and six holes (Fig. 44, B). One ring is placed in the opening of the jaw of the clamp (Fig. 44, C) and is held in place by closing the clamp. The prongs project upward and will pass into the holes of the opposite ring at the time of the anastomosis. To orient the prongs of one clamp with the holes of the other ring, the rings are rotated until a notch on the ring lies opposite a scored mark on the jaw of its holding clamp. With a small hook provided for this purpose, the cleaned end of the vessel is drawn through the ring and everted over the prongs (Fig. 44, D). This most difficult step of the procedure requires practice in the laboratory. It is facilitated by gently dilating the end of the vessel with a small hemostat. The edges of the vessel must be forced down over each prong of the ring individually, using the fine tissue forceps. The vessel may be more firmly fixed on the prongs by a stylet of appropriate size. The other end of the anastomosis is similarly fixed to the ring in the other holding clamp.

The ends of the vessel are joined when the jaws of the two clamps are approximated (Fig. 44, E). The projections on the face of one clamp fit into indentations in the other clamp. A small clip holds the two clamps together. A special pliers is applied to the ends of the clamps so that its notched jaws surround the projecting vessels. This pliers is closed very firmly to drive the prongs of each ring through the opposite vessel into the holes of the other ring. The prongs are bent as they are pressed against the plate of the holding clamp. The pliers and clip are removed and the clamps opened to free the rings (Fig. 44, F). The anastomosis may be made more watertight by further compressing the rings with a strong hemostat throughout their circumference.

An end-to-side or side-to-side anastomosis may be constructed by drawing the edges of an opening in the side of a vessel through the hole of the ring and everting over the prongs in the same manner.

With practice, the anastomosis can be accomplished in about half the time required to suture vessels of the same size. The intimal surface is uniformly smooth and free of foreign material since the rings and traumatized vessel edges lie outside the lumen. The union is strong and seldom leaks. Reloading is simple and rapid. Other rings may be sterilized separately and inserted into the clamps at the operating table.

There are three important limitations of the stapler:

1. The eversion over the prongs requires that the vessel edges be pliable.
2. The anastomosis is permanently surrounded by a rigid ring that prevents

---

*Devised by Prof. Komei Nakayama, Chiba University Medical School in Japan. The instrument and staples are available in the United States from V. I. Mueller & Co., Chicago, Ill. The Nakayama stapler has been used extensively with great success on more than fifty canine renal transplants by Dr. Thomas Sheridan in our laboratory.

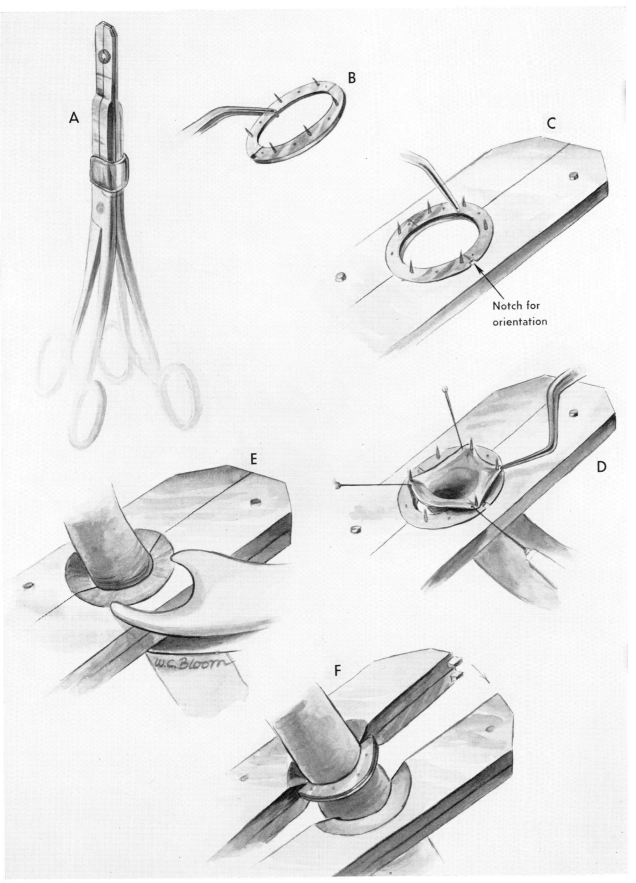

Fig. 44. Nakayama stapler for anastomosis of a small vessel. **A,** Nakayama clamps. **B,** Stapling rings. **C,** Stapling ring recessed in clamp. **D,** End of vessel drawn through ring and everted over prongs. **E,** Approximate two clamps to join two ends of vessel. **F,** Open clamp to free ring anastomosis.

Notch for orientation

expansion and growth. Dr. Nakayama reports observing aneurysmal dilatation of the vessel distal to the ring in some dogs. The staple rings are scored for the purpose of being fractured by bending after completion of the anastomosis to make expansion possible. However, this often results in unacceptable leaking.

3. In our experience, the apparatus is not useful for ureteral or bile duct anastomosis because of stricture formation. The lumen of the thick-walled tube (such as a dog ureter) is narrowed where the entire circumference must pass through the circle. This is less significant for thin-walled tubes.

The apparatus has been very useful in renal artery anastomosis in dog kidney transplants and clinically for anastomosis of the radial and ulnar arteries.

Chapter 9

Operations on the superior mesenteric artery

SUDDEN OCCLUSION

Sudden occlusion of the superior mesenteric artery produces gangrene of the major portion of the small intestine. A few patients may survive such a disaster after massive resection of the infarcted intestine. However, it is obviously preferable to salvage the ischemic tissues by early diagnosis, early operation, and treatment to restore the arterial flow. Unfortunately, early diagnosis is difficult.

Sudden occlusion is usually embolic or thrombotic in origin. Chronic occlusion (discussed below) is more likely to present problems in diagnosis and treatment. Both embolectomy and aortic–superior mesenteric artery bypass are performed in the accessible portion of the superior mesenteric artery after it emerges beneath the pancreas.

Symptoms

The initial symptoms are vomiting, abdominal pain, and at times severe and bloody diarrhea. After a quiescent period the signs and symptoms of peritonitis usually appear, but at this time gangrene of the intestine is well established.

Diagnosis

The diagnosis is perhaps most easily made when fibrillation or a recent myocardial infarct alerts the physician to the possibility of embolism. Early laboratory work can be equivocal, although a markedly elevated white blood cell count is not infrequent. We have demonstrated an early and marked elevation of serum lactic dehydrogenase in most of the patients. At times infarction of the intestine is observed without organic occlusion, usually in conjunction with shock or some other form of cardiovascular failure and particularly in conjunction with aortic insufficiency. Mesenteric vascular occlusion may occur in children. This may be primarily arterial, primarily venous, or combined. In most of the patients no specific etiological factor could be identified.

Treatment

In acute occlusion of the superior mesenteric artery, early correct diagnosis and abdominal exploration will make possible the restoration of pulsatile blood flow by embolectomy or endarterectomy. The point of narrowing is usually 0.25 to 1 cm. distal to the aortic orifice of the superior mesenteric artery. About one-half of the fresh occlusions are confined to the superior mesenteric artery with normal distal branches and are therefore correctable by operation. If operation is done very early, the bowel may appear normal but without pulsation of the superior mesenteric artery. If the bowel is dark and discolored, viability may still be retained. In such cases, if blood flow can be successfully restored, careful postoperative observation and reexploration in twenty-four to forty-eight hours is advised to detect and resect any segment of intestine that has not recovered.

MESENTERIC ANGINA

In addition to the acute occlusions of the superior mesenteric artery, partial obstruction may result in cramping pain, particularly following meals. Such pain is analogous to the ischemic work pain of intermittent claudication in skeletal muscle. Usually both the celiac axis and the superior mesenteric artery must be affected by occlusive disease to produce symptoms. The collateral circulation is so abundant that surgical treatment may be limited to revascularization of the superior mesenteric artery by aortic–superior mesenteric artery bypass with a Dacron prosthesis or with an autogenous vein graft.

Symptoms

Symptoms include abdominal pain following meals, constipation, and weight loss. The pain is cramping in nature, develops shortly after ingestion of food, and lasts one or two hours. The patients have malabsorption and exhibit a high-fat content in the feces and occult blood in the stools. Physiologically, the deficiency in blood flow to the small intestine may be confirmed by the decreased absorption of D-xylose. The cause is usually atherosclerotic occlusion or narrowing of the superior mesenteric and celiac arteries.

Diagnosis

The diagnosis is made either by translumbar or by retrograde percutaneous aortography. It may be helpful and necessary to take films in the lateral decubitus position to better visualize the celiac axis and its branches. To do this by the translumbar route, it is safer to introduce a flexible Teflon catheter than to use a rigid needle. A confirmatory sign of superior mesenteric occlusion is the finding of an enlarged meandering inferior mesenteric and/or left colic artery bringing collateral circulation to the ischemic superior portion of the intestine.

Treatment

In chronic cases of intestinal angina, bypass of the superior mesenteric artery obstruction with a vascular prosthesis is employed to revascularize the intestine. The celiac axis need not be revascularized. The superior mesenteric artery is best vascularized by a direct bypass from the aorta. Endarterectomy is more difficult and unnecessary.

SURGICAL EXPOSURE

Anesthesia

General anesthesia or high spinal anesthesia is satisfactory. For this surgery high in the abdomen, adequate relaxation is essential.

Procedure

Exposure of superior mesenteric artery for embolectomy or bypass

The following procedure exposes enough of the superior mesenteric artery to perform an adequate embolectomy. The usual site for lodgment of an embolus is at the origin of the middle colic artery. The superior mesenteric artery narrows considerably at this branch. When further exposure of the superior mesenteric artery is necessary, the extended exposure procedure may be used, or the balloon catheter may be passed into the proximal superior mesenteric artery to extract proximal emboli.

1. Open the abdomen through a long left paramedian or a midline incision (Fig. 45, A).

2. Retract the transverse colon upward and retract the most proximal portion of the jejunum to the left. When retracting, make certain that tension has been placed on the middle colic artery. This maneuver both elevates and fixes the superior mesenteric artery and facilitates the subsequent dissection. (See Fig. 45, B.)

3. Pick up the parietal peritoneum just to the right of the duodenojejunal flexure with a fine thumb forceps. Make a longitudinal incision in the peritoneum approximately 4 cm. long. The superior mesenteric artery will appear in the fatty tissue immediately beneath the incision and can be kept relatively superficial by continued traction on the colon and the jejunum (Fig. 45, C and D). Isolate the artery by blunt dissection with small rolls of umbilical tape. When the artery has been visualized, dissection can be carried along its anterior aspect, exposing 3 or 4 cm. of the vessel.

Exposure of retropancreatic portion of superior mesenteric artery

1. Expose the distal portion of the superior mesenteric artery as detailed in the preceding procedure.

2. Beginning at the top of the peritoneal incision, extend the incision in the parietal peritoneum to the left along the lower border of the pancreas for 6 to 8 cm.

3. Gently and carefully divide the peritoneal attachment of the duodeno-jejunal flexure and the ligament of Treitz so that the duodenojejunal flexure can be retracted inferiorly. Retraction should be gentle to protect the first jejunal branches that enter the bowel from the superior mesenteric artery at this point.

4. Clamp, ligate, and divide the *inferior* mesenteric vein.

5. Dissect along the anterior surface of the mesenteric artery carefully, tunneling under the pancreas. The inferior pancreatic artery may be divided. As the dissection proceeds, place a narrow Deaver retractor under the inferior edge of the pancreas, rolling the pancreas anteriorly and exposing the origin of the superior mesenteric artery from the front of the aorta.

Restoration of blood flow

The principles and techniques of embolectomy, including balloon catheters, patch angioplasty, localized endarterectomy, and bypass grafting, are described

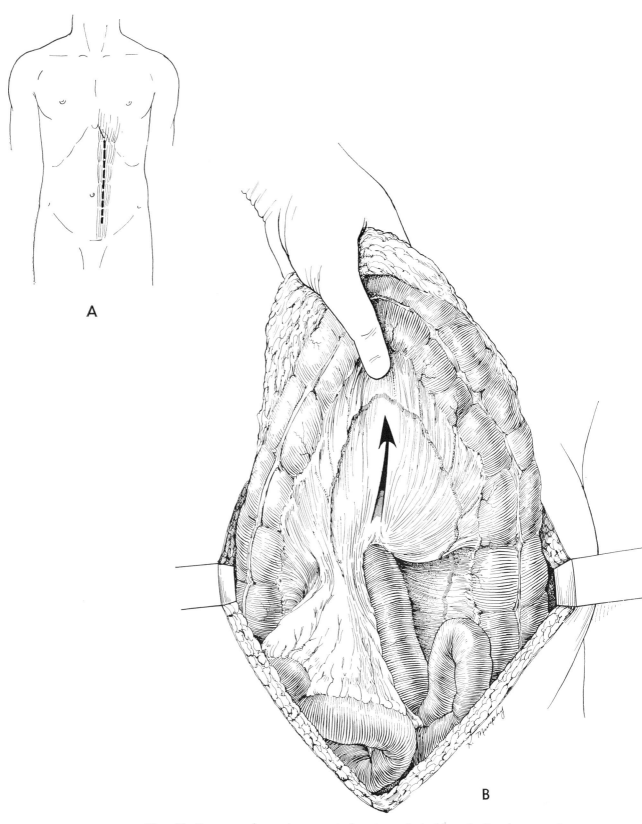

Fig. 45. Exposure of superior mesenteric artery. **A,** Incision. **B,** Traction on colon, meso-colon, and midcolic artery.

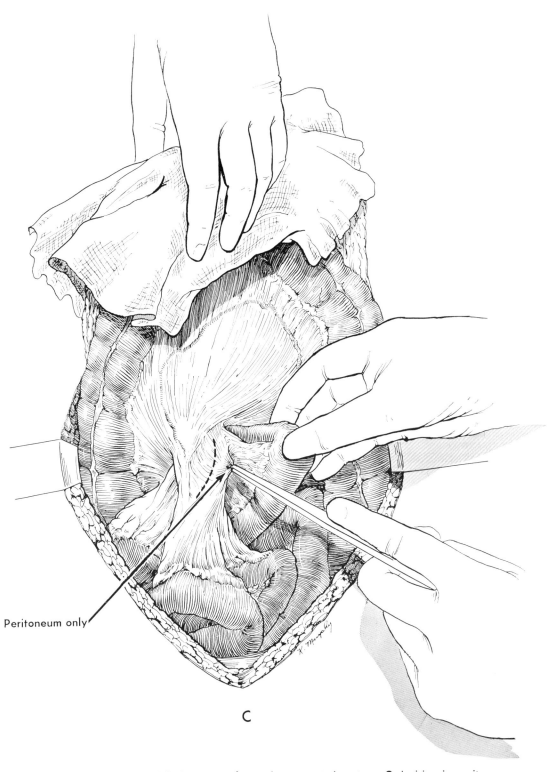

Peritoneum only

C

Fig. 45, cont'd. Exposure of superior mesenteric artery. **C,** Incision in peritoneum.

Continued.

161

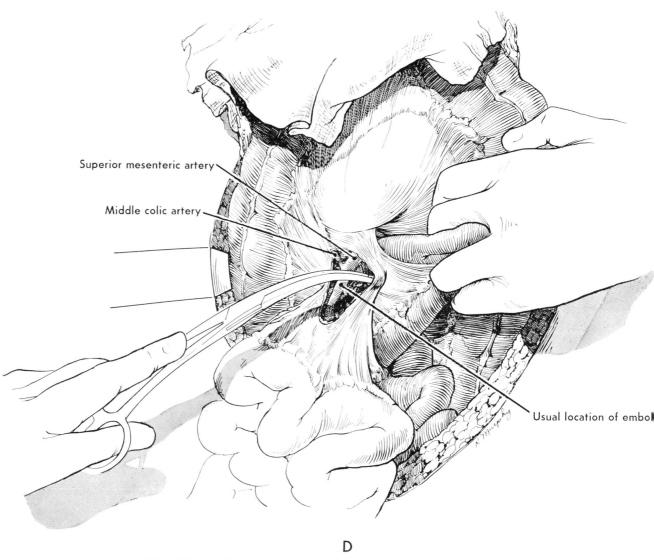

Superior mesenteric artery

Middle colic artery

Usual location of embol

D

Fig. 45, cont'd. Exposure of superior mesenteric artery. **D,** Artery has been freed from surrounding tissues.

elsewhere in this book. The bypass prosthesis must be at least 8 mm. in diameter and connect the side of the superior mesenteric artery to the side of the aorta or to the side of another prosthesis. Saphenous vein grafts deserve a trial in this site as bypass tubes or for patch angioplasty.

AORTIC–SUPERIOR MESENTERIC ARTERY BYPASS
Procedure

1. Prepare and expose the superior mesenteric artery as for thrombectomy or embolectomy (Fig. 45, A-D).

2. Expose the anterior surface of the aorta by enlarging the incision in the mesentery of the small intestine or by reflecting the mesentery to the right and incising the posterior peritoneal reflection over the aorta.

3. Select a site on the anterior wall of the aorta that is relatively free of

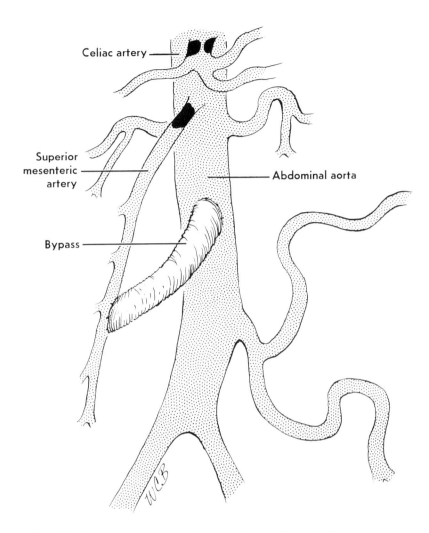

Celiac artery

Superior
mesenteric
artery

Bypass

Abdominal aorta

Fig. 46. Aortosuperior mesenteric artery bypass for occlusion of superior mesenteric artery with narrowing of celiac artery.

atherosclerosis and calcification. This may be quite high. Prepare about 4 to 6 cm. of the anterior aortic wall for anastomosis by stripping it of perivascular lymphatics, etc. Circumferential exposure is not necessary.

4. Place a curved partially occluding clamp on the anterior aortic wall. Make a small anterior incision, rinse with heparinized saline solution, and attach a vein graft or Dacron prosthesis by the usual end-to-side suture technique using 4-0 arterial polyethylene or Tevdec.

Comment: *Monofilament sutures glide easily through the thin-walled superior mesenteric or renal arteries.*

5. Adjust the length of the graft or prosthesis. If the aorta was exposed to the left of the root of the mesentery, a tunnel must be made through the mesentery to the superior mesenteric artery.

6. Temporarily occlude the superior mesenteric artery with tapes or vascular clamps. Make a short longitudinal incision on the posterior or lateral wall of the artery, rinse with heparinized saline solution, and again proceed with end-to-

163

side anastomosis. Before completing the last few stitches, check back bleeding from the mesenteric side and then flush from the aortic side. Complete the anastomosis (Fig. 46). Before closing, check the arterial supply of the small intestine for pulsation.

Comment: *If the operation is performed for acute mesenteric occlusion in which the viability of bowel is still in doubt, take a "second look" twenty-four hours after revascularization. The delay permits further recovery of viable bowel and the demarcation of the doubtful bowel. At reoperation, bowel resection will be safe and less extensive.*

Chapter 10

Surgical treatment of renovascular hypertension

RENAL HYPERTENSION

Reconstructive vascular procedures can restore blood flow and can usually correct hypertension caused by renal artery obstruction. In such patients hypertension is the clinical counterpart of the renal hypertension first demonstrated by Goldblatt, who induced hypertension experimentally by restricting renal blood flow. Humoral substances (the renin-angiotensin system) are released by the ischemic kidney under certain circumstances. Measurement of these factors is not yet practical for the diagnosis of renovascular hypertension. Renal ischemia is probably a relatively uncommon cause of elevated blood pressure. However, as many as 25% of hypertensive patients are said to have varying degrees of renal arterial pathology.

In screening hypertensive patients for conditions that are correctable surgically, renal ischemic lesions should be suspected in association with the following circumstances:

1. When long-standing hypertension suddenly becomes severe
2. When malignant hypertension arises suddenly, particularly in a middle-aged or older patient
3. When signs or symptoms of renal infarct precede the development of hypertension (a history or findings of unilateral renal pain and hematuria are suggestive)
4. When a hypertensive patient is unusually young and does not have a family history of hypertension

When hypertension of renal origin is suspected, excretory urography with certain modifications is the most readily available test of renal function. Films taken one to three minutes after injection may show a delay in excretion by the involved kidney. In some instances an increase in the filtration factor on the affected side has resulted in the contrast medium appearing in greater density in the affected kidney fifteen to thirty minutes after injection. If the physiology of this situation is not kept in mind, the diagnosis may be missed. The affected kidney may be somewhat smaller than the normal one.

Separated renal function tests are helpful when carefully performed and

165

evaluated. When blood flow to the kidney is impaired, the glomerular filtration rate and the effective renal plasma flow are correspondingly reduced. On the constricted side, the output of sodium and of water will be reduced. In unilateral pyelonephritis or partial infarction of the kidney, the urinary sodium levels usually remain the same. It should not be forgotten that arterial stenosis can protect the parenchyma of the kidney distal to the stenosis, so that even though this organ shows decreased function compared to its mate, it may actually be histologically healthier and as a consequence superior in functional potential once the arterial obstruction is corrected.

Renal arteriograms are the most important study for accurate location and confirmation of the diagnosis. The method of percutaneous retrograde catheterization described in Chapter 2 is usually applicable, although for patients with associated occlusive lesions of the aorta or iliac arteries we prefer translumbar aortography. A sequence of films of the kidneys obtained with the changer is useful but not essential.

Renal ischemia and constriction may result from atherosclerotic plaques, thrombosis, embolism, congenital or acquired stenosis, thromboangiitis, external pressure by aneurysm, fibrous bands, tumors, or trauma. Of those named, atherosclerosis is the most common cause in older adults, and fibromuscular hyperplasia of the renal artery is the lesion most commonly encountered in young patients.

Surgical procedures

The purpose of surgical reconstruction is to restore normal pulsatile blood flow to the affected kidney. The ideal surgical candidate is a relatively young recently hypertensive patient who has no atherosclerotic disease in the coronary or cerebral arteries. When reconstruction of the artery is not feasible, nephrectomy is performed. Nephrectomy is elected when the renal artery is completely occluded or the kidney is very atrophic. Various procedures to restore flow may be used according to the situation encountered.

The procedures for atherosclerotic stenosis (Fig. 47, A, C, E, and F) are quite different than the operations for fibromuscular dysplasia (Fig. 47, B and D) because the latter is usually more diffuse and distal. Thromboendarterectomy, excision of the fibrous constriction with end-to-end anastomosis, bypass prosthesis or vein graft, splenorenal anastomosis on the left side, or implantation of the renal artery into a new site on the aorta may each be appropriate. In doubtful cases, the pressure in the renal artery distal to the stenosis should be measured at exploration. If significant pressure difference cannot be demonstrated across the suspicious area, the correction of stenosis is only prophylactic.

Of all the surgical procedures mentioned, direct aortorenal bypass grafting is probably the most useful and the most widely applicable. In elderly patients with atherosclerotic disease, this procedure may be done bilaterally or may be combined with prosthetic replacement of the aorta or with aortofemoral bypass procedures.

Anterior approach to kidney

For patients with atherosclerotic occlusions, the anterior approach must be employed, since it allows inspection of both kidneys, better exposure of the proximal renal vessels, and access to the aorta. The most useful exposure is through a long midline or paramedian incision.

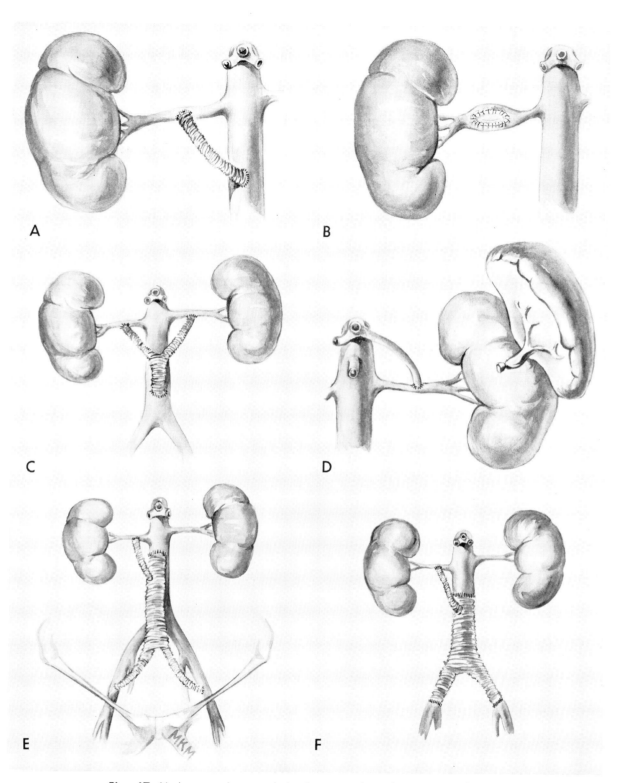

Fig. 47. Various renal revascularization operations. **A,** Aortorenal bypass prosthesis. **B,** Patch angioplasty. **C,** Bilateral aortorenal bypass prosthesis. **D,** Splenorenal arterial anastomosis. **E,** Renal artery bypass from aortoiliac bypass prosthesis. **F,** Renal artery bypass from prosthesis for aortic resection.

Exposure of both kidneys is facilitated by several adjuncts: (1) a small sandbag beneath the eleventh and twelfth ribs and the flank to push the kidney forward, (2) an additional assistant to retract the costal margin, and (3) elevation of the renal arteries by the special renal artery clamps.

Anterior approach to proximal portion of renal arteries

Atherosclerotic lesions involve the proximal part of the artery. The exposure is an upward continuation of the exposure of the lower abdominal aorta (Fig. 11).

1. Make a long midline incision (Fig. 48, A). Mobilize the small bowel to the right, divide the ligament of Treitz, and reflect the duodenum to the right (Fig. 48, B).

2. Divide the inferior mesenteric vein where it crosses the aorta at the inferior border of the pancreas.

3. Isolate and lift the left renal vein with umbilical tape, and ligate and divide the adrenal and ovarian or spermatic veins (Fig. 48, D and E).

4. Retract the mesocolon upward and laterally.

5. Divide the inferior mesenteric artery if it is necessary to retract the left mesocolon laterally.

6. For access to the proximal part of the right renal artery, between the inferior vena cava and the aorta, dissect the inferior vena cava free so that the medial edge can be rolled laterally and held with a narrow Deaver retractor (Fig. 48, E).

7. Mobilize the proximal portion of the renal arteries and uncover the front and sides of the nearby aorta preparatory to clamping it. The origin of the superior mesenteric artery will be visualized just above the renal arteries emerging beneath the pancreas.

8. Palpation of the renal arteries, possibly measurement of the arterial pressure in the aorta and renal arteries, and review of the arteriograms are helpful in choosing the correct operation.

9. After choice of the operation, whether endarterectomy or bypass grafting, arterial clamps of appropriate size and shape are chosen so that when applied they leave the renal artery anteriorly and hold the inferior vena cava and left renal vein aside (Fig. 48, F).

Bilateral renal endarterectomy

Bilateral renal endarterectomy is employed when the obstructing plaques are only in the proximal part of the renal arteries. The endarterectomy may include adjacent plaques in the aorta. It is seldom, if ever, necessary to suture distal intima after removal of short plaques because the distal intima will be normal. If the plaques extend farther than 1 cm. into the renal artery, bypass is preferred so that the renal arteriotomy can be short.

Choice of incisions for the endarterectomy are illustrated. If an incision extends onto the origin of the renal artery, close it with a patch angioplasty.

The approach and surgical exposure is via the anterior midline approach previously described and illustrated in Fig. 48.

1. Clamp the aorta below the left renal vein with a coarctation or angle clamp applied vertically.

2. Inject heparin above and below this clamp (a total of 50 mg.).

3. Clamp the aorta above the renal arteries in the same fashion.

4. Temporary occlusion of the lumbar arteries posteriorly is obtained by the proper application of coarctation or angle clamps with the tips close together posteriorly or by the use of the S-shaped Craaford clamp inferiorly applied as illustrated in Fig. 21.

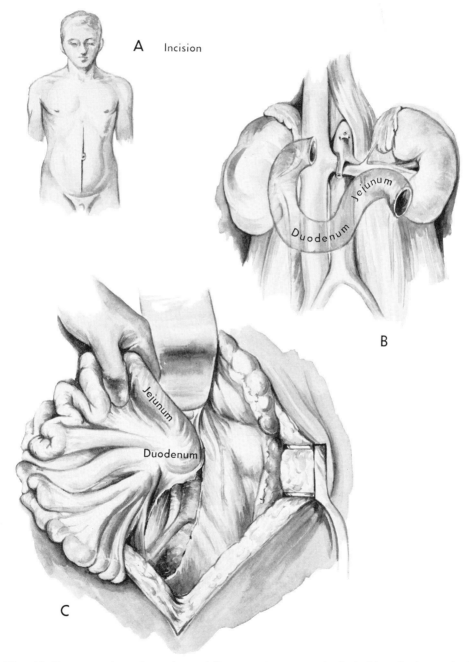

Fig. 48. Exposure of renal arteries—midline anterior approach. **A,** Incision. **B,** Anatomical relationships of structures overlying renal arteries. **C,** Peritoneal incision and division of ligament of Treitz.   *Continued.*

169

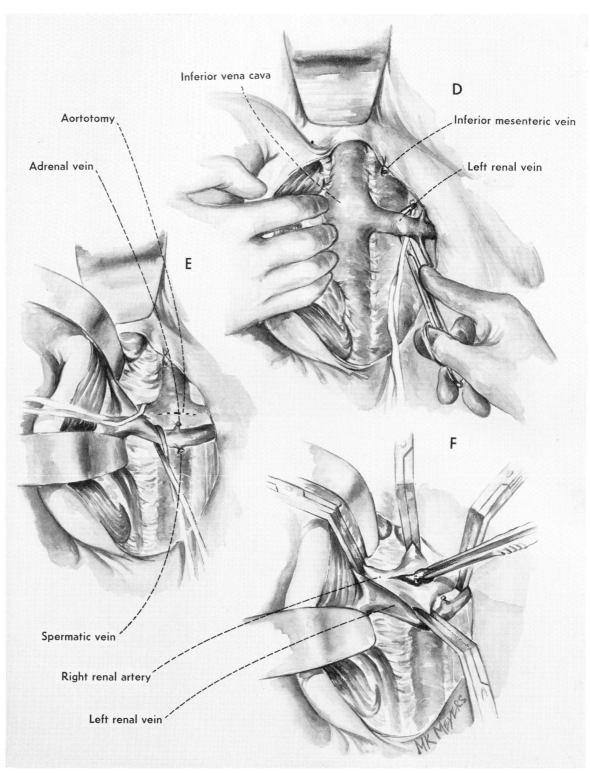

Inferior vena cava

Aortotomy

Adrenal vein

Inferior mesenteric vein

D

Left renal vein

E

F

Spermatic vein

Right renal artery

Left renal vein

MK MEYERS

Fig. 48, cont'd. Exposure of renal arteries—midline anterior approach. **D,** Mobilization of left renal vein. **E,** Aortotomy at origin of both renal arteries. **F,** Endarterectomy of orifices of both renal arteries.

5. Aortotomy is begun with the No. 15 blade, and the incision is lengthened with the Potts vascular scissors after it has been ascertained that the aortic clamps have control (Fig. 48, E).

6. Apply the spring-handled renal artery clamp distally on the renal artery with the tip of the clamp 1 to 2 cm. deeper than the artery, which is thereby held forward and more accessible. The clamp also holds the inferior vena cava or renal vein aside (Fig. 48, F).

7. Endarterectomy is performed by finding the plane of cleavage at the edge of the arteriotomy or aortotomy and developing this plane around the orifice of and into the proximal renal artery. The plaque teases out. Inspect the tip of the plaque which is removed. If it is thin, the distal intima is most likely normal. However, if in doubt, the incision should be extended onto the renal artery to permit inspection of the distal intima, which must be sutured if it is loose.

8. Irrigate the arteriotomy with dilute heparin to flush out detritus and reveal loose tags of intima. The beaded cannula and syringe are useful to instill heparin in the renal arteries.

9. Ascertain the diameter of the renal artery with Bakes dilators if in doubt about the caliber.

10. Release the proximal and distal aortic clamps momentarily to flush out any small clots, etc.

11. Suture the aortotomy with 4-0 or 5-0 arterial suture. If the incision extended onto the renal artery, close it with a patch angioplasty to avoid narrowing the renal artery (Fig. 48). Uncrimped plastic prosthesis sews easily and is preferred.

12. Cover the arteriotomy with Gelfoam and apply gentle pressure while you release first the distal aortic clamp, then the proximal aortic clamps, and finally the renal artery clamps.

Bypass operations for renal artery stenosis

Bypass procedures are preferred when atherosclerotic plaques occupy more than the proximal 1 cm. of the renal artery. During a bypass procedure the renal artery need be occluded only briefly because the renal arteriotomy for bypass procedures never exceeds 8 mm. Local endarterectomy and patch angioplasty in such cases require longer arteriotomies.

The varieties of bypass procedures are illustrated in Fig. 47. The renal anastomosis is always distal to the arteriosclerotic plaque and the aortic anastomosis is inferior. Turbulence does not appear to be a problem, no doubt because the grafts are short. The aortic anastomosis may be to the side of the aorta or to the side of an aortic prosthesis if such is needed to replace the abdominal aorta.

Congenital anomalies and fibromuscular dysplasia require special techniques because of their unique location and the longer life expectancy of the patients. These are discussed later.

Right renal artery bypass

The midline anterior approach was previously described and illustrated (Fig. 48). Good exposure of the proximal 2 to 3 cm. of the right renal artery is obtained by retracting the inferior vena cava to the right and the left renal vein inferiorly. Deep and narrow Deaver and Harrington retractors are essential.

1. Determine whether bypass or endarterectomy is necessary. Use a bypass if an endarterectomy would require arteriotomy longer than 10 mm.

2. Cut the end of an 8 mm. fine-knitted DeBakey or Weaveknit prosthesis obliquely, and preclot it by filling it with blood.

3. Prepare the site for the aortic anastomosis of the bypass graft. Although sidewise clamping of the aorta is theoretically advantageous, it is usually easier and preferable to cross clamp the aorta for the fifteen to twenty minutes needed to anastomose the graft.

4. Cross clamp the aorta with vertical clamps.

5. Inject 20 mg. of heparin proximally and distally.

6. Incise the anterolateral aspect of the aorta or aortic prosthesis vertically for a distance of 10 mm.

7. Empty the preclotted graft and suture it to the aortotomy, using a double-armed 4-0 monofilament arterial suture.

8. Flush out the distal aorta by releasing the distal clamp and reapplying it momentarily. Release the proximal clamp to flush out the proximal aorta via the bypass tube.

9. Restore flow through the aorta after the graft is clamped close to the anastomosis. When the aortic clamps are released, any slight bleeding from the suture line is controlled by Gelfoam and gentle pressure.

10. Cut the distal end of the graft transversely at a length that reaches the renal artery without tension.

11. Lift the right renal artery with the tape around it preparatory to heparin injection and clamping. Have renal artery clamps ready.

12. Inject 10 mg. of heparin into the right renal artery.

13. Quickly apply the distal clamp with the artery held up and the inferior vena cava retracted far to the right. Apply the clamp at 30 degrees to the perpendicular so that it can be rotated superiorly for better access to the posterior row of sutures.

14. Apply the proximal renal artery clamp in the same fashion.

15. Make the arteriotomy 8 mm. long distal to the obstruction and on the anteroinferior aspect of the renal artery. Place small retracting stitches into the renal artery first. Hold these up while incising the renal artery with a No. 11 blade. Complete the arteriotomy with the angled Potts scissors.

16. Begin with the posterior row of sutures to anastomose the end of the bypass graft to the side of the right renal artery. Use 5-0 arterial or polyethylene monofilament sutures, which glide easily through the thin-walled renal artery. Turn the handles of the renal artery clamps superiorly to rotate the posterior edge of the renal arteriotomy more anterior and make it more accessible.

17. Start the double-armed arterial suture at one end of the arteriotomy and pass the needle through the artery and graft separately. Then pull the stitch into place, approximating the edges, using your forceps to guide the suture and edges and avoid tearing the renal artery. A blunt nerve hook is useful.

18. Complete the posterior row and continue the same suture anteriorly. Flush and fill the prosthesis before tying the last suture. Flush and fill the prosthesis by releasing the proximal renal artery clamp. Then tie the last suture.

19. Release the distal renal artery clamp. Control of minor bleeding at the suture line with gentle pressure and Gelfoam must not obstruct the renal artery.

Slowly release the clamp at the aortic end of the graft to restore full flow to the kidney. Then remove the proximal clamp on the renal artery.

20. Cover the prosthesis with soft tissue of the mesentery of the colon so that the duodenum is not in contact with the graft. This procedure prevents graft-enteric fistulas.

RENOVASCULAR HYPERTENSION DUE TO FIBROMUSCULAR DYSPLASIA

Fibromuscular dysplasia of the renal arteries is a rare cause of renovascular hypertension, but it is particularly troublesome because the disease usually involves most of the renal artery, may extend distally into the branches of the renal artery, and is frequently bilateral.

The disease has been recognized in various essential peripheral arteries such as the renal, coronary, internal carotid, cerebral, and popliteal. It doubtlessly occurs elsewhere but is asymptomatic in areas in which the collateral circulation is adequate.

The renal arteriograms (Fig. 49) show multiple short areas of stenosis with intervening dilation, giving a "beaded" appearance. The stenotic areas may not be obvious at operation, but the "beaded" areas are small aneurysms whose walls may be so thin that the blood may be seen swirling inside. In the thin bulging areas the media and internal elastic lamina are degenerated or absent. In the stenotic areas the media is thickened by loose myxomatous tissue, or the stenosis may be due mainly to intimal thickening (Fig. 50). Periarterial fibrosis is seldom troublesome.

The arteriographic appearance is characteristic. There is no evidence of atherosclerosis elsewhere. The patients are young (with an average age of 35 years) and frequently have an audible murmur over the upper abdomen and flank.

Many operations have been utilized because of the extent and variety of pathology encountered. The difficulties for the surgeon arise because the disease usually extends to the bifurcation of the renal artery. The maneuvers to expose the distal renal artery at the hilum of the kidney are illustrated in Fig. 51. Access to the distal portion of the left renal artery seldom requires reflection of the colon because the inferior mesenteric vein can always be divided and the mesocolon can be divided a considerable distance without encountering the arterial supply to the colon (Fig. 51, A). Access to the distal right renal artery frequently requires reflection of the hepatic flexure of the colon and the duodenum and head of the pancreas.

The natural history of the disease is unknown, but because the patients are young and the arteries are small, autogenous vein or artery is the preferred graft material. Vein bypass from the aorta to the renal artery resembles the technique described earlier for prosthesis except the anastomosis may be at the hilum of the kidney. The splenic artery can be readily divided distally and anastomosed to the left renal artery without sacrifice of the spleen (Fig. 49, B). The body and tail of the pancreas are elevated anteriorly to gain access to the splenic artery without mobilizing the spleen or sacrificing it.

When accessory renal arteries are involved, partial nephrectomy or, in other inoperable situations, total nephrectomy is regrettable but necessary. In occa-

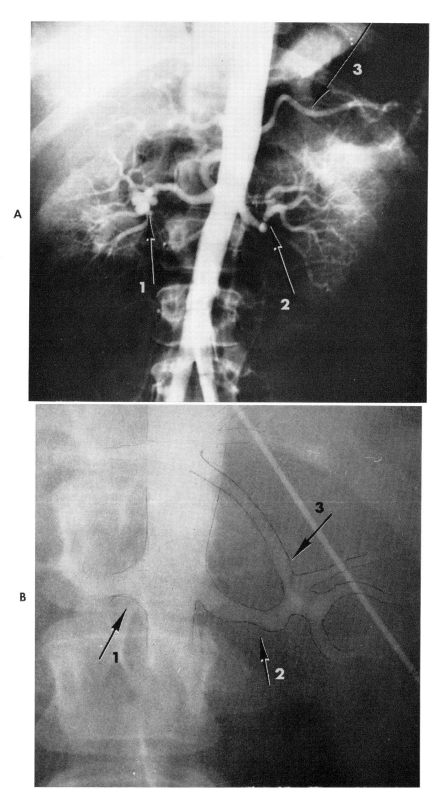

Fig. 49. Renal arteriograms in fibromuscular dysplasia. **A,** Preoperative film: **1,** multiple aneurysms in right renal artery; **2,** stenosis in left renal artery; **3,** splenic artery. **B,** Postoperative splenorenal arterial anastomosis: **1,** right renal artery; **2,** left renal artery; **3,** splenorenal anastomosis.

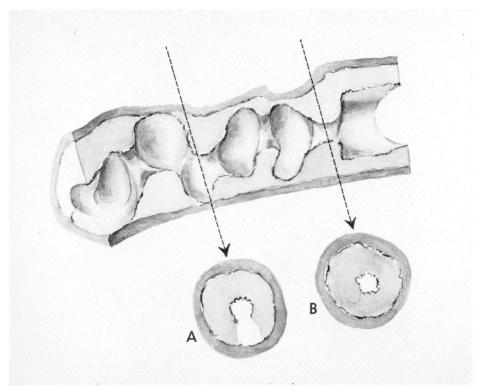

Fig. 50. Fibromuscular stenosis of renal artery with multiple microaneurysms (cross section **A**) and intervening fibromuscular thickenings with narrowings of lumen (cross section **B**). (Redrawn from Bernatz, Philip E.: Arch. Surg. **85:**608-616, 1962.)

sional patients suspension of the kidney (nephropexy) to straighten the course of the renal artery is said to relieve the pressure gradient. In one patient we widened the lumen of two stenotic primary branches of the renal artery with a vein patch in the shape of a Y whose base extended onto the main renal artery.

Extended approach to distal renal arteries by anterior approach

The anterior midline transperitoneal approach is preferable to the flank approach. The anterior approach gives access to the aorta for bypass grafting or to the other renal artery for bilateral lesions.

Reflection of the colon is illustrated but is seldom needed to expose the full length of the left renal artery. The proximal part of the left renal artery and vein are uncovered alongside the aorta as described on p. 169 and illustrated in Fig. 51. The inferior mesenteric vein is divided with impunity, and the medial part of the mesentery of the splenic flexure covers the hilum of the kidney. The mesentery is avascular between the left colic and middle colic arteries for at least several inches. The incision in the mesentery can be extended along the inferior border of the pancreas.

Reflection of the splenic flexure and descending colon gives access to the kidney for inspection and biopsy, as well as full exposure of the distal renal vessels. It also facilitates splenorenal arterial anastomosis.

1. The long midline incision has been made, and usually the proximal part of the renal artery and abdominal aorta are exposed as described on p. 169.

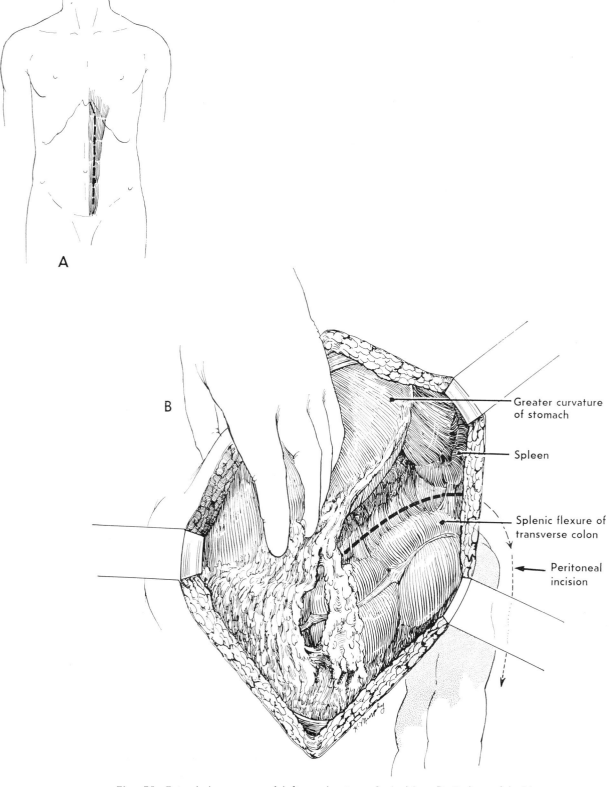

Fig. 51. Extended exposure of left renal artery. **A,** Incision. **B,** Peritoneal incision to uncover left kidney.

Greater curvature of stomach

Spleen

Splenic flexure of transverse colon

Peritoneal incision

A

B

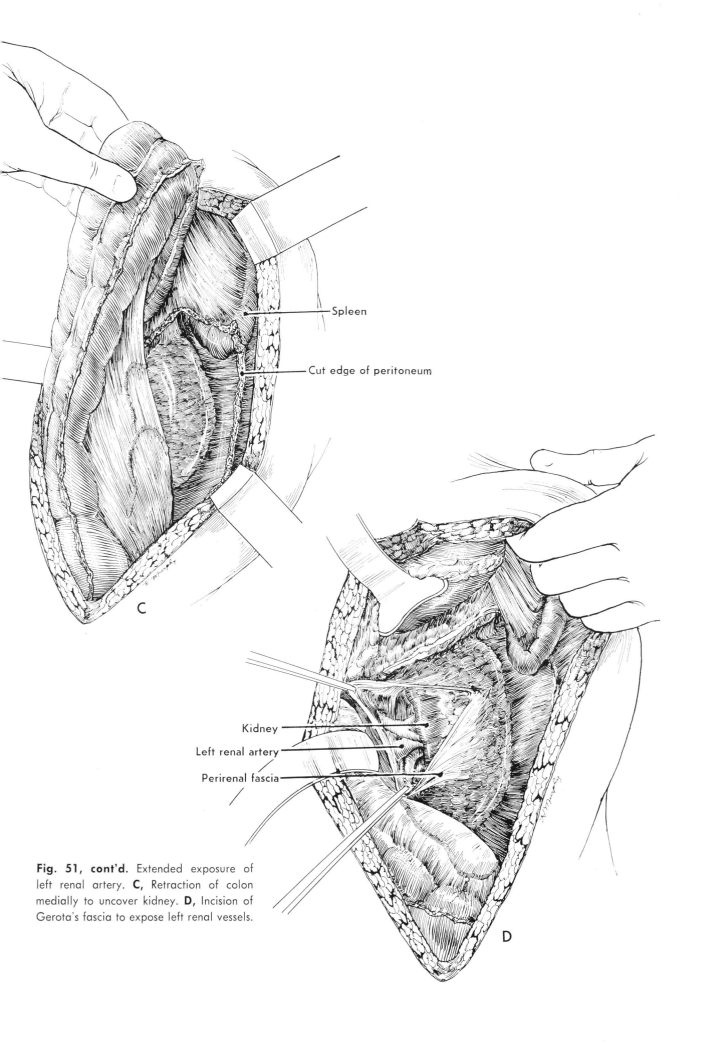

Spleen

Cut edge of peritoneum

C

Kidney

Left renal artery

Perirenal fascia

D

Fig. 51, cont'd. Extended exposure of
left renal artery. **C,** Retraction of colon
medially to uncover kidney. **D,** Incision of
Gerota's fascia to expose left renal vessels.

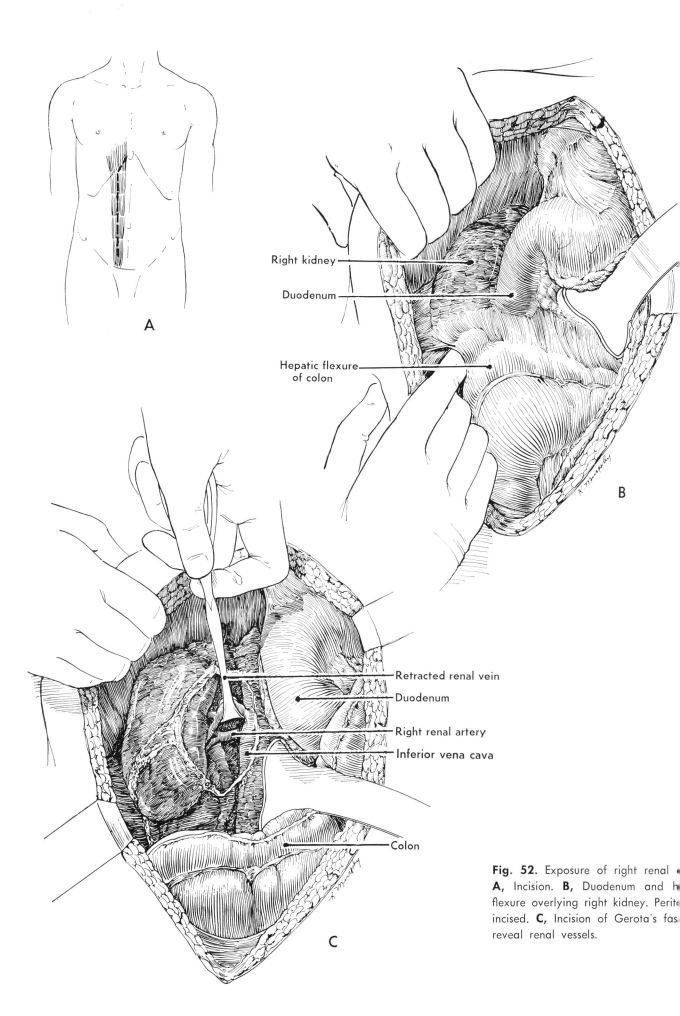

Right kidney

Duodenum

Hepatic flexure
of colon

A

B

Retracted renal vein

Duodenum

Right renal artery

Inferior vena cava

Colon

C

Fig. 52. Exposure of right renal
A, Incision. **B,** Duodenum and h
flexure overlying right kidney. Perit
incised. **C,** Incision of Gerota's fas
reveal renal vessels.

2. Incise the posterior parietal peritoneum in the left gutter. It may be necessary to continue this up and medially to reflect the splenic flexure.

3. Uncover the kidney by retracting the splenic flexure and descending colon anteriorly and to the right (Fig. 51, *B*). Identify the ureter and renal pelvis.

4. Incise Gerota's fascia to expose the kidney and its hilum (Fig. 51, *C* and *D*).

5. If the aorta has not already been uncovered by the midline approach, it is easily accessible by further mobilization of the mesocolon. The inferior mesenteric vein may be divided if it is in the way, or the surgeon may lift it anteriorly and tunnel beneath it to the origin of the renal artery from the aorta.

Extended anterior approach to distal right renal artery and kidney

1. Make a long right paramedian or midline incision (Fig. 52, *A*).

2. Divide the avascular attachment of the hepatic flexure of the colon (Fig. 52, *B*) and retract it downward.

3. Mobilize the duodenum and head of the pancreas medially after incising the peritoneum to the right of the second portion of the duodenum (Kocher maneuver).

4. Dissect free the lateral (right) border of the inferior vena cava and the right renal vein. The right renal vein lies over the renal artery and is shown retracted in Fig. 52, *C*. The proximal right renal artery is accessible between the inferior vena cava and the aorta.

5. Access to the distal aorta for a bypass may be obtained by tunneling under the mesentery of the small bowel and uncovering the distal aorta as illustrated in Fig. 11 and described on pp. 36-38.

Chapter 11

Cerebral arterial insufficiency

Introduction

Cerebral symptoms from localized occlusive lesions of the innominate, common carotid, internal carotid, subclavian, or vertebral arteries can usually be corrected. Most often the underlying disease is atherosclerosis, either at the origins of the great vessels from the aortic arch or distally in the neck. The more common sites of atherosclerotic disease are illustrated in Fig. 53. The best surgical results are obtained in patients with intermittent symptoms, partial occlusions, and no persistent neurological defect.

Medical success in treating hypertension has brought about a marked decrease in hemorrhagic stroke and a corresponding increase in the number of "strokes" that are due to occlusive vascular disease and/or thrombosis. Currently, the stroke victim usually must be regarded as nonhemorrhagic and a possible candidate for surgery. We can give no exact figure for the time during which hemiparesis can be successfully reversed by surgical means and, in addition, cannot predict which patients with strokes from occlusive disease will recover without surgery. However, when patients are seen within the first twenty-four hours, we believe surgical treatment should be considered after an arteriographic survey.

Signs and symptoms

Signs and symptoms are variable, and the correlation of symptoms and specific arteriographic findings has proved most difficult. At one end of this spectrum are the patients in whom major cerebral arterial occlusion, even of several major arteries, produces a minimum of symptoms, and at the other end are the more numerous patients who cannot tolerate major arterial occlusion without significant neurological damage.

It is difficult sometimes to associate specific occlusion with specific symptoms. Any neurological sign may result from generally deficient cerebral blood flow, and any arterial obstruction must be relieved surgically if possible to restore cerebral blood flow, prevent strokes, and relieve ischemic attacks.

With internal carotid artery occlusion the classical picture of homolateral visual disturbance and contralateral sensory and motor disturbance is rather

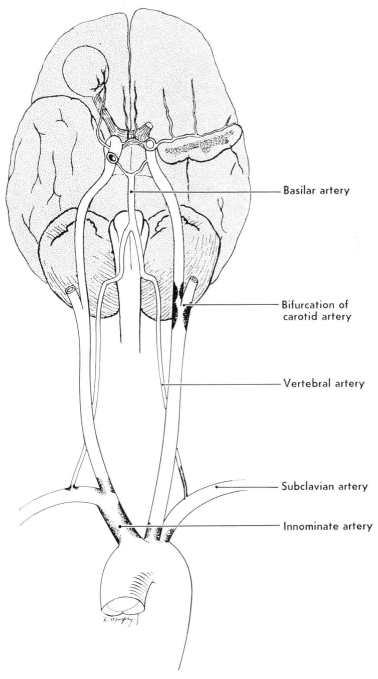

Basilar artery

Bifurcation of
carotid artery

Vertebral artery

Subclavian artery

Innominate artery

Fig. 53. Usual sites of extracranial occlusive disease affecting cerebral circulation.

rare. When atherosclerosis affects the origins of the vertebral arteries, the "basilar artery syndrome" may be produced—cortical visual loss, cerebellar and cranial nerve symptoms, and bilateral motor and sensory symptoms. As a rule, interference with the circulation from both vertebral arteries is necessary to produce this picture, provided that there is no disease in the intracranial portion of the vertebral arteries or the basilar artery itself. If arteriography shows one vertebral artery to be normal, visualization of the opposite vessel is probably not necessary.

Arterial insufficiency involving the aortic arch or the carotid vessels produces recurrent hemiplegia, aphasia, paresthesias, syncope, and visual disturbances that may be unilateral or bilateral. When the aortic arch is involved, decreased pulses and decreased blood pressures in the arms may be noted. Claudication in the arm is rare. Systolic murmurs referable to the areas of narrowing may be audible. Pressure on the opposite carotid artery usually produces syncope. Palpation of the internal carotid pulse in the tonsillar fossa is unreliable.

Arteriograms are essential to demonstrate extracranial occlusions and offer the best estimate of the degree of obstruction. A 20 mm. Hg pressure gradient across the stenotic area is clinically significant, and such a significant fall in the pressure gradient may be predicted if there is a 50% reduction in the arterial lumen as seen on the preoperative arteriogram. The method of arteriographic survey by right transbrachial-cerebral combined with left carotid arteriography is described in detail in Chapter 2.

The pathological causes of extracranial occlusions or narrowing are usually atheromatous plaques at the major bifurcations. Tortuosity of the internal carotid artery may cause symptoms by kinking. Vertebral occlusions may result from external pressure by osteophytic spurs, constricting bands, etc. Compression of the opposite carotid artery usually causes prompt slowing of the waves on the electroencephalogram. Compression can be released before untoward symptoms or alarming attacks develop. These tests and complete neurological work-up are essential. A coincidental brain tumor was found in several of our patients with extracranial arterial occlusion.

Subclavian steal syndrome

In special instances, attacks of basilar artery insufficiency are induced by exercise of the arm. In these patients, occlusion of the subclavian artery, or, on the right, the subclavian and/or innominate artery may be found. Exercise involving the arm on the affected side causes retrograde flow in the vertebral artery on that side, inducing the cerebral symptoms. The simplest solution, if the innominate artery is not involved, is ipsilateral common carotid–subclavian arterial shunt using a Dacron prosthesis. (See Fig. 54, D.)

Reconstructive procedures and choice of operation

The best results from arterial vascular reconstruction of the extracranial portions of the cerebral circulation are obtained in patients with intermittent neurological signs and symptoms and no residual neurological damage. Surgical attempts to restore flow should not, however, be denied to patients with recent and progressing stroke due to occlusive vascular disease. The results of a current cooperative clinical study may clarify indications or contraindications in patients with progressing or completed strokes.

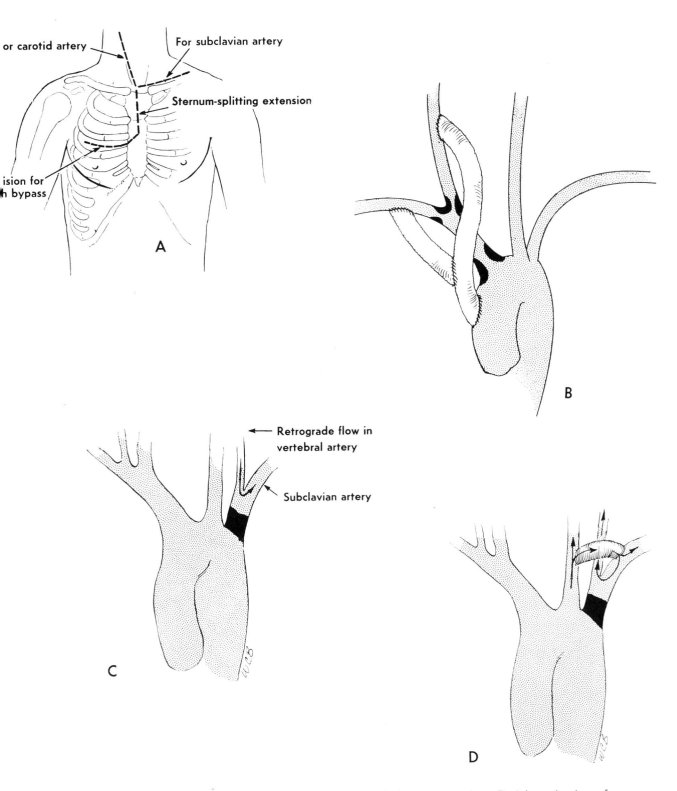

Fig. 54. A, Incisions for various types of arch bypass operations. **B,** Schematic view of arch bypass procedure. **C,** Subclavian steal syndrome. Retrograde flow of blood from subclavian artery occlusion. **D,** Carotid-subclavian artery bypass for subclavian steal.

183

The surgical procedures currently in use are endarterectomy, patch angioplasty, and bypass grafting. The bypass method is most applicable when obstruction involves the origins of the great vessels at the aortic arch, whereas endarterectomy is more applicable to the common and internal carotid arteries. The preferred procedure for localized plaque at the origin of the internal carotid artery is localized endarterectomy with patch angioplasty.

Narrowing at the origins of the vertebral arteries may be treated by endarterectomy of the subclavian and patch angioplasty at the origin of the vertebral arteries.

Operations for tortuosity, external compression, etc. are improvised according to the situation encountered. Symptoms referable to tortuosity may be relieved by nothing more than surgical mobilization. In some patients the internal carotid artery may be detached and reimplanted at a lower level.

It has been widely held that a completely occluded internal carotid artery is inoperable. This is frequently true. However, we believe that recent occlusions with definite contralateral symptoms should be explored. Particularly when embolism may be the cause of the occlusion, we have employed the Fogarty balloon catheter, passing it distally as far as the carotid siphon. By this method, otherwise inaccessible clots can be extracted. In some instances excellent back bleeding from the distal internal carotid artery has been obtained.

Special measures to support the cerebral circulation are not necessary during short periods of carotid artery occlusion, particularly with general anesthesia. The anesthetist should maintain blood pressure and ensure adequate oxygenation. An internal shunt allows longer periods of occlusion with safety (Fig. 58), and clamps and plastic tubing suitable for shunting are always included in the surgical setup.

OPERATIONS FOR OCCLUSIVE DISEASE OF AORTIC ARCH AND ITS BRANCHES
Signs, symptoms, and indications

Various bypass procedures are useful when occlusive disease involves the aortic arch and the origins of the major branches to the head and arms. Occlusion may be complete or incomplete, and multiple sites of involvement are frequent. A nonspecific arteritis (Tokayasu's disease, pulseless disease) occurs in young women, with obliteration of the subclavian or innominate arteries or both. Otherwise the etiology of obstructive lesions is usually atherosclerosis. Signs and symptoms referable to interference with blood supply to the brain are reviewed on p. 180. Corrective surgery is contraindicated in patients who are poor risks for major surgical procedures that include thoracotomy.

In some patients, however, bypass from carotid artery to carotid artery or from subclavian artery to carotid artery may be accomplished in the neck without resection of the clavicle and without entering the chest. Fig. 54, C and D, illustrates such a procedure for correction of the subclavian steal syndrome.

Choice of operation

Endarterectomy should be employed only for very localized and readily accessible plaques. The bypass procedures described may usually be accomplished without splitting the sternum, and the small right anterior thoracotomy is well

184

tolerated. In general, endarterectomy in the branches close to the aortic arch is more difficult, requires wider exposure, and carries a higher mortality rate than the bypass procedures. Endarterectomy of vessels with obliterative panarteritis should not be attempted. The general plan of all arch bypass procedures is much the same. The proximal end of the prosthesis is sutured to the side of the ascending aorta and is brought through a tunnel formed by blunt dissection beneath the sternum and anterior to the great veins. The distal anastomosis in the neck past the occlusions may require anastomosis to one or both carotid arteries, to the subclavian artery, or to some combination. (See Fig. 54, B.)

Preoperative preparation

Satisfactory arteriograms are necessary. Neurological consultation and medical evaluation of the cardiopulmonary status are very helpful. Preoperative digitalization is advisable.

Anesthesia

Since the chest will be opened, general endotracheal anesthesia must be employed. Blood pressure and adequate oxygenation must be maintained to ensure adequate cerebral blood flow during the short peroid of occlusion.

Choice of incision

The ascending aorta is exposed through an incision in the right third intercostal space (Fig. 55, A). The subclavian arteries are exposed through supraclavicular incisions, rarely aided by subperiosteal resection of the clavicle. A vertical incision along the anterior border of the sternocleidomastoid muscle offers ready access to the carotid artery (Fig. 55, A). At times a larger transverse cervical incision or a combination incision may be necessary. Exposure of the vertebral artery is discussed on pp. 196-198.

Procedure

Exposure of ascending aorta

1. Make an incision in the right third intercostal space extending from the lateral border of the sternum laterally to the anterior axillary line (Fig. 55, A). Split the pectoralis major muscle. Divide the cartilages of the third and fourth ribs. Splitting the sternum is not necessary. Tilt the table to the patient's left, and enlarge the incision with the aid of a rib spreader (Fig. 55, B).

2. Retract the apex of the lung inferiorly.

3. Identify the superior vena cava and the phrenic nerve nearby beneath the parietal pleura.

4. Incise the pleura anterior to the superior vena cava, and clean the subpleural fatty tissue from the underlying pericardium.

5. Incise the pericardium longitudinally over the ascending aorta, and retract the cut edges of the pericardium with sutures (Fig. 55, B).

6. Identify the right lateral edge of the innominate artery arising from the aorta.

Selection and suture of prosthesis

Bifurcation prostheses used in the abdomen are too large and might compress the great veins in the upper mediastinum. Any type of bypass prosthe-

185

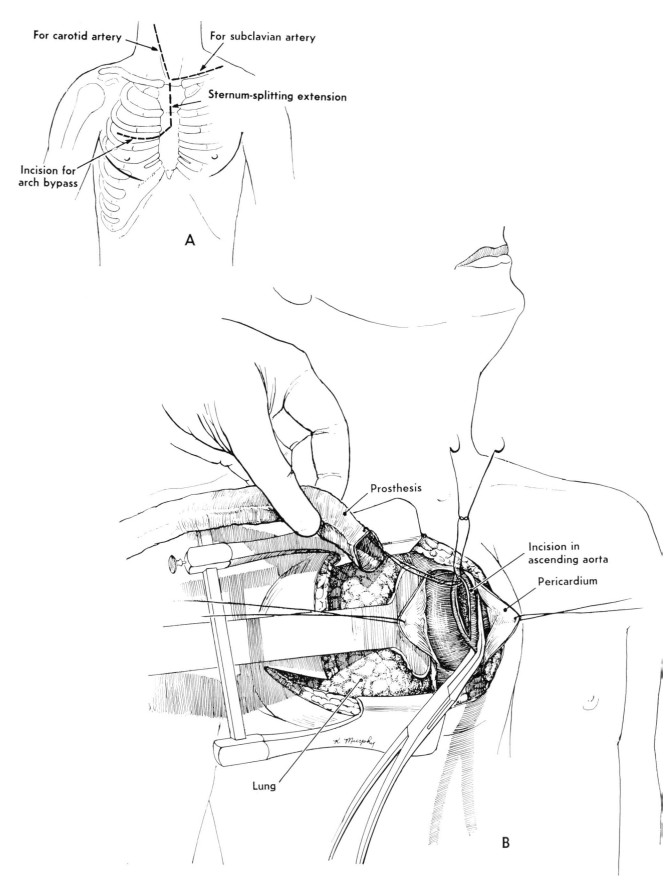

Fig. 55. Arch bypass. **A,** Incisions. **B,** Exposure of ascending aorta for proximal anastomosis of arch bypass.

sis can be fashioned from knitted Dacron tubes. The Y prosthesis is made by suturing a 12 mm. tube to a 10 mm. tube to form the necessary Y with an appropriate angle and shape. The fine-knitted prosthesis is preclotted with blood drawn from the superior vena cava or the surgical field.

Aortic anastomosis

1. Select a tangential occlusion clamp for the aorta. The jaw must be long enough to isolate a sufficient length, wide enough to hold the pulsating aorta securely, and deep enough to provide edges to attach the graft (Fig. 55, B).

2. Apply the clamp to the anterolateral surface of the ascending aorta, just proximal to the innominate artery. The back edge of the clamp must be readily accessible, and there must be an ample edge for anastomosis.

3. Incise the aorta with a scalpel, and complete the aortotomy with Potts angled scissors. The aortic wall is 2 to 3 mm. thick.

4. Cut the 12 mm. stem of the Y graft obliquely at the correct length (Fig. 54, B).

5. Begin the anastomosis with a mattress suture placed at the superior end of the aortotomy, using 3-0 arterial Dacron suture material with a needle at both ends (Fig. 55, B).

6. Start the posterior row with a very snug over-and-over continuous suture, sewing from prosthesis to aorta and placing the needle 2 to 3 mm. from the edge of the aortotomy.

7. Continue the posterior row of sutures around the inferior end of the aortotomy, and carry it superiorly along the anterior side of the anastomosis.

8. Complete the anterior row of sutures in the middle, joining the suture lines begun both inferiorly and superiorly.

9. Loosen the clamp *slightly* to preclot the prosthesis again, this time under pressure. Tighten the clamp immediately, and empty the prosthesis of any clotted blood.

Cervical incision and exploration of outflow tract

Make the appropriate neck incision to expose the carotid and subclavian arteries distal to the occlusion.

Substernal tunnel

Use the tip of a finger to bluntly dissect between the great veins and the sternum. Pass the fingers both from below upward and from above downward. Draw the prosthesis through the tunnel without twists or kinks.

Distal anastomosis

Appropriate arterial clamps with jaws and handles of a convenient size and shape should be on hand, and every possible detail should be prepared in advance to minimize carotid occlusion time. The principles and technique of end-to-side anastomosis are identical to those described in detail for bypass grafting of the abdominal aorta, with insertion of the distal limb of the prosthesis into the side of the iliac artery (p. 75). Occlusion time for the cerebral circulation should not exceed ten to fifteen minutes.

Restoration of circulation

Check for back bleeding and expel air and clots before completing the distal anastomosis.

Closure

1. Employ an anterior chest tube attached to water-seal drainage.
2. Close the intercostal incision with pericostal sutures of No. 1 chromic catgut.
3. Close the cervical incision without drainage.

Postoperative care

No anticoagulants are used. Digitalis is continued. The chest tube is removed when the lung has reexpanded and oscillations have ceased, usually one or two days postoperatively.

CAROTID ENDARTERECTOMY
Indications, signs, and symptoms

Carotid endarterectomy may be employed to remove atherosclerotic plaques at the carotid bifurcation and thereby restore normal pulsatile blood flow in the internal carotid artery, relieve cerebral arterial insufficiency, and prevent internal carotid artery thrombosis. The usual indication is localized stenosis at the carotid bifurcation, producing a narrowing of 50% or more in one arteriographic view. The signs and symptoms are discussed at greater length on p. 180 and in general comprise intermittent motor weakness, paresthesia, aphasia, and visual disturbance. Arteriographic visualization of the cerebral circulation is best accomplished by right transbrachial-cerebral arteriograms combined with arteriography of the left common carotid artery. It must be demonstrated that the partial stenosis is symptomatic and that the atherosclerotic block is extracranial. Neurological consultation is helpful and has revealed coincidental tumors. Carotid compression during electroencephalography is a safe and significant test of flow through the opposite carotid and cross cerebral collateral adequacy. When compression of a normal carotid artery causes slowing of the alpha waves in the electroencephalogram, it signifies significant obstruction of the cerebral flow from the opposite side.

Occasionally, a complete unilateral carotid occlusion will be found without significant neurological defect. Operation should not be advised if there is generalized cerebral arteriosclerosis or if complete occlusion of the internal carotid artery has been present for more than one week.

Anticoagulant treatment has been used by some in preference to surgery. However, anticoagulants do not remove the obstruction and frequently fail to relieve the symptoms. Patients with intracerebral occlusions or thromboses may benefit from anticoagulant therapy.

Anesthesia

Careful light general anesthesia is preferred to maintain blood pressure and consequent cerebral blood flow across areas of "critical stenosis" (p. 14). Based upon measurements of oxygen saturation studies in the jugular sinuses, the suggestion has recently been offered that the addition of carbon dioxide to the

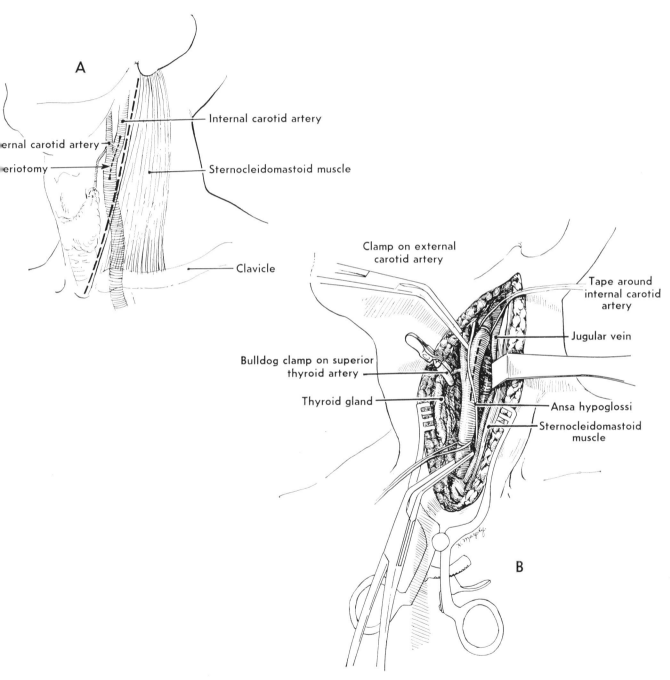

A

Internal carotid artery

ernal carotid artery

eriotomy

Sternocleidomastoid muscle

Clavicle

Clamp on external
carotid artery

Tape around
internal carotid
artery

Jugular vein

Bulldog clamp on superior
thyroid artery

Thyroid gland

Ansa hypoglossi

Sternocleidomastoid
muscle

B

Fig. 56. Carotid endarterectomy with patch angioplasty. **A,** Incision. **B,** Exposure of carotid bifurcation.

anesthetic mixture will result in additional cerebral vasodilation and total blood flow. At this time, we prefer routine internal shunting. This step takes only a few minutes and allows unhurried meticulous surgery, long arteriotomy, and patch angioplastic closure. Improved catheters, techniques, and special clamps have simplified the shunt procedure (Fig. 58).

Procedure

Place the patient in the supine position, turning his head slightly away from the side to be operated upon. Avoid hyperextension of the head and neck if there is associated basilar artery insufficiency.

Exposure

1. Incise the skin along the anterior border of the sternocleidomastoid muscle (Fig. 56, A). In short necks, carry the incision to the mastoid process.

2. Retract the sternomastoid muscle and the external jugular vein laterally. Divide the anterior facial vein and the cervical fascia.

3. Open the sheath of the common carotid artery near the bulb. Infiltrate the tissue near the bifurcation with local anesthetic.

4. Expose the front of the common carotid artery for about 2 cm. below the bifurcation. Employ careful perivascular dissection and separate the artery from the internal jugular vein and vagus nerve. Pass a tape around the carotid artery below the plaque area. Divide or retract the ansa hypoglossi.

5. Expose the internal carotid artery up to the parotid gland. Expose several centimeters of the external carotid artery as well. Ligate or occlude with a bulldog clamp the superior thyroid artery. Identify the hypoglossal nerve. Pass a tape about the internal carotid artery (Fig. 56, B).

Comment: *The amount of exposure necessary varies according to the length of the atherosclerotic plaque. It is not necessary to free the entire artery except where clamps will be applied. If the plaques are long, the hypoglossal nerve must be retracted upward.*

Preparation of Dacron prosthesis patch

1. Cut a strip of knitted Dacron prosthesis, preferably flat material, about 5 to 10 mm. in width and several centimeters longer than the intended arteriotomy.

2. Tag the lower end with a 2-0 black silk suture, and round the corners of the opposite (upper) end.

3. Place a double-needle 4-0 arterial suture through the upper tip of the patch.

4. Preclot the patch with a small amount of blood drawn from the jugular vein or present in the wound.

Arteriotomy and insertion of internal shunt

1. Inject 50 mg. of heparin in 1 ml. of saline solution into the common carotid artery, and immediately clamp the common and external carotid arteries.

Comment: *The DeBakey angled clamps are ideal for this purpose, since the handles lie flat and out of the way of the operator.*

190

2. Incise the anterolateral aspect of the internal carotid and the common carotid arteries for the full length of the plaque to be removed and an additional 5 mm. The incision normally divides the plaque close to its edge. Check for back bleeding from the internal carotid artery.

Comment: *If there is no back bleeding, endarterectomy alone will probably be ineffective and the distal portion of the internal carotid artery should be explored with a small Fogarty balloon catheter.*

3. Insert the internal shunt as diagramed in Fig. 57, A, and secure it in place with Javid clamps. If these special clamps are not available, loops of umbilical tape secured by a short length of plastic tubing and a hemostat may be improvised.

Comment: *For internal shunts, cut a piece of the tapered U510 Travenol hemodialysis catheter with the correct diameter at the upper end so that it fits the internal carotid easily. Other soft, thin-walled polyvinyl tubing, 10-14 F. in diameter, can also be used. Prior to its insertion, tie a stout suture at the upper end of the internal shunt for use in its removal later.*

4. Restore flow to the internal carotid artery via the shunt by removal of occluding clamps on the carotid arteries.

Endarterectomy

1. Develop a plane of cleavage between the plaque and the media of the artery. Tease the plaque away from the arterial wall, and dissect with a Freer elevator. The circular muscular fibers of the arterial media appear beneath the plaque as it is removed.

2. Free the plaque until it is attached superiorly by thin, normal intima. Lengthen the arteriotomy if necessary. With blood flowing through the internal shunt, there is no hurry and thickened intima superiorly almost always can be removed. It is almost never necessary to leave loose thick intima which formerly needed to be reattached and held in place with sutures.

3. Free the plaque inferiorly down into the carotid bulb, and tease it out of the orifice of the external carotid artery. One can readily work around the internal shunt.

Comment: *The arteriotomy can be lengthened superiorly, but it is never necessary to extend it more than 1-2 cm. inferiorly. A small strip of thickened intima is safely left proximally in the common carotid artery.*

4. Irrigate the lining of the artery with heparinized saline solution and inspect it carefully to wash out debris or tease out fragments still attached.

Closure of arteriotomy by patch angioplasty

The internal shunt has restored cerebral blood flow during meticulous endarterectomy and closure. We use this patch angioplasty for secure closure of all arteriotomies of the internal carotid or other arteries this size. Secure closure requires a large bite of the arterial wall, including adventitia 1 to 2 mm. from the edge of the arteriotomy. This may appear crude externally, but when the suture is pulled snug, the inside is very smooth. The wide cuff necessary for a secure closure narrows the internal carotid lumen unless a patch is interposed between the edges of the arteriotomy.

1. Irrigate and remove all debris and clots from the arterial lumen.

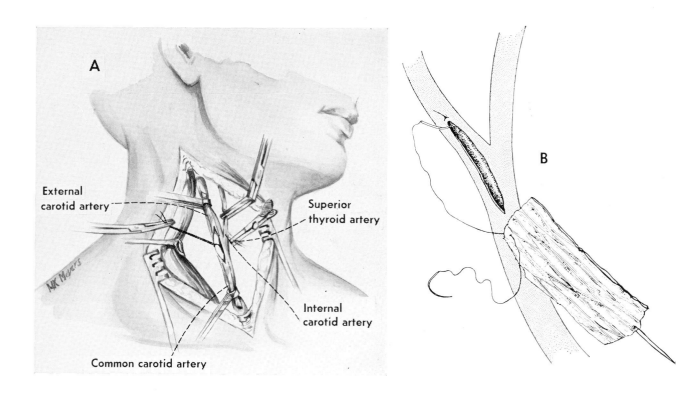

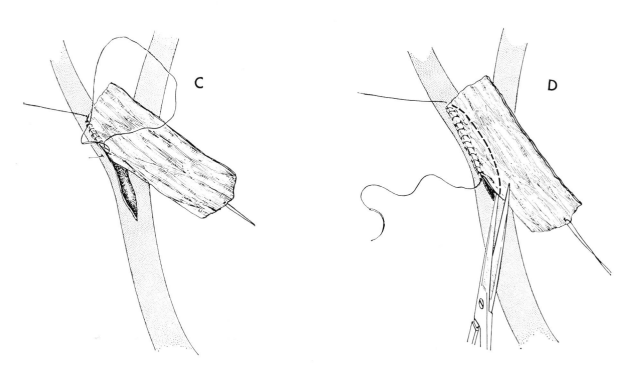

Fig. 57. Closure of endarterectomy with prosthetic patch (patch angioplasty). **A,** Operative exposure for carotid endarterectomy showing arteriotomy of internal and common carotid arteries. **B,** First suture. **C,** Posterior row of sutures. **D,** Trim patch to size and shape. (**A,** From Polin, S. G., and Hershey, F. B.: Amer. J. Surg. **111:**296-297, 1966.)

2. For the first stitch, pass one of the needles out of the superior end of the arteriotomy, and secure by tying with a square knot to hold the apex of the patch in place (Fig. 57, B). The schematic drawings of the patch angioplasty do not show the internal shunt tube in place.

3. Sew the patch to the posterior edge of the arteriotomy, proceeding from above downward with an over-and-over stitch passing from the prosthesis to the artery (Fig. 57, C). The assistant must hold the suture taut so as to pull up the edges for ready access and rapid placement of the sutures. The second assistant pulls the inferior edge of the patch downward with the previously attached silk suture, holding it steady and in place.

4. Trim the patch to correct size and shape as the posterior suture line is completed (Fig. 57, D).

5. Begin the anterior closure by continuing the posterior row around the bottom of the patch, ascending on the anterior side of the arteriotomy, and then sewing downward from above with the other limb of the double-armed suture. Do not complete suturing of the inferior end of the anterior edge of the patch Leave an aperture for removal of the shunt.

Removal of internal shunt and completion of patch angioplasty

1. Suture the portion of the patch on the internal carotid artery, leaving an aperture inferiorly for removal of the internal shunt tube (Fig. 58, A). This aperture should be on the common carotid inferior part of the arteriotomy.

2. Loosen the clamps or tapes on the internal shunt and slide the shunt inferiorly in the artery by traction on the tie at the tip of the shunt (Fig. 58, A).*

3. With a small tangential occluding clamp in place (Fig. 58, B), draw the tip of the shunt out. It will spurt vigorously, so quickly pull it out of the artery and close the clamp (Fig. 58, C) close to the edge of the arteriotomy. Flow is now restored through the internal carotid artery, and the patch angioplasty can be completed (Fig. 58, C and D).

4. Complete the process of suturing the patch in place. Apply a pad of Gelfoam soaked in topical thrombin to the patch if it oozes or leaks at suture holes.

5. Tie the final suture, release the tangential clamp, and apply the Gelfoam sponge to the remainder of the Dacron patch for complete hemostasis.

Closure of incision

1. Suture the carotid sheath over the vessels and the patch.
2. Close the cervical fasciae, platysma, and skin in layers.
3. A drain is advisable in some patients.

Postoperative care

Anticoagulants are unnecessary unless the occlusion was embolic. A liquid diet during the first few days will prevent undue discomfort during swallowing.

Comment: *The internal shunt is simple, it conducts a large flow, it requires*

---

*This maneuver with the tie at the superior tip of the shunt was suggeested by Dr. Richard Lennahan.

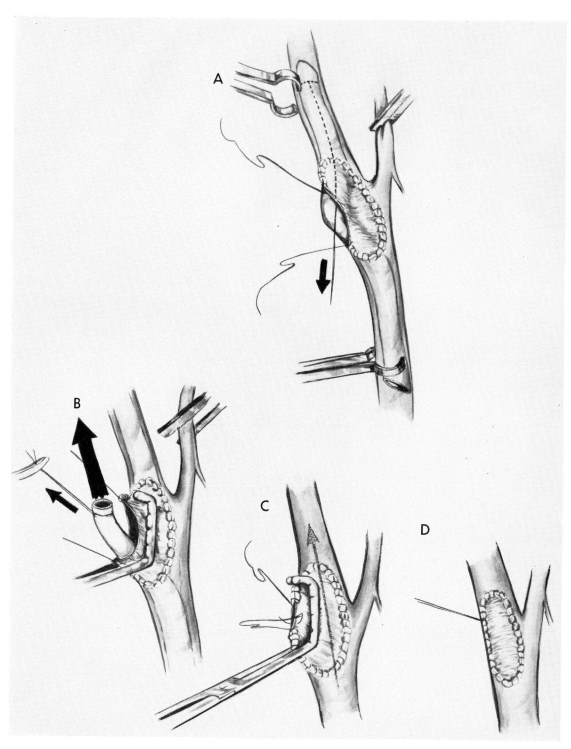

Fig. 58. Removal of internal shunt and completion of patch angioplasty. **A,** Withdrawal of internal shunt from internal carotid artery. **B,** Withdrawal of internal shunt from common carotid artery. **C,** Flow restored through internal carotid artery during completion of patch angioplasty. **D,** Patch angioplasty completed. (From Polin, S. G., and Hershey, F. B.: Amer. J. Surg. **111:**296-297, 1966; **A** and **B** slightly modified.)

no additional needle punctures, etc. The internal shunt permits ample operating time for a long arteriotomy, complete endarterectomy, careful reattachment of the intima, and secure closure. It also permits safe operation on patients under general anesthesia.

VERTEBRAL ARTERY OCCLUSION
Diagnosis and indications

Vertebral arterial insufficiency usually gives rise to the symptoms of the basilar artery syndrome, that is, visual disturbance, cerebellar symptoms, and bilateral mixed cranial nerve and spinal nerve, motor, and sensory symptoms. The usual peripheral cause is atherosclerosis at the origin of the vertebral artery from the subclavian artery. Unilateral occlusion is seldom symptomatic, and repair of only one artery is an adequate surgical procedure. Other causes of occlusion are tortuosity and compression by osteophytic spurs. Diagnosis must be made by arteriograms. If intracranial occlusive disease is severe, extracranial surgical procedures will not be successful. Carotid insufficiency is frequently associated, and both lesions may be surgically treated at the same time through an appropriately designed or modified incision. Sometimes restoration of flow in the carotid arteries relieves basilar symptoms and operation on the vertebral artery is not always necessary or possible.

In the subclavian "steal" syndrome, the vertebral artery is open, and symptoms of basilar insufficiency are due to cerebrifugal or retrograde flow down the vertebral artery, which now supplies collateral circulation to the arm around an occluded subclavian artery (Fig. 54, *C* and *D*). Symptoms due to the subclavian steal may be more severe than those from occlusion. Occasionally, the same syndrome is due to occlusion of the innominate artery.

When carotid stenosis is associated with symptoms of basilar artery insufficiency, surgical relief of carotid stenosis may, at times, be all that is possible or necessary. Since any increase of cerebral circulation in the circle of Willis may relieve basilar symptoms, surgery correcting carotid occlusions is usually helpful.

In all patients a preoperative radiographic survey, including transbrachial-cerebral arteriography on the right and common carotid arteriography on the left, should be made.

Surgical approach

Usually the origin of the vertebral artery may be approached through an incision along the upper border of the clavicle. However, extended exposure or exposure in thick-necked persons may require splitting the upper part of the sternum in the midline and extension of the incision into the third intercostal space on the affected side. The vertebral artery is visualized during the approach to the stellate ganglion, which will be described as a portion of supraclavicular cervical sympathectomy (pp. 227-232). The origin of the vertebral artery and other branches of the first portion of the subclavian artery may be visualized by a continuation of this procedure and blunt dissection downward along the subclavian. To expose the vertebral artery, the deepest layer (prevertebral or prescalene layer) of the cervical fascia must be divided medial to the scalenus anticus muscle and the phrenic nerve. It is necessary to divide the anterior scalene muscle. The phrenic nerve, the recurrent laryngeal nerve, and the thoracic duct are contiguous structures that must be protected. Extended exposure of the vertebral artery is seldom necessary. Descriptions of the surgical approaches to the upper portions of the vertebral artery in its extracranial course can be found in other publications.

Choice of operative procedure

For localized plaques at the origin of the vertebral artery, local endarterectomy with or without patch angioplasty is the best treatment. No operative procedure is indicated for partial occlusion of only one vertebral artery, since the collateral supply to the basilar artery is excellent.

Anesthesia

Because the pleura may be inadvertently opened, general endotracheal anesthesia is advisable.

Procedure—vertebral endarterectomy

1. Place the patient in the supine position, the neck extended and slightly rotated away from the side to be operated upon.

2. Make either a supraclavicular or a cervicothoracic incision, whichever appears indicated (Fig. 59, A and B).

Exposure

For more details and drawings of the following steps, review pp. 228-232.

1. Divide the clavicular head of the sternocleidomastoid muscle if the cervical approach is employed. Divide the entire insertion of the sternocleidomastoid muscle if the cervicothoracic incision is employed.

2. Divide the omohyoid muscle.

3. Retract the prescalene fat pad laterally.

4. Retract the jugular vein and carotid artery medially.

5. Identify the phrenic nerve or nerves on the anterior surface of the anterior scalene muscle.

6. Divide the anterior scalene muscle. Retract the phrenic nerve medially. The prevertebral layer of deep cervical fascia is divided in the direction of the phrenic nerve and is retracted medially, holding this and the other structures in the carotid sheath medially.

7. Identify and spare the thoracic duct on the left. If the duct is injured, ligate it to avoid a troublesome lymph fistula.

8. Ligate and divide the thyrocervical trunk at its origin from the subclavian artery.

9. Dissect along the subclavian artery bluntly, using a finger or small dissecting sponge, until the innominate artery is reached on the right or the aortic arch on the left.

10. Divide the vertebral vein if necessary. Inferiorly, this lies anteriorly and laterally, but near the entrance of the vertebral artery into its foramen in the transverse process of the sixth cervical vertebra, the vertebral vein covers the artery.

11. Depress the pleura. It need not be freed laterally or anteriorly.

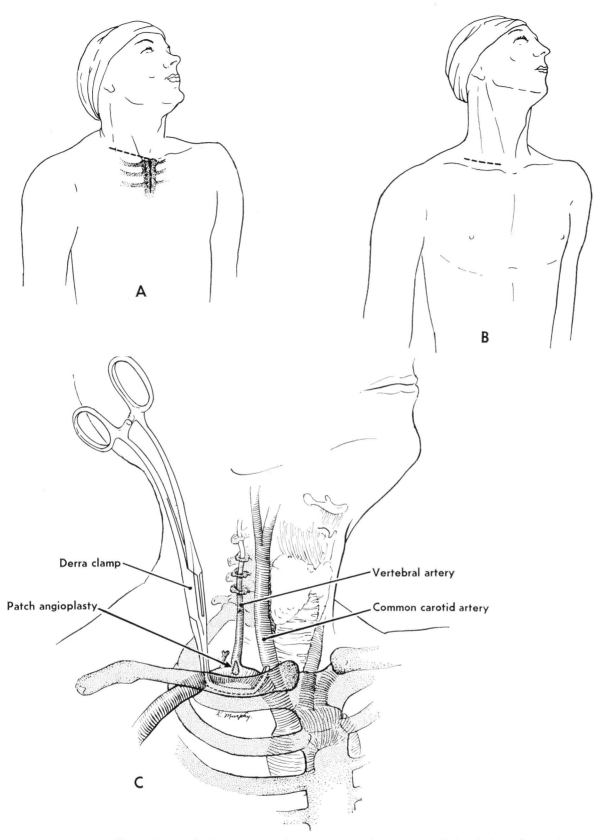

Fig. 59. Vertebral artery—patch angioplasty. **A,** Sternum-splitting incision for patients with thick necks or low origin of vertebral artery. **B,** Usual incision. **C,** Patch angioplasty completed.

Derra clamp

Patch angioplasty

Vertebral artery

Common carotid artery

A

B

C

197

Comment: *The internal mammary artery may be visualized anteriorly with the phrenic nerve close behind or anterior to it.*

Proximal and distal control

1. Select a single deeply curved partially occluding clamp. The Derra clamp is ideal. This will serve as a handle and permits traction upward on the subclavian artery, allowing ample room for the arteriotomy (Fig. 59, *C*).

2. Inject 30 mg. of heparin in 30 ml. of normal saline solution into the subclavian artery while the clamp is held in position ready to close.

3. Close the Derra clamp to obtain proximal and distal control of the subclavian artery as illustrated in Fig. 59, *C*.

4. Obtain distal control of the vertebral artery just proximal to the sixth cervical vertebra with a delicate clamp. Separate and ligate the fragile vein, if necessary.

Arteriotomy and endarterectomy

1. Make a vertical arteriotomy in the proximal vertebral artery, and extend it upward distal to the vertebral plaque and also into the subclavian artery.

2. Momentarily release the distal clamp to check for back bleeding.

3. Remove only a circumferential or ulcerated plaque. If endarterectomy proves unnecessary, only enlargement of the arterial lumen by patch closure (below) is done.

4. Suture the intima in the vertebral artery if it seems loose and might occlude the lumen.

5. Irrigate the area and flush out clots.

Patch closure of arteriotomy

The technique of patch angioplasty is described in detail and illustrated on pp. 191-193. Interposition of a triangular patch between the edges of the arteriotomy permits secure placement of sutures in the adventitia 1 to 2 mm. from the edge of the arteriotomy and enlarges the lumen of the vertebral artery. A prosthetic patch is essential because a vein patch may dilate in vessels of large diameter.

Closure of incision

Lungs and pleura are reexpanded with positive pressure and by aspiration. For details, see the closure following cervicothoracic sympathectomy, p. 232. Complete expansion of the lung is obtained by suction on an *extra*pleural catheter. If the sternum has been split, it is reapproximated with wire.

Chapter 12

Portal hypertension

Several procedures have been devised for the treatment of portal hypertension. Usually the portal vein or a large tributary such as the splenic vein is anastomosed to the inferior vena cava or the left renal vein. Anastomosis of the inferior vena cava to the superior mesenteric vein may also be accomplished.

The main purpose of the venous shunts is relief of pressure in esophageal varices and prevention of bleeding from esophageal varices. Ascites caused by hepatic outflow block may also be decreased by relieving the intrahepatic pressure. The shunt procedures do not improve liver function and, indeed, may impair it in some patients.

Portal hypertension in children is usually the consequence of thrombosis of the portal vein. The block is extrahepatic, the liver function is usually normal, and the surgical approaches are quite different.

PERCUTANEOUS SPLENOPORTAL VENOGRAPHY

Splenoportal venography is useful in the diagnosis of bleeding of the upper gastrointestinal tract and for choosing an operation to relieve portal hypertension. Rarely, the portal vein is occluded and splenorenal anastomosis is performed. If splenic pulp pressure is not elevated and venograms show no gastroesophageal collateral circulation, bleeding from esophageal varices is unlikely and at laparotomy a peptic ulcer or other cause for bleeding will be found. If there is portal cirrhosis, the venogram will show numerous collateral channels. In patients with obstruction of the extrahepatic portal vein, no contrast medium enters the portal vein and the abundant collateral circulation arising from the spleen or the splenic vein is the main feature of the splenoportogram. Fig. 60, *A*, depicts an early stage in the filling of the portal system, and Fig. 60, *B*, depicts the flow of contrast medium into collateral channels six seconds later. The splenic vein is large, and esophageal varices are seen. Portal systemic connections are diagramed in Fig. 60, *C*.

Splenic puncture is contraindicated in patients who have a bleeding tendency, thrombocytopenia, or prothrombin times of under 50%. After splenic puncture, slight intraperitoneal hemorrhage is common, but copious hemorrhage is rare. When portacaval shunt is contemplated, it is our custom to perform spleno-

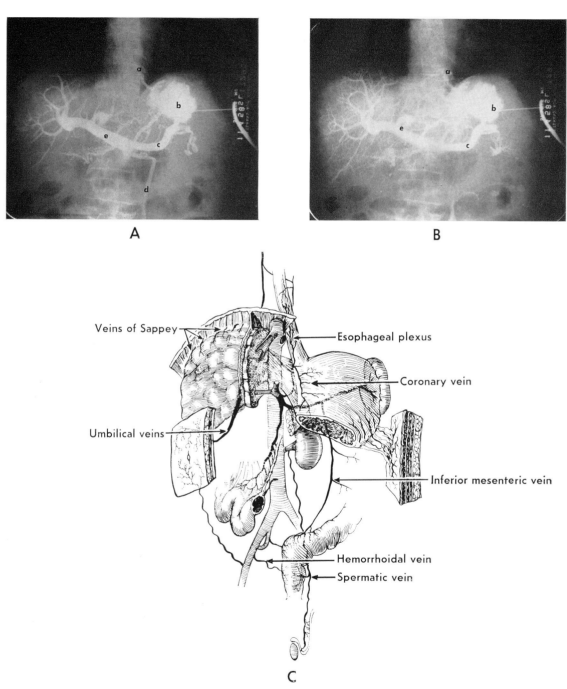

Fig. 60. Splenoportogram with early film, **A,** and late film, **B,** showing **a,** esophageal varices; **b,** deposit of media in splenic pulp; **c,** splenic vein; **d,** inferior mesenteric vein. **C,** Artist's drawing of portal-systemic connections.

200

portography on the morning of surgery. At exploration we have noted no unusual bleeding from the spleen. Splenoportography may be omitted provided the clinical diagnosis is certain.

Anesthesia

Adequate preoperative sedation and local anesthesia are best. If the patient is at all apprehensive or is to be operated upon at once, light general anesthesia is preferable.

Preparation

The large bowel is prepared by preliminary enemas and by the administration of 1 Gm. of neomycin every four hours for twenty-four hours. The patient should be tested with a small intravenous dose of contrast medium to determine the possibility of hypersensitivity. If local anesthesia is contemplated, premedication should include sodium phenobarbital.

Procedure

1. Place the patient in the supine position on the x-ray table. A sandbag under the left upper quadrant may be helpful in elevating the spleen (Fig. 61, A).

2. Prepare and drape the skin of the lower left lateral chest wall.

3. Insert a 6-inch No. 15 Rochester needle or similar Teflon catheter snugly fitted over a needle (this device consists of a flexible plastic cannula enclosing a long No. 18 needle) in the midaxillary line of the ninth or tenth intercostal space at about the level of the xiphoid, depending upon the size of the spleen and the depth of the costophrenic sinus (Fig. 61, B). A sensation of firmness will be discerned as the needle enters the splenic pulp. Direct the needle approximately in the direction of the umbilicus and somewhat backward.

4. Before plunging the needle farther into the spleen, instruct the patient to make a maximum expiratory effort and to hold his breath. If general anesthesia is employed, the anesthesiologist maintains an apneic state.

5. Advance the needle into the spleen. A slow flow of dark blood will drip from the needle. Withdraw the metal needle, leaving the flexible plastic sheath in the splenic pulp. The patient can then be permitted to breathe lightly.

6. Inject a trial dose of 5 to 10 ml. of Conray 600 and take a survey x-ray film to confirm the position of the needle.

7. Measure the splenic pulp pressure to confirm the diagnosis of portal hypertension: (a) First, inject 1 or 2 ml. of normal saline solution to flush the plastic tube. (b) Connect the spinal manometer, a three-way stopcock, and a syringe filled with saline solution. (c) Fill the manometer with saline solution and turn the stopcock to connect the manometer and spleen. If the patient has portal hypertension, the column of saline solution will not fall and the pressures will usually exceed 250 mm. of water. Normal pressures are usually 40 to 80 mm. of water. Three readings are taken while the scout film is being developed. The zero point for calculation of the portal pressure is the level of the right atrium, which is 10 cm. from the table.

8. Inspect the scout radiograph. If the needle is lodged correctly in the spleen, a small irregular radiopaque spot will be seen at the needle tip. Frequently the proximal part of the splenic vein may be seen faintly. If the tip is

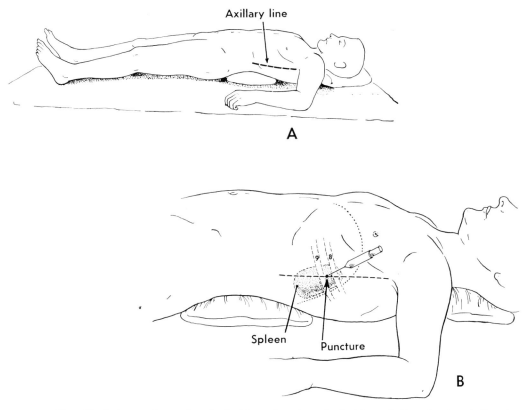

Fig. 61. Splenoportography. **A,** Position of patient. **B,** Position of skin wheal and direction of needle.

close to the capsule, a thin dense curved subcapsular line of radiopaque medium can be noted. If the needle is not in correct position, a repeat puncture with another needle may be made. Multiple punctures are not desirable. If the colon is punctured, discontinue the procedure to avoid contamination of a sub-diaphragmatic hematoma.

9. Connect a 50 ml. syringe filled with Conray 600 to the needle. Inject the contrast medium forcibly over a period of five or six seconds. Proportionately less contrast medium is used for children.

10. Take the first film at the end of the injection and withdraw the needle. The collateral veins and portal vein fill more slowly. Therefore, multiple films are necessary. The Sanchez-Perez cassette changer should be loaded to take six to eight exposures at the rate of one per second. Film cassettes may be changed by hand every few seconds if there is ample help and good teamwork.

Interpretation of splenoportograms

Various patterns of venous collateral circulation may be seen. In bleeding varices due to portal hypertension, the varices will always be seen, and abundant collateral circulation via the coronary and azygos veins will be apparent in the upper abdomen. These collateral pathways will be seen to fill before or at least simultaneously with the portal vein. This confirms the diagnosis. Visualization of large portal and splenic veins gives the surgeon a choice of operation.

Nonvisualization of the portal vein is rare but occasionally misleading. "Streaming artifacts" or "fading phenomena" in the opacification of the portal vein occur at the entrance of large tributaries, almost always the superior mesenteric vein. Complete thrombosis of the portal vein is rare. The ground-glass appearance of the vein on the films is sometimes due to delay and dilution of the dye in patients with severe portal hypertension in whom there is reduced blood flow into the liver. If at laparotomy the foramen of Winslow is open to the palpating finger, the portal vein is open or rare thrombi are small and non-occluding.

Portal venograms during laparotomy

Portal venograms can be made during laparotomy by injecting contrast medium through a small polyethylene catheter fastened into any accessible and sufficiently large vein that drains into the portal system. This is an extremely useful procedure if information is necessary at the time of operation or if the spleen has been previously removed. When splenectomy has been performed, portovenography is done through a small incision into which a loop of jejunum or the omentum is delivered for the procedure.

Complications

Complications of splenic puncture for x-ray visualization of the portal system include untoward amounts of bleeding from the spleen, infection in the subdiaphragmatic space, false puncture with extravasation of the contrast medium, pleuritis, referred pain in the left shoulder, and allergic response to the contrast medium. For the most part it should be possible to avoid these complications by observing adequate precautions, that is, administration of a test dose of contrast medium, careful aseptic technique, use of the Rochester or similar plastic needle, and avoidance of excessive motion and consequent laceration of the spleen following the puncture.

OPERATIONS FOR PORTAL HYPERTENSION

The end-to-side portacaval shunt may be the only operation feasible when the portal vein is very short (Fig. 62, A). The side-to-side shunt is now preferred (Fig. 62, B) by some surgeons.

The side-to-side shunt is chosen when the pressure on the hepatic end of the portal vein rises with temporary occlusion of the pancreatic side of the portal vein. After side-to-side shunts, the pressure in the liver and the hepatic end of the portal vein does not increase, as it may after the end-to-side shunt, in which the hepatic end of the portal vein is sutured shut. The hemodynamics in patients with cirrhosis of the liver with portal hypertension and esophageal varices is not completely understood, and the mechanisms of ascites in these patients likewise is complicated. When the ascites is due to outflow block in the cirrhotic liver, the hepatic decompression with the side-to-side portacaval shunt is helpful, but the presence of ascites without portal hypertension and esophageal varices is a contraindication to operation.

For emergency shunts the Valdoni midline approach is quickest and best (Fig. 62, C). Splenorenal shunts are usually possible. They decompress the liver like a small side-to-side portacaval shunt if the portal vein is open, but

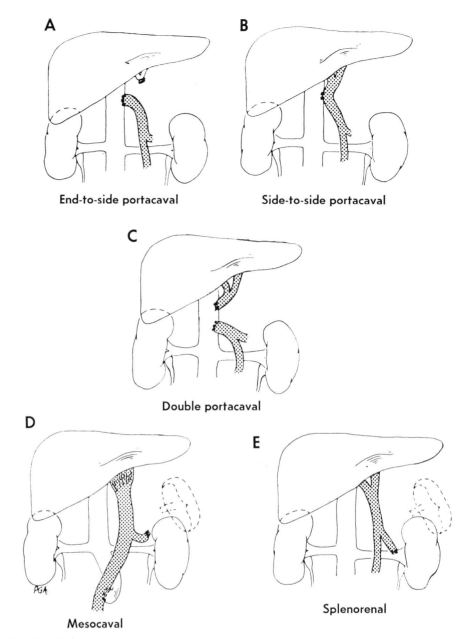

A End-to-side portacaval

B Side-to-side portacaval

C Double portacaval

D Mesocaval

E Splenorenal

Fig. 62. Common types of portal-systemic shunts. All types of portacaval anastomoses will decompress the collateral circulation and the esophageal varices, lessening the danger of fatal esophageal hemorrhage. Recently, various investigators have compared the merits of end-to-side versus side-to-side shunts. The arguments revolve about the problem of decompression of the hepatic outflow tract. If flow in the portal vein is toward the liver, then all agree that end-to-side shunt is best. The side-to-side anastomosis is advocated when there is hepatofugal flow in the portal system, because the side-to-side anastomosis decompresses the portal system on the hepatic side. An hepatic artery-portal-systemic shunt is thus preserved. The question arises whether such decompression benefits hepatic function, improves or reduces hepatic blood flow, or relieves ascites or whether it is better that such flow be directed into the hepatic veins by the end-to-side anastomosis. There is little data on the effect of these two shunts on liver function in human beings with disease. Our present policy is to use small (1.5 cm.) side-to-side shunts when portal pressure measurements indicate an hepatic outflow block. (From McDermott, William V., Jr.: Surgery of the liver and portal circulation. In Welch, Claude E., editor: Advances in surgery, vol. 1, Chicago, 1965, Year Book Medical Publishers, Inc.)

these splenorenal anastomoses are small and distal (Fig. 62, *D*). If the splenic vein is small or thrombosed or if there has been a previous splenectomy, a shunt of the proximal inferior vena cava to the superior mesenteric vein should be considered (Fig. 62, *E*). The inferior vena cava is divided just above the iliac veins, and several inches are mobilized so that the superior end of the inferior vena cava can be implanted into the side of the superior mesenteric vein through a tunnel in the mesentery. Various other procedures have proved unsatisfactory. Division of the superior mesenteric vein and implantation into the inferior vena cava is not advised because it is difficult and is a small shunt. Ischemia or gangrene of the small bowel may result. Side-to-side anastomosis of the superior mesenteric vein and vena cava in the retropancreatic area is extremely difficult technically. Experimentally, synthetic grafts for portal-systemic shunts exhibit a high rate of thrombosis.

Indications

Because of the poor liver function of patients with portal hypertension, elective operation is to be preferred to an emergency procedure. In patients who are bleeding, operative mortality is high and improved methods of controlling the bleeding are urgently needed. Possibly intragastric hypothermia may be useful. A twelve- to twenty-four-hour trial of a Sengstaken-Blakemore tube is advisable and may arrest the hemorrhage.

Operative mortality, in general, is closely related to liver function, and the best surgical results are obtained in patients with good liver function evidenced by serum albumin of 4 gm.% or over, Bromsulphalein retention of less than 35%, and no clinical jaundice.

Contraindications

Contraindications to elective surgery are jaundice, poor or deteriorating liver function, hypoprothrombinemia that does not respond to administration of vitamin K, ammonia intoxication, and other forms of hepatic coma.

Preparation for portacaval anastomosis

Preoperative preparation includes medical treatment to improve liver function and preparation of the intestine with intestinal antibiotics such as Sulfasuxidine or neomycin. Nasogastric tubes should be avoided to prevent possible abrasion of varices. At least six units of blood should be available.

Splenoportography is done the day before or the morning of surgery to establish the patency of the portal vein and to measure portal pressure.

Anesthesia

Light general anesthesia should be employed. Hepatotoxic anesthetic agents should be avoided. Ample oxygenation and removal of carbon dioxide should be ensured. The dosage of Pentothal and muscle relaxants should be kept small. When the chest is open, a cuffed endotracheal tube is necessary. If the patient is actively bleeding or has recently bled, there is some danger of vomiting and aspiration during the induction period. To avoid this, insert the endotracheal tube under topical anesthesia with the patient awake. Once inserted, the cuffed tube prevents aspiration of blood, clots, or other gastric contents.

Incision

Either an abdominal or thoracoabdominal approach may be employed. Each incision is illustrated with one of the procedures that follows, and either incision may be used. The long subcostal abdominal incision is best for most patients. If the liver is very large, the thoracoabdominal incision is needed to displace the liver into the chest. In the presence of ascites, incision through the diaphragm invites the complication of pleuroperitoneal fistula.

Postoperative care

The diseased liver must receive maximum support. A gastrostomy is preferable to a nasogastric tube and may be used initially for decompression and later for medication and supplementary feedings. Introduce a polyethylene catheter into the cephalic vein so that the tip lies in the subclavian vein. We have found that the constant administration of 10 to 25% glucose is essential to support hepatic function in the immediate postoperative period. Arginine glutamate infusions (Modumate) are also helpful. Vitamins are added to the infusion. If large amounts of dextrose appear in the urine, fructose may be tried or small amounts of insulin may be added to the infusion. Excessive fibrinolysis sometimes develops preoperatively or postoperatively, and epsilon aminocaproic acid (Amicar) may be helpful.

End-to-side portacaval anastomosis
Preparation and anesthesia

See discussion on p. 203 and drawings on p. 204.

Procedure

1. Place the patient in the supine position with a small pillow under the right shoulder and another under the right hip.

2. Apply a strap across the hips and a brace under the opposite axilla.

3. The position may then be further improved by tilting the operating table to the patient's left (Fig. 63, *A*).

Exposure—thoracoabdominal approach

1. Commence the incision at the costal margin at the tenth intercostal space. Carry it downward and obliquely across the abdomen toward the umbilicus. Occasionally the rectus sheath must be divided anteriorly and posteriorly, but it is not necessary to divide the rectus muscle. (See Fig. 63, *B*.) Explore the abdomen.

Comment: *The porta hepatis, gastrohepatic ligament, foramen of Winslow, and other landmarks should be identified. Dense adhesions in the foramen of Winslow suggest old or recent portal thrombosis. If the precaution of spleno-portography has not been taken, portal venography may now be done. Bleeding from the splenic puncture for the recent splenoportogram is seldom more than a few hundred milliliters. In patients with portal hypertension of the intrahepatic type, there may be mild ascites. The posterior peritoneum and liver capsule are frequently edematous and thickened and appear whitish gray or frosted. Examine the pancreas, the pyloric area, the stomach, and the gallbladder.*

2. Extend the incision between the tenth and eleventh ribs. It is unnecessary to divide the costal margin.

3. Divide the diaphragm between medium-sized Pean clamps. Horizontal mattress sutures of No. 2 silk are placed, tied, held, and later tied together to close the diaphragmatic incision (Fig. 63, B).

Comment: *When the liver is small, a radial incision as far as the central tendon of the diaphragm may be sufficient and does not denervate too much of the diaphragm. Do not divide the triangular ligament. Larger livers can be tilted upward into the chest only after more extensive division of the diaphragm. For patients with larger livers, divide the diaphragm in a circumferential fashion, about 1 inch from the costal margin, and continue the incision until the liver can be displaced into the chest with the anterior edge of the liver above the costal margin. The undersurface of the liver and the hilum are then readily accessible.*

4. Mobilize the duodenum and head of the pancreas using the Kocher incision (Fig. 63, C). Obtain access to the vena cava by retracting the duodenum and head of the pancreas anteriorly and medially with a Deaver or Harrington retractor.

Comment: *There is an abundant venous collateral circulation, not normally seen, in the peritoneum in this area and in the omental adhesions. In uncovering the inferior vena cava and in exposing the portal vein, the surrounding peritoneum and connective tissue should be divided between clamps and hemostasis should be obtained with suture-ligatures of catgut on atraumatic needles.*

5. Dissect the front of the inferior vena cava free, and expose it from the level of the renal vein inferiorly to a point high up beneath the liver. Mobilize the hepatic flexure of the colon if necessary.

Dissection and exposure of portal vein

The portal vein lies posterior and slightly medial to the common bile duct and the hepatic artery. The posterior approach keeps the surgeon away from these structures. The vein is concealed by a mass of fat and lymph nodes in the edge of the gastrohepatic ligament. Rarely an anomalous hepatic artery originating from the superior mesenteric artery is encountered.

1. Define the foramen of Winslow. Have the operating table tilted 30 degrees to the patient's left, and palpate the tense portal vein posteriorly. Pick up the peritoneal reflection at the posterior edge of the gastrohepatic ligament and incise it (Fig. 63, D). The vein lies just beneath the peritoneum posteriorly, and this approach avoids lymph nodes and collateral veins. It is not necessary to identify the common duct or the hepatic artery, which lie anteriorly and medially. Do not divide any large artery in this region. The hepatic artery may be anomalous and may lie directly in front of the portal vein.

2. The portal vein lies in a tunnel of loose areolar tissue and is relatively sturdy and thick walled. Carefully work around it and pass a ¼-inch umbilical tape around it. Draw the vein laterally and posteriorly, and continue mobilization with small "peanut" sponge dissectors or with the suction tip. Mobilize the vein for a distance of 4 to 5 cm. between the pancreas and the liver. The first proximal tributary is the pyloric vein (rarely seen). The first distal tributary is a small anteromedial branch to the quadrate lobe.

3. Measure the portal pressure. A free connection through a No. 18 needle is satisfactory. Measurements are made with the inferior vena cava level as a

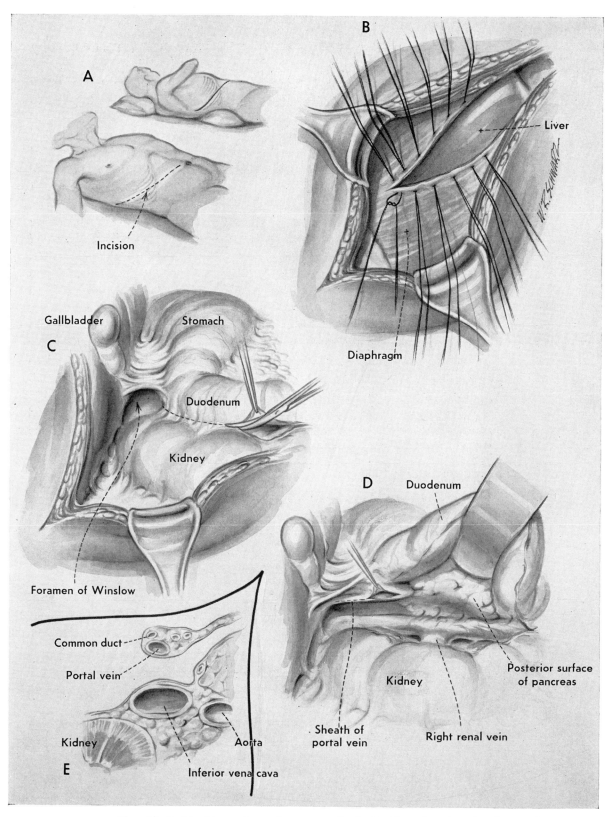

Fig. 63. End-to-side portacaval anastomosis. **A,** Position of patient for thoracoabdominal incision. **B,** Thoracic part of incision showing traction sutures in diaphragm. **C,** Liver tilted up into chest. Incision in peritoneum to mobilize duodenum. **D,** Duodenum lifted to gain access to portal vein and inferior vena cava. **E,** Cross section of gastrohepatic ligament.

Continued.

zero or reference point, first with the vein occluded between the manometer and the liver and then with the vein occluded between the manometer and the pancreas. A rubber-shod bulldog clamp is useful for occlusion. If the portal pressure on the hepatic side of the bulldog clamp remains high after occlusion, side-to-side anastomosis is preferred.

Resection of caudate lobe

At times a large caudate lobe is interposed between the portal vein and the inferior vena cava. A wedge of the caudate lobe of the liver must be resected to gain access to the inferior vena cava.

1. Place a large No. 1 chromic catgut mattress suture through the liver substance along the proposed line of excision, using a swedged-on atraumatic needle. Cut the liver as far as the ligature will permit. The fibrous liver holds sutures well. Rarely, oxidized cellulose (Surgicel) is also needed.

2. Place a second mattress suture, overlapping the first, and continue the resection so as to uncover sufficient inferior vena cava for anastomosis.

Comment: *Resection of the caudate lobe is unnecessary with the Valdoni approach for side-to-side portacaval shunt (pp. 217-221).*

Anastomosis—end-to-side

Side-to-side shunts are preferred whenever they are technically feasible.

1. Divide the portal vein. Apply a patent ductus clamp transversely to the portal vein near the hilum of the liver (Fig. 63, *F*) and apply a modified Bethune clamp or a Potts right-angled forceps about 1.5 cm. proximally, placing the jaw parallel to the inferior vena cava. Divide the portal vein about 2 mm. below the hilar clamp, oversew the cuff with 4-0 arterial silk (Fig. 63, *G*), and remove the clamp. This maneuver conserves the full length of the portal vein to reach the inferior vena cava.

2. Apply the tip of a fine Adson hemostat to the site selected for anastomosis on the anterior and medial aspect of the inferior vena cava. Place the stoma close to the liver so that the portal vein will not be kinked when the anastomosis is completed. With slight traction on the hemostat, place a toothed Satinsky clamp on the inferior vena cava (Fig. 63, *H* and *I*), occluding one-fourth to one-third of the lumen.

3. Excise a window in the inferior vena cava (Fig. 63, *I*). This should be elliptical in shape. Cut the back side of the ellipse no longer than one-half the circumference of the portal vein. Leave the lateral side of the ellipse attached for traction (Fig. 63, *J*). Place a fine arterial suture for traction on the ellipse and to hold the edges of the inferior vena cava apart.

4. Place two everting 4-0 mattress sutures at each end of the anastomosis (Fig. 63, *J* and *K*). The sutures are Tevdec or monofilament polyethylene and double-armed. These sutures should be closely placed, about 1 mm. apart and 1 to 2 mm. from the edge of the stoma. Hold but do not tie the ends. Do not attempt to approximate the portal vein and inferior vena cava until the row of sutures has been completed (Fig. 63, *L*).

5. Place the back row of everting mattress sutures from within the lumen. While placing the back row of sutures, the assistant holds the portal vein steadily about 1 cm. from the inferior vena cava, so that the back edge of the vein can

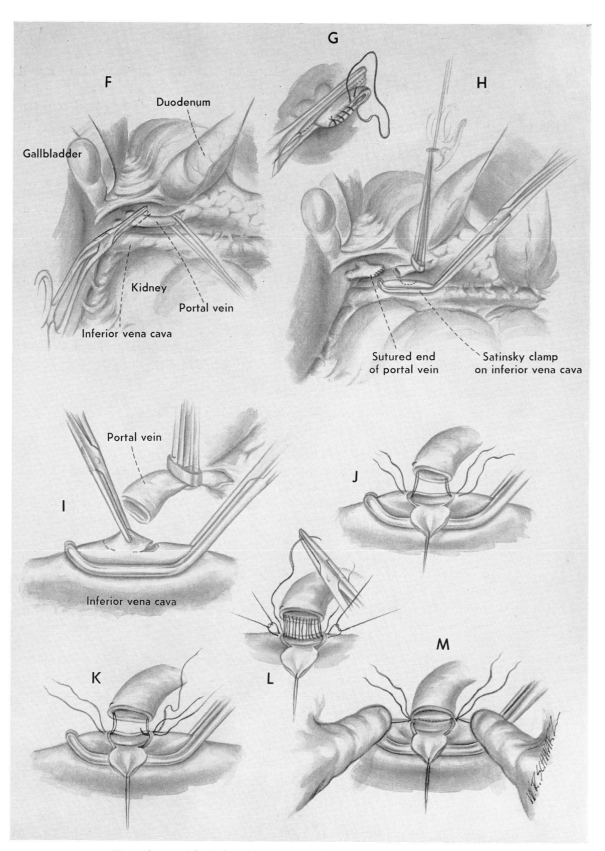

Fig. 63, cont'd. End-to-side portacaval anastomosis. **F,** Patent ductus clamp at site of division of portal vein. **G,** Suture hepatic end of portal vein. **H,** Site of anastomosis to inferior vena cava. **I,** Cut ellipse from inferior vena cava. **J,** Everting mattress sutures at each end of anastomosis. **K,** Begin back row of continuous everting mattress sutures. **L,** Complete back row of continuous everting mattress sutures. **M,** Draw edges of back row of sutures together.

be manipulated for accurate placement of the sutures. Start the back row by passing the needle from the outside into the lumen of the inferior vena cava about 1 mm. from the end mattress suture. Pass the needle and suture inside the lumen to the back edge of the portal vein, and pierce the portal vein from within outward next to the end mattress suture. Reenter the portal vein from without inward 1 to 2 mm. farther along the lumen. Cross to the caval side within the lumen. Repeat the everting mattress suture on the caval side.

To complete the back row, end the suture outside the lumen on the side of the inferior vena cava. Hold the inferior vena cava and portal vein in approximation with clamps. Draw the suture straight so that it is snug and seals the posterior edges. The suture should be correctly placed and be pulled straight with the tips of the index fingers (Fig. 63, M). Tie the mattress sutures, and tie the ends of the posterior row to one of the ends of the mattress suture at each end.

6. Use one of the ends of the mattress sutures to close the anterior portion of the anastomosis. Fig. 63, N-P, shows an everting mattress suture similar to the posterior row. However, a simple over-and-over stitch gives equally good results and is more rapid because the edges of the portal vein and inferior vena cava are now in close approximation.

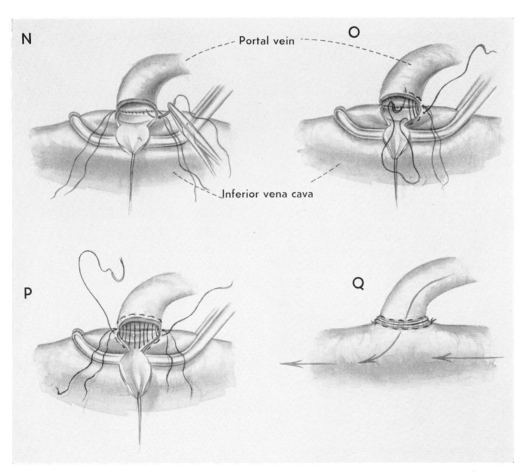

Fig. 63, cont'd. End-to-side portacaval anastomosis. **N,** Begin anterior row of sutures. **O** to **Q,** Completion of anterior row of sutures. A simple over-and-over suture pulled snug with each stitch can also evert the edges easily and quickly.

7. Slowly release the Satinsky clamp. There is seldom any bleeding or leakage. Remove the occluding clamp on the portal vein and measure pressure in the portal vein and the inferior vena cava.

Comment: *The aggravating high-pressure capillary oozing from the operative field stops promptly after the anastomosis is completed and the clamps are released. Do not waste time attempting capillary hemostasis. Complete the anastomosis.*

Closure

1. Close the diaphragm by tying the previously placed silk mattress sutures. Large suture material (No. 2) should be used so that the sutures do not tear the diaphragm.

2. A chest tube is brought out in the midaxillary line in the seventh or eighth interspace and connected to water-seal drainage. If the lung is expanded under positive pressure before closure, an anterior tube is unnecessary.

3. Dovetail the costal margins and close them with No. 24 steel wire sternotomy suture. This is not necessary when the costal margin has not been divided. Close the intercostal incision with pericostal sutures of No. 1 catgut.

4. Place a Stamm gastrostomy using a No. 24 Hurwitt gastrostomy catheter in the fundus of the stomach along the greater curvature before closing the abdominal incision. Draw the tube out through a hole in omentum, suture the anterior wall of the stomach to the peritoneum, and snub the catheter to the skin with a sturdy silk suture so as to prevent leakage of ascitic fluid. The gastrostomy tube can be used for feeding later as well as for decompression in the early postoperative period.

Side-to-side portacaval anastomosis
Introduction

Side-to-side anastomosis is preferred for most patients with portal hypertension since the liver is also decompressed by this procedure. Side-to-side anastomosis can be accomplished if the veins can be mobilized and held in serrated arterial clamps as illustrated in Fig. 64, C. The ideal size for side-to-side shunts is still unknown. Present policy is 1.5 to 2 cm.

The purposes, indications, anesthesia, and preoperative and postoperative care are given on pp. 203-206.

The subcostal approach is illustrated with this procedure. This incision may be used for either type of shunt and is most satisfactory when the costal arch is not too narrow. Thoracoabdominal incisions should be avoided in patients with ascites because of the possibility of pleuroperitoneal fistulas through the diaphragmatic suture line. See the preceding discussion of end-to-side anastomosis for details of the thoracoabdominal incision, as well as greater detail concerning abdominal exploration, isolation of the inferior vena cava and portal vein, and resection of the caudate lobe.

Procedure—side-to-side portacaval shunt

1. Place the patient in the supine position with sandbags under the lower right thorax and right hip (Fig. 64, A).

2. Make a long subcostal incision extending from far out in the right flank

upward, across both rectus muscles (Fig. 64, *A* and *B*). Divide the round ligament between clamps and ligatures.

3. Mobilize the duodenum and head of the pancreas using the Kocher incision. Detach the hepatic flexure of the colon if necessary. Retract the duodenum and pancreas medially and inferiorly.

Comment: *There is an abundant venous collateral circulation, not normally seen, in the peritoneum in this area and in the omental adhesions. In uncovering the inferior vena cava and in exposing the portal vein, the surrounding peritoneum and connective tissue should be divided between clamps and hemostasis should be obtained with suture-ligatures of catgut on atraumatic needles.*

4. Locate the common bile duct. Retract it anteriorly and medially. Tilt the table to the left. Incise the peritoneal reflection over the posterolateral aspect of the portal vein at the foramen of Winslow. Pass an umbilical tape about the portal vein, and with traction on the tape carefully dissect the portal vein free. Avoid dissection of the vascular lymphatic tissue in the free edge of the gastrohepatic ligament.

5. Free the portal vein from the hilum of the liver to the pancreas, visualizing the tributary to the quadrate lobe. Divide the pyloric vein and the pancreatoduodenal vein so that the portal vein can be mobilized from its tunnel in the pancreas. Measure the portal venous pressure.

6. Expose the anterior surface of the inferior vena cava, and apply the toothed Satinsky clamp (Fig. 64, *C*). Apply patent ductus clamps to the portal

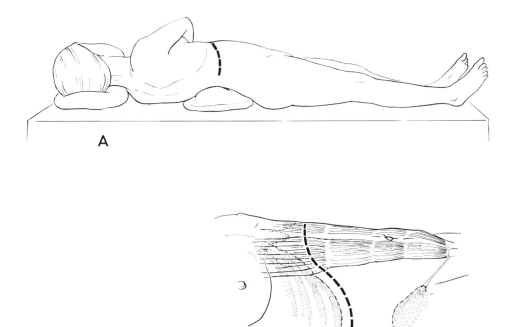

Fig. 64. Side-to-side portacaval shunt. **A,** Position of patient. **B,** Subcostal incision.

Continued.

213

vein, the distance between them being slightly longer than the proposed length of the anastomosis. These clamps are applied at a 60-degree angle to the sagittal plane and are rotated toward the sagittal plane to gain access to the posterior row of sutures.

Comment: *The three-bladed clamp is useful also. The clamp and the technique of anastomosis is similar to the description and drawings of the Valdoni technique (pp. 216-220).*

Resect a wedge of caudate lobe if it prevents close approximation of clamps and an ample length of vein.

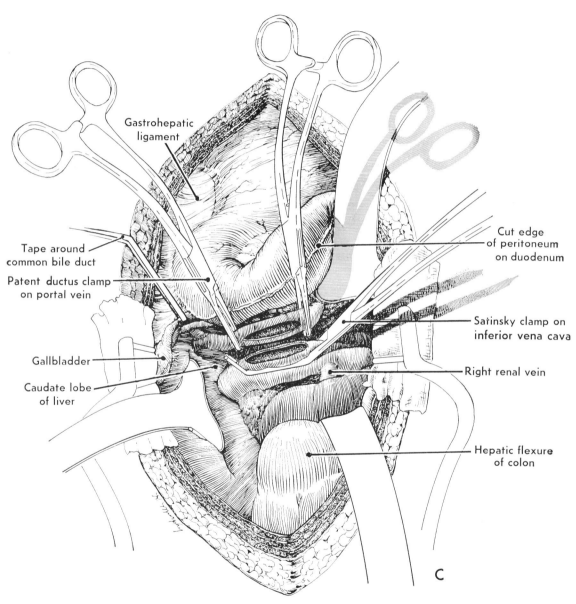

Gastrohepatic ligament

Tape around common bile duct

Patent ductus clamp on portal vein

Gallbladder

Caudate lobe of liver

Cut edge of peritoneum on duodenum

Satinsky clamp on inferior vena cava

Right renal vein

Hepatic flexure of colon

C

Fig. 64, cont'd. Side-to-side portacaval shunt. **C,** Exposure for side-to-side portacaval anastomosis. Shunt is unnecessarily large in this drawing. From 1.5 to 2 cm. is sufficient. Extra large shunts appear to impair liver blood flow.

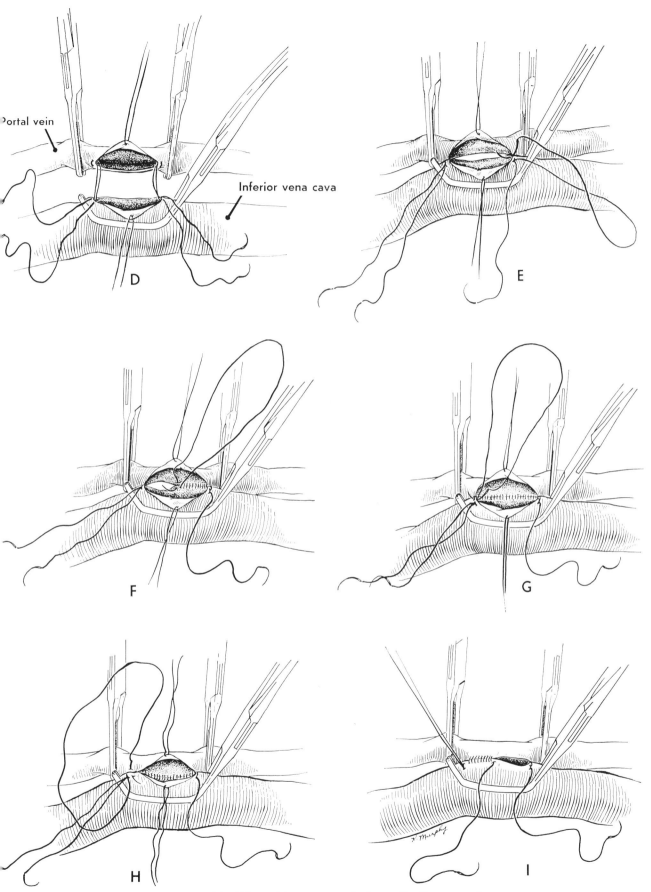

Portal vein

Inferior vena cava

D

E

F

G

H

I

Fig. 64, cont'd. Side-to-side portacaval shunt. **D,** Place everting mattress sutures at each end. **E,** Hold veins together with clamps. Begin posterior row of sutures. **F,** Posterior row of continuous over-and-over sutures. **G,** End posterior row. **H,** Begin anterior row. **I,** Completing anterior row.

If necessary, cut the posterior portion of the pancreas between the portal vein and the vena cava in order to approximate them.

7. Cut the openings in the portal vein and inferior vena cava (Fig. 64, C). Do this by first tenting the vein with a fine-pointed Adson forceps. The opening in the portal vein is on the posterior side and that in the inferior vena cava on the anteromedial side. The Potts 90-degree scissors is employed to excise a narrow ellipse from each vein, the length of the opening being 1½ to 2 cm.

Comment: *The size of the shunt in the drawing is larger than necessary. From 1.5 to 2 cm. is adequate.*

8. Lift the inferior vena cava with the Satinsky clamp. Push the clamps on the portal vein toward the inferior vena cava. Place a retracting suture (Fig. 64, D) on each side of the anastomosis in order to visualize the posterior row of sutures. Place a mattress suture across the anastomotic site on each end, using a double-armed 4-0 monofilament or Tevdec arterial suture.

9. Tie the mattress sutures. Enter the inferior vena cava posteriorly and from the outside with one of the sutures (Fig. 64, E). Suture the back side of the anastomosis with a running over-and-over stitch placed 1 to 2 mm. from the edge and 1 to 2 mm. apart (Fig. 64, F).

10. At the hepatic end of the anastomosis pass the needle outside the inferior vena cava and tie the suture to one end of the adjacent mattress suture (Fig. 64, G).

11. Use the remaining mattress suture to suture the front row of the anastomosis with an over-and-over continuous stitch. Hold the suture taut to evert the edges (Fig. 64, H and I). Emerge next to the first mattress suture and tie to one limb of it.

12. When the anastomosis is complete, release the caval clamp first. There is usually little bleeding. Release the clamps on the portal vein. Take postoperative portal pressure, and close the abdomen without drainage. Insert a gastrostomy tube through a separate stab wound as described on p. 212. Because of ascites, special care must be taken to seal the gastrostomy with omentum and to suture the stomach to the peritoneum around the tube.

Emergency portacaval shunt through midline incision—medial approach to portal vein and inferior vena cava
Preoperative control of hemorrhage

Patients bleeding from esophageal varices require an emergency operation if the Blakemore-Sengstaken tube (Fig. 65) does not stop the hemorrhage or if hemorrhage recurs when the tube is decompressed or removed in twenty-four to forty-eight hours. If the tube does not control the hemorrhage, varices may not be the source of the bleeding. Obviously patients who were denied elective shunts because of poor liver function cannot survive emergency operations.

The Sengstaken tube must have traction applied in order to draw the gastric balloon up and compress varices at the esophageal hiatus as well as compress them with the esophageal balloon. The Preston traction helmet* is the most satisfactory device to maintain alignment of the tube. Two constant-tension spring devices on the lightweight padded helmet maintain three-fourths or one and one-half pounds of traction as selected.

---

*Manufactured by E. J. T. Industries, 8439 W. Sunnyside Ave., Chicago, Ill. 60631.

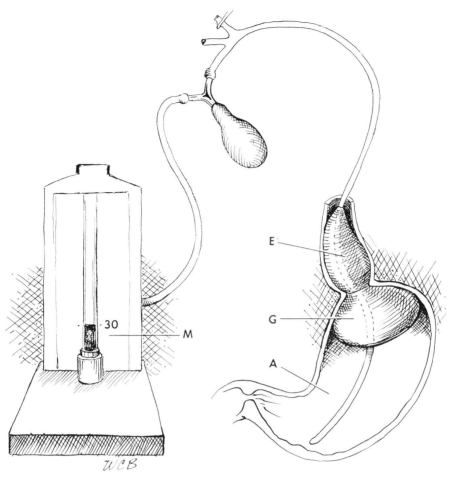

Fig. 65. Sengstaken tube to arrest hemorrhage from esophageal varices. **E,** Esophageal balloon. **G,** Gastric balloon. **A,** Aspirating or feeding tip in stomach. **M,** Manometer used to set pressure in balloons.

Ammonia intoxication results from the deamination of blood proteins in the bowel. Prevention and treatment of this and other aspects of preoperative and postoperative care have been discussed previously.

Introduction

The emergency portacaval shunt through a midline incision mobilizes the portal vein and the inferior vena cava medial to the hepatic artery after opening the gastrohepatic ligament at this site. The veins are very close to each other, and the caudate lobe does not intrude. The dissection is less extensive so the blood loss is small and operating time is short. The special three-bladed Valdoni clamp is essential. It fits nicely into the small operative field. Our experience with this technique is still small, but it appears so promising we include it here.*

---

*Valdoni, P.: Complementary surgical technique in portal caval anastomosis, J. Cardiov. Surg. 3:26-31, 1962; Portal hypertension—personal experience of the surgical treatment, Proc. Roy. Soc. Med. **56:**261-263 (section of surgery, pp. 9-11), 1963.

Procedure

1. Make a midline incision from the xiphoid to below the umbilicus (Fig. 66, *A*). Explore the abdomen. Palpate the foramen of Winslow.

2. Open the gastrohepatic omentum widely and palpate the hepatic artery at the superior border of the pancreas and its ascending portion overlying the portal vein. Divide the right gastric artery to free the pyloric end of the stomach and retract it inferiorly (Fig. 66, *B*).

3. Expose the ascending portion of the hepatic artery, pass an umbilical tape about it to lift it, and retract it laterally (Fig. 66, *C*).

4. Expose the portal vein beneath the hepatic artery and resect the lymphatic tissue and fat along its medial border. The vein is thick walled and lies in a tunnel of areolar tissue. Pass a tape around the portal vein to lift it (Fig. 66, *C*).

5. Expose the front of the inferior vena cava directly posterior by incising and excising the peritoneum that overlies it (Fig. 66, *D*).

6. Prepare the portal vein and inferior vena cava for anastomosis by resection of intervening lymphatic tissue. This is not an extensive dissection. Take portal pressure.

7. Apply the three-bladed Valdoni clamp to the posteromedial aspect of the portal vein by seizing that part of the wall of the vein with a fine-pointed long hemostat and tenting it up anteriorly to place and close the clamp. This is the part of the vein that lies close to the front of the inferior vena cava.

8. Pick up the center of the intended anastomotic site on the inferior vena cava with another long fine-pointed hemostat and apply the other side of the Valdoni clamp (Fig. 66, *F*).

9. Excise an ellipse from both veins (Fig. 66, *G, 1*). Save at least a 2 mm. edge in the clamp for secure anastomosis. Place retracting sutures in the outside edges of the veins to hold them apart.

10. Start the anastomosis at the most accessible end (that is, inferior end) and tie the knot of the double-armed Tevdec or polyethylene monofilament suture outside (Fig. 66, *G, 2*). Pass the needle inside and suture the edges of the veins snugly together with an over-and-over suture, progressing superiorly.

11. At the superior end of the anastomosis, pass the needle outside and suture the anterior edges together with an over-and-over suture or everting mattress sutures as shown in Fig. 66, *G, 2*, progressing inferiorly.

12. Complete the anastomosis by tying the two sutures together outside (Fig. 66, *G, 3,* and *H*).

13. Release the portal vein from the three-bladed clamp and then release the inferior vena cava. Depress the clamp posteriorly and then slide the middle blade out from behind the anastomosis carefully.

14. Take postoperative portal pressures.

15. Perform a Foley or Hurwitt catheter gastrostomy to decompress the stomach and avoid a tube in the esophagus. Place the tube through a purse-string suture high on the greater curvature of the stomach. Draw the tube out through a hole in the omentum and a separate snug stab incision in the left upper quadrant. Suture the stomach wall to the parietal peritoneum. The tube may be useful for supplementary feedings in the postoperative period or for antacid medication.

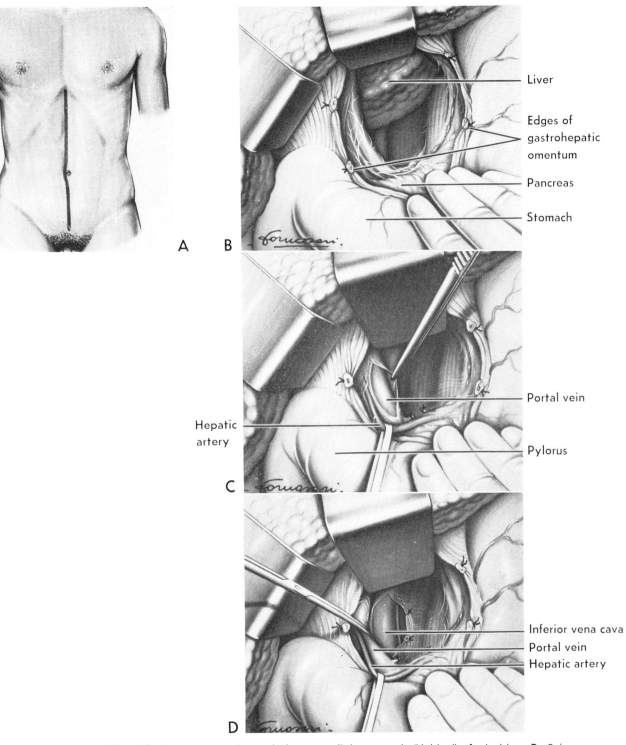

Fig. 66. Emergency portacaval shunt—medial approach (Valdoni). **A,** Incision. **B,** Relationship of hepatic artery, portal vein, and inferior vena cava after opening the gastrohepatic omentum. **C,** Retracting the hepatic artery and exposing the portal vein. **D,** Exposing the inferior vena cava.

Continued.

219

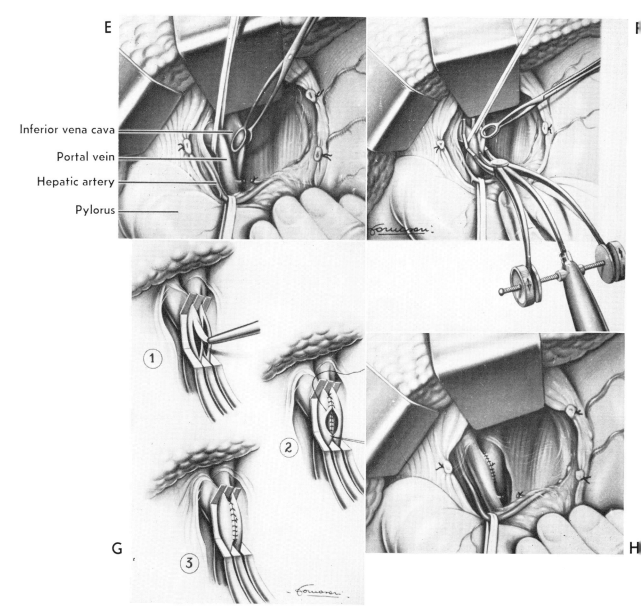

Inferior vena cava
Portal vein
Hepatic artery
Pylorus

E

F

G

H

Fig. 66, cont'd. Emergency portacaval shunt—medial approach (Valdoni). **E,** Portal vein and inferior vena cava at site of anastomosis. **F,** Apply the three-bladed clamp (Valdoni). **G,** Side-to-side portacaval anastomosis: **1,** excise ellipse; **2,** completed posterior and beginning anterior anastomosis; **3,** completed anastomosis. **H,** Clamp removed. (Courtesy Prof. Pietro Valdoni, Surgical Clinic, University of Rome, Rome, Italy.)

Extrahepatic portal block—mesocaval shunt

For extrahepatic portal block, mesocaval shunt may be the only operation feasible. The portal system is decompressed by attaching the divided end of the inferior vena cava to the side of the superior mesenteric vein (Fig. 62, *E*). It is most useful in children with the extrahepatic obliteration of the portal vein because many of them have had splenectomy or the splenic vein is small. It has been used in adults not only for extrahepatic block, but also for portal hypertension due to cirrhosis of the liver.

The inferior vena cava is divided at the confluence of the iliac veins and sufficient tributaries up to the renal veins are divided to permit the cava to reach the superior mesenteric vein, and a terminolateral anastomosis is made. The inferior end of the inferior vena cava is sutured shut (Fig. 62, *E*).

The papers of Gliedman,* Clatworthy, Wall, and Watman,† and Marion‡ furnish further detail and illustrations.

---

*Gliedman, M. L.: The technique of the side-to-end superior mesenteric vein to inferior vena cava shunt for portal decompression, Surg. Gynec. Obst. **121**:1101, 1965.

†Clatworthy, H. W., Jr., Wall, T., and Watman, R. N.: New type of portal-to-systemic venous shunt for portal hypertension, Arch. Surg. **71**:588, 1955.

‡Marion, M. P.: Anastomose spléno-rénale, anastomose mésentérico-cave, pour obstructions portales extra-hépatiques, Jour. Chir. **76**:698, 1958.

Chapter 13

Sympathectomy

Introduction

Sympathectomy will release vasomotor tone and will increase blood flow through collateral arterioles. Therefore, it has been widely used in the treatment of patients with occlusive and vasospastic diseases of the extremities. The dilation of collateral vessels is helpful when arterial insufficiency is not very severe and when ischemic lesions are superficial. Dilation of collateral arterioles is never sufficient to save extremities with established gangrene caused by major arterial occlusions. The dilation or development of collateral vessels is seldom sufficient for an adequate arterial supply during exercise, although the intermittent claudication may improve. The new techniques of arterial reconstruction are the only effective ways to restore normal or near normal flow in such patients.

Sympathectomy is often a useful procedure. Some of the arterial reconstructive procedures performed in the legs occlude again and, of course, have higher morbidity and mortality rates than sympathectomy.

Good results from sympathectomy require proper selection of patients. Good results are expected if the main symptom has been intermittent claudication. Superficial or localized necrosis of toes will be improved, but ischemia of the entire forefoot, severe pain at rest, atrophy of skin or muscle, or other signs of severe arterial insufficiency cannot be arrested or improved solely by sympathectomy.

We recommend denervation of the entire extremity, releasing vasomotor tone in the thigh as well as distally. This requires removal of the sympathetic chain from the twelfth dorsal to the fifth lumbar vertebra. Unless the first lumbar ganglion is preserved on one side, there may be difficulty with ejaculation in males. The high sympathectomy is more certain to interrupt the aberrant pathways that occasionally occur. An extended sympathectomy is also advised for the arm (pp. 227-232).

Shortly after operation the extremity will be warm and dry. A few days later the vasodilation decreases temporarily and then stabilizes, but the extremity seldom regains its initial warmth and color. Failure to achieve significant vasodilation generally means that the patient was not a suitable subject or the opera-

222

tion was inadequate. Inadequate denervation may occasionally result from the anomalies and variations in the sympathetic system, particularly from crossover of nerve fibers from the other side and from ganglionic cells and sympathetic outflow in the ventral nerve roots and spinal nerves. Patients have been observed in whom bilateral sympathectomy was necessary before maximum effects of denervation appeared on the first side.

Long-term survival or limb survival may be frustrated by progression of the underlying occlusive disease in the visceral arteries as well as in the limbs. Patients with diffuse arteriosclerosis in the affected limb or in the heart, kidneys, or brain have a poor prognosis. Diabetic patients likewise have a poor prognosis. There is little evidence for regeneration of the nerves, sensitization to norepinephrine, etc.

Sympathectomy is helpful for Buerger's disease if the patient stops smoking. It is useful for Raynaud's disease and other vasospastic diseases that do not respond to medical therapy. It is of no value as treatment for varicose ulcers unless accompanied by arterial insufficiency. It aggravates lymphedema. It is recommended for acute frostbite only if performed early, that is, before twenty-four to forty-eight hours.

Sympathectomy will relieve disabling hyperhidrosis or causalgia caused by major nerve injury. Reflex sympathetic dystrophy is a difficult diagnostic and therapeutic problem best treated conservatively. Specialized scientific papers and textbooks should be consulted for further details.

LUMBAR SYMPATHECTOMY

The lumbar portion of the sympathetic chain, like the rest of the vegetative nervous system, is subject to great anatomical variation. Because of the structural variation and interconnections and because some sympathetic fibers are probably contained in the spinal nerves and do not traverse the sympathetic chain or its ganglia, it is probably impossible to do an anatomically complete sympathectomy. For clinical purposes, however, removal of the sympathetic ganglia does seem efficacious. Functional tests of skin resistance and sweating ability, if done routinely, will usually establish the fact of sympathetic interruption, the effects of which persist for many years.

Lumbar sympathectomy need not affect sexual function. When sympathectomy is unilateral, no complication is anticipated. When sympathectomy is performed bilaterally, it is advisable to preserve the first lumbar ganglion on one side. Otherwise, ejaculation may not be normal.

Plan of operation

The plan of operation is to remove the lumbar sympathetic ganglionated nerve from at least the first to the fifth lumbar vertebra, including afferent and efferent rami to the chain and the terminal portion of the sympathetic trunk. If sympathectomy is to be bilateral, the first lumbar ganglion should be removed on only one side.

Anesthesia

General endotracheal anesthesia is desirable since there is some chance of entering the pleural cavity superiorly.

223

Position

Place the patient in the lateral position with the side to be operated upon upward. The area between the twelfth rib and the pelvic crest should be centered over the break in the operating table or over the kidney rest. The lower leg is flexed for stability, and the upper leg is half flexed to provide relaxation of the psoas muscle (Fig. 67, *A*). For muscle-splitting incisions it is advantageous to rotate the patient's hips toward the operator. Otherwise, no rotation is necessary.

Procedure

1. Begin the skin incision at the tip of the twelfth rib (Fig. 67, *B*). Carry it downward and medially to meet the lateral border of the rectus sheath at a point approximately 2 cm. below the umbilicus or roughly at the level of the anterior superior spine. If the distance between the twelfth rib and the iliac crest is relatively short, the incision should include 3 or 4 cm. of the tip of the twelfth rib, which will be resected. If the space between the twelfth rib and the iliac crest seems ample, the incision may be brought 1 or 2 cm. below the twelfth rib without removing it.

2. Incise the external oblique and internal oblique muscles in the direction of the skin incision. This will require cutting across the fibers of these structures.

3. The transversus abdominis may usually be incised in the direction of its fibers. Properitoneal fat and peritoneum are found directly under the transversus muscle anteriorly. In the lateral part of the incision the retroperitoneal fat is encountered.

4. Retract the edges of the divided transversus abdominis, and bluntly dissect the peritoneal sac and its contents medially. As this dissection is performed, the psoas muscle and other structures in the retroperitoneal area will come into view (Fig. 67, *C*). Avoid the groove behind the quadratus lumborum muscle.

5. Identify the anatomical landmarks. The sympathetic chain is identified by palpating the chain with its characteristic ganglia in the position indicated on the vertebral bodies. Visualization of the chain frequently requires division of the prevertebral fascia, although in many patients this is not a particularly strong structure.

6. Hold the sympathetic chain taut with the nerve hook, and trace it upward and downward. Divide rami as they are encountered. Remember that the chain has many anatomical variations (Fig. 68, *A-C*). As the chain is traced upward, the tendinous arc of the diaphragmatic crus must be divided and the muscle fibers separated at the first lumbar vertebra or beyond (Fig. 68, *F* and *G*). Tilt the patient's head down, and spread the crus with the dissecting scissors before division. The crus may be inserted as low as the third or fourth lumbar vertebra (Fig. 68, *D*). When the top of the sympathetic chain is reached, apply several silver clips for identification and divide the chain (Fig. 68, *G*). The nerve runs behind the pleural reflection at this level, but a small nick need not be sutured and is covered when the retracted crus is released.

7. Grasp the superior portion of the sympathetic chain with a hemostat. Trace the chain downward. One or more lumbar veins are encountered. They are usually posterior to the chain, which is gently dissected from them. If the chain goes behind the veins, it may be easier to isolate and divide the veins.

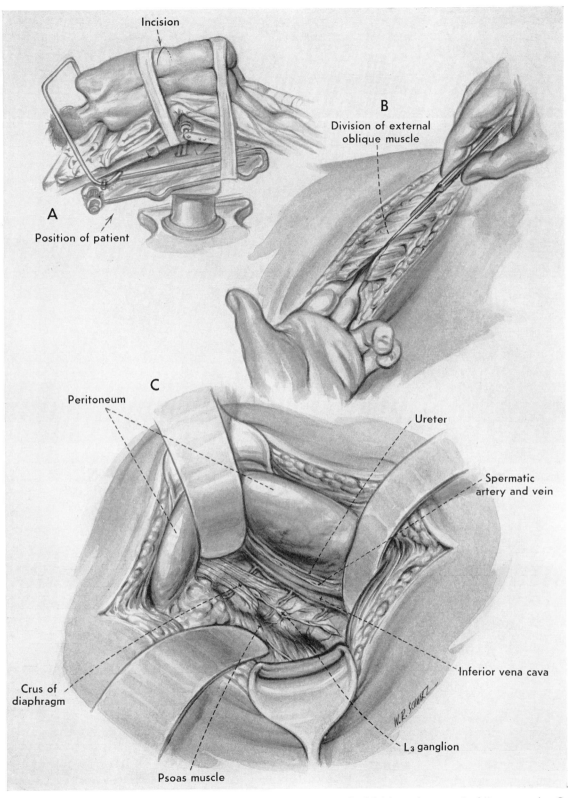

Fig. 67. Lumbar sympathectomy. **A,** Incision. **B,** Division of external oblique muscle. **C,** Exposure of lumbar sympathetic ganglia.

Labels on figure:

A — Incision, Position of patient

B — Division of external oblique muscle

C — Peritoneum, Ureter, Spermatic artery and vein, Inferior vena cava, L₃ ganglion, Psoas muscle, Crus of diaphragm

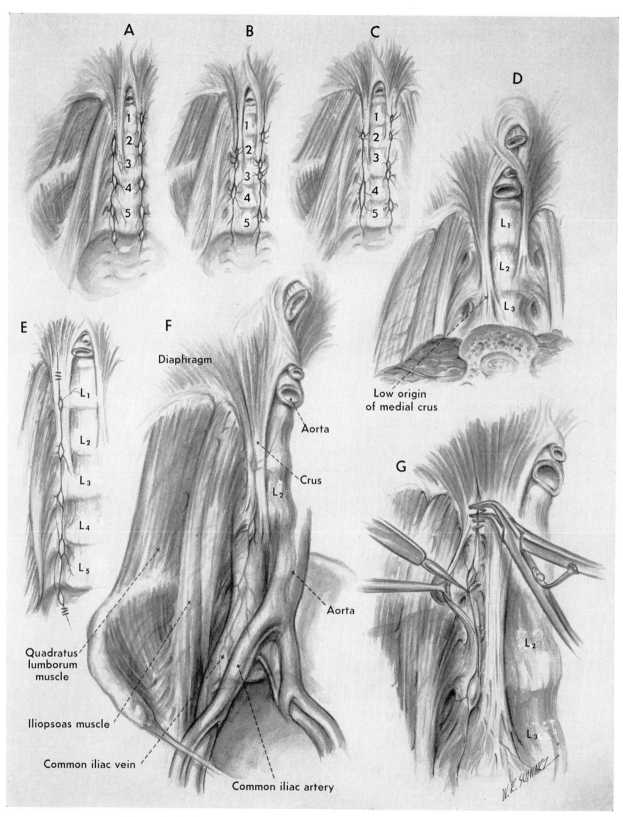

Fig. 68. Lumbar sympathectomy. **A** to **C,** Variations of lumbar sympathetic ganglia. **D,** Variations in origin of crus of diaphragm. **E,** Extent of resection of ganglionated nerve marked with silver clips. **F,** View of retroperitoneal structures in relation to sympathetic ganglia. **G,** Crus split to show upper limit of resection marked with clips.

226

The inferior portion of the sympathetic chain lies under the iliac vessels and should be carefully dissected out. It is unnecessary to attempt to follow the chain beyond this level. Usually at the level of the iliac vessels, the sympathetic chain has divided into two or three terminal branches. Apply silver clips to these and divide the chain inferiorly (Fig. 68, E).

8. Close the incision in layers.

Postoperative care

No special care is necessary. As a rule, the skin of the sympathectomized extremity will become warm and dry almost immediately. The use of a supporting binder for several weeks postoperatively adds comfort during the postoperative period.

Complications

Aside from the ordinary complications of wound healing, those complications peculiar to lumbar sympathectomy can, for the most part, be avoided. The ureter and the genitofemoral nerve must not be mistaken for the sympathetic chain.

Following lumbar sympathectomy, nausea and ileus are rare complications, even when the peritoneal cavity has been opened. Neuritis of the ilioinguinal or genitofemoral nerve may occur. This is manifested by pain in the ilioinguinal region and the anterior medial portions of the thigh. The condition is self-limited, and pain disappears in three to six weeks.

CERVICODORSAL SYMPATHECTOMY BY SUPRACLAVICULAR APPROACH

Vasospastic disease of the upper extremities that does not respond to medical treatment may be treated by cervicodorsal sympathectomy. The cervicodorsal sympathetic chain is removed from the level of the sixth cervical vertebra inferiorly to the fourth thoracic ganglion. The supraclavicular approach as described provides a more extensive sympathectomy than the ordinary dorsal sympathectomy performed extrapleurally after resection of the proximal portions of the third rib. The Horner's syndrome that results from this is of cosmetic significance only, and the more conservative operations that avoid it are less satisfactory.

The operation is of no lasting value to patients with collagen diseases such as scleroderma. Intractable and disabling hyperhidrosis of the hands requires only stellate ganglionectomy. The extended operation we describe is advisable for causalgia of the arm.

Anesthesia

Because the pleural cavity may be entered, endotracheal general anesthesia with a cuffed tube is essential.

Procedure

Incision and surgical approach

1. Place the patient in the supine position with the head turned away from the side of the incision and the neck somewhat hyperextended. Make the incision above and parallel to the clavicle from the midportion of the sterno-

cleidomastoid muscle laterally to the anterior edge of the trapezius muscle (Fig. 69, A).

2. Divide the platysma and the clavicular head of the sternocleidomastoid muscle (Fig. 69, B).

3. Divide the omohyoid muscle near its clavicular origin (Fig. 69, C).

4. Retract the prescalene fat pad laterally, retract the jugular vein medially, and identify the phrenic nerve overlying the anterior scalene muscle.

Dissect out the phrenic nerve, leaving an abundant amount of perineural connective tissue about it. Pass a tape around the phrenic nerve and retract it medially. Divide the anterior scalene muscle close to its attachment at the first rib (Fig. 69, D).

Comment: *Dissection and retraction of the phrenic nerve should be gentle. Otherwise hiccough or partial phrenic paralysis may occur. The operator may encounter and should spare any accessory phrenic nerves. Bilateral operation at one stage is not advisable because of possible interference with phrenic nerve function.*

Identification of stellate ganglion and cervical sympathetic trunk

1. Identify and expose the subclavian artery, and ligate and divide the thyrocervical arterial trunk (Fig. 69, E). Beware of the thin vertebral vein that lies along the vertebral column and adjacent to the sympathetic chain. Palpate the stellate ganglion as it lies on the neck of the first rib lateral to the vertebral artery and in close proximity to the vertebral vein.

2. Lift the stellate ganglion with a nerve hook, and with gentle, blunt, and sharp dissection identify its "dumbbell" shape and its various rami. Trace the sympathetic chain upward as far as convenient, usually the transverse process of the sixth cervical vertebra where the vertebral artery dips posteriorly to enter the foramen in the transverse process. Fig. 69, F, represents the relationships of the stellate ganglion and shows the relationship of the sympathetic chain to the vertebral artery and vein, the cervical plexus, the cupola of the lung, and the subclavian vessels.

Exposure and removal of sympathetic ganglia—first to third dorsal inclusive

1. With sharp and blunt dissection, mobilize the pleura from the entire circumference of the first rib. Posteriorly, the attachments are more dense (Sibson's fascia). Detach the apical pleura from the upper dorsal vertebras and the subclavian artery, and push it downward (Fig. 69, G). Dissection is in the extrapleural space.

Divide the highest intercostal artery if it is present. The artery crosses the thoracic inlet after the pleura over the cupula of the lung has been pushed downward. Hold the pleura laterally with a narrow Deaver or a narrow malleable retractor, and continue extrapleural dissection, peeling the pleura away from the dorsal vertebras and the necks of the first four ribs. If the thoracic inlet through the circle of the first rib is large, the pleura can be mobilized as far as the azygos vein on the right side and the fourth or fifth dorsal vertebras on the left side. Divide the insertion of the posterior scalene muscle if necessary to enlarge the thoracic inlet.

2. Place a nerve hook under the sympathetic chain, and lift it from the

228

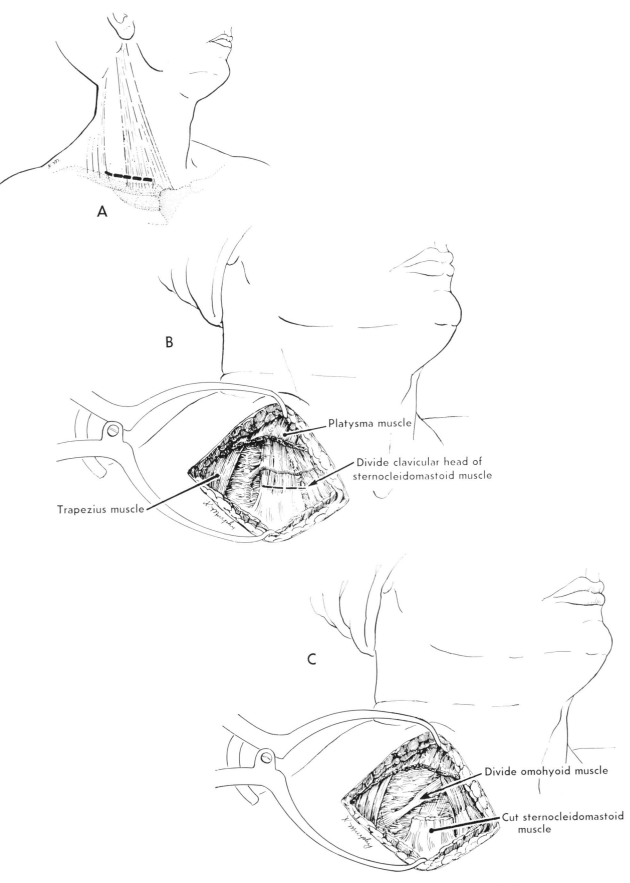

Fig. 69. Supraclavicular cervical sympathectomy. **A,** Incision. **B** and **C,** Successive steps in surgical approach.

Continued.

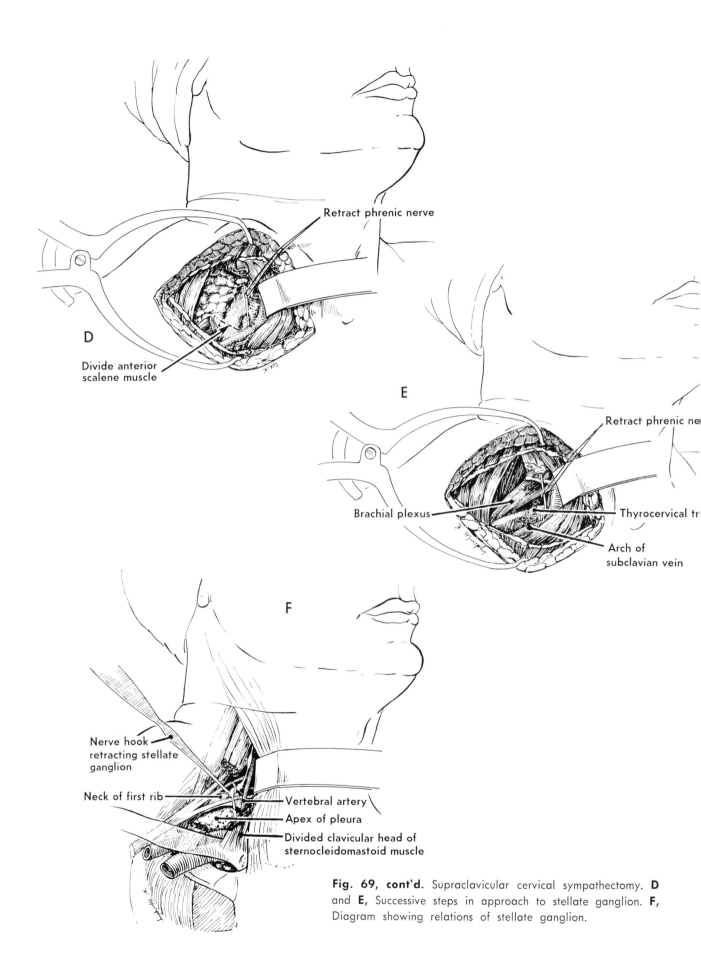

D

Retract phrenic nerve

Divide anterior
scalene muscle

E

Retract phrenic ne[rve]

Brachial plexus

Thyrocervical tr[unk]

Arch of
subclavian vein

F

Nerve hook
retracting stellate
ganglion

Neck of first rib

Vertebral artery

Apex of pleura

Divided clavicular head of
sternocleidomastoid muscle

Fig. 69, cont'd. Supraclavicular cervical sympathectomy. **D** and **E**, Successive steps in approach to stellate ganglion. **F**, Diagram showing relations of stellate ganglion.

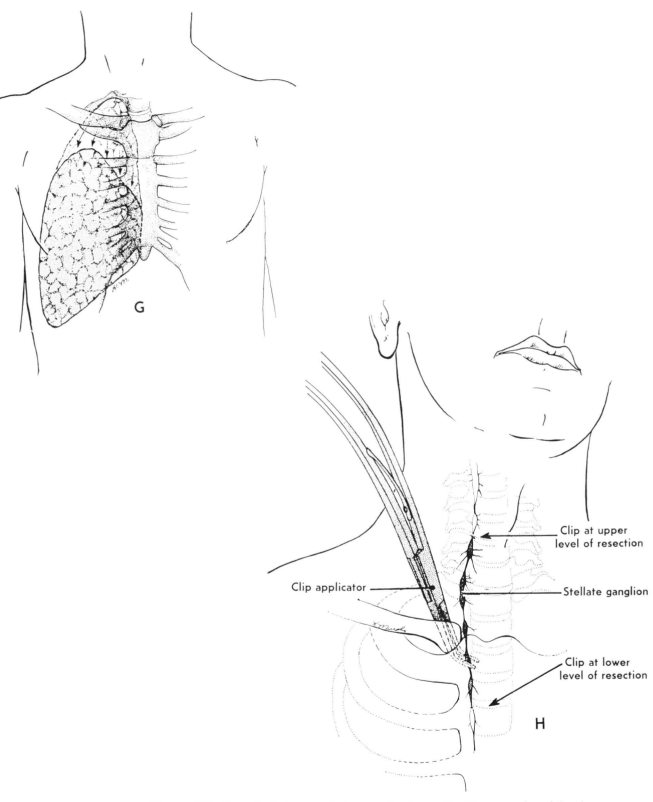

Fig. 69, cont'd. Supraclavicular cervical sympathectomy. **G,** Diagram of mobilized pleura, dropping inferiorly. **H,** Diagram of extent of sympathectomy.

vertebras. Identify and clip the various rami with silver clips. At the lower end of the resection, place several clips across the chain to mark the inferior limit of the resection. (See Fig. 69, *H*.)

Divide the chain inferiorly below the third dorsal ganglion or lower when feasible, then trace it superiorly, dividing the rami of the stellate ganglion, and mark the upper extent of the resection with silver clips.

Closure

1. Leave a No. 20 catheter in the extrapleural space along the spine until closure of the skin is airtight.

2. Suture the clavicular head of the sternocleidomastoid muscle. Do not attempt suture of the scalene or the omohyoid muscle.

3. Suture the platysma with fine silk.

4. After a correct sponge count, close the skin airtight around the catheter.

5. Aspirate the catheter while the anesthesiologist applies positive pressure to the lungs. This inflates the lung and prevents dead space.

6. Withdraw the catheter slowly with continuous suction.

Comment: *The morbidity of the extended cervicothoracic sympathectomy by this approach is very low.*

Adequate exposure, careful hemostasis, and the precautions emphasized in the text will prevent disturbances of the phrenic nerve or opening of the pleural cavity. The various rami of the sympathetic chain are clipped before they are divided and hemostasis is ensured. Endotracheal anesthesia ensures that an inadvertent perforation of the pleura will cause no serious difficulty. The vertebral vein is frequently fragile and may have to be ligated. To divide the anterior scalene muscle, a small curved clamp is carefully passed behind it and the fibers are incised a few at a time so as to identify and ligate several small blood vessels that course in the substance of the muscle. The operation described will result in Horner's syndrome with anhidrosis of the affected side of the face and neck, the entire upper extremity, the upper part of the chest, and part of the axilla.

UPPER DORSAL SYMPATHECTOMY BY ANTERIOR TRANSTHORACIC APPROACH
Indications and choice of operation

Sympathectomy by the transthoracic route removes the dorsal sympathetic chain usually from the first to the fifth dorsal vertebra, including the cardiac rami or nerves. The upper part of the stellate ganglion is not accessible by this approach and is usually left or incompletely removed, depending upon whether or not it is fused with the first dorsal ganglion. Indications for the transthoracic approach are vasospasm or arterial insufficiency of the upper extremity that relapses after stellate or cervical ganglionectomy, angina pectoris,[*] or paroxysmal auricular tachycardia refractory to all medical therapy.[†] In general, the anterior approach through the thorax has a lower morbidity rate and produces better

---

[*]Palumbo, L. T.: Anterior transthoracic approach for upper dorsal sympathectomy, Arch. Surg. **72**:659, 1955.
[†]White, J. C., Smithwick, R. H., and Simeone, F. A.: The autonomic nervous system, New York, 1952, The Macmillan Co.

232

exposure than the dorsal extrapleural method through the beds of the second and third ribs as advocated by White, Smithwick, and Simeone. Although the extended cervical thoracic sympathectomy by the supraclavicular approach (pp. 227-232) is probably best for vasospastic disease of the arm or causalgia, this procedure must occasionally be supplemented by this approach.

Anesthesia

General endotracheal anesthesia is necessary.

Procedure

1. Place the patient in the supine position with the arm elevated and supported (Fig. 70, A). Tilt the table away from the side to be operated upon.

2. Make a long incision in the third intercostal space, extending from the sternum laterally to the anterior axillary line (Fig. 70, B, which shows the operation on the right side).

3. Incise the pectoralis major muscle in the direction of its fibers.

4. Incise the intercostal muscles and pleura widely to permit spreading the ribs. Rarely it may be necessary to divide the second costal cartilage. Insert the rib spreader.

5. Free the lung if necessary, and retract it inferiorly, holding it in place with a Harrington retractor.

6. Tilt the table to the left about 15 degrees, and visualize the superior vena cava and phrenic nerve. The mediastinal structures will be retracted medially (Fig. 70, B). On the left side the aorta and subclavian artery are seen.

Removal of sympathetic nerve and ganglion

1. Identify the ganglionated chain beneath the parietal pleura on the vertebral bodies close to the necks of the ribs.

2. Incise the pleura overlying the sympathetic chain, and place three dural clips on the chain (Fig. 70, B) to mark the distal end of the resection for radiographic identification at a later date. This will be at the level of the hilum of the lung, normally about the level of the fifth dorsal vertebra.

3. Remove the sympathetic chain from below upward, dividing the rami connecting it to the spinal nerves as they are encountered (Fig. 70, C).

4. Identify the neck of the first rib and the first dorsal ganglion, that is, the lower part of the stellate ganglion. The upper part of the stellate ganglion will not be completely visualized from this approach.

5. Mark the upper extent of the resection with a dural clip, and divide the chain between the ganglia on the neck of the first rib. Measure and diagram the specimen.

Comment: *Anatomically, exposure is excellent, and the underlying intercostal veins usually cause no difficulty. Comparisons of anatomy on the right and left are shown in Fig. 71, A and B. The large cardiac rami course anteriorly. The nerve of Kuntz may occasionally be noted. Sometimes the first intercostal vein passes anterior to the sympathetic chain in the upper portion of the thorax. The first thoracic ganglion may be independent or fused to the inferior cervical ganglion to form the stellate ganglion. The latter arrangement is more common. The second thoracic ganglion may be similarly fused. Below the second thoracic*

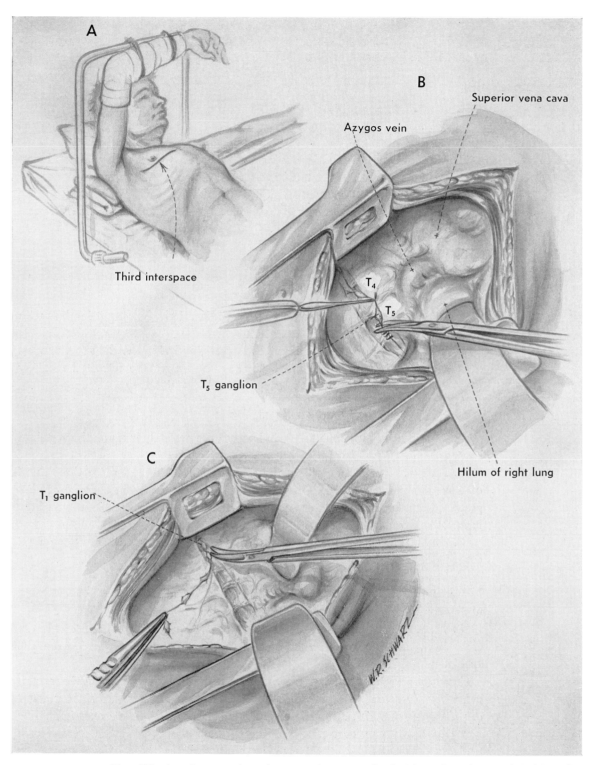

Fig. 70. Anterior transthoracic sympathectomy. **A,** Position of patient and incision. **B,** View of sympathetic ganglion at inferior limit of resection. **C,** View of sympathetic ganglion (T₁) at superior limit of resection.

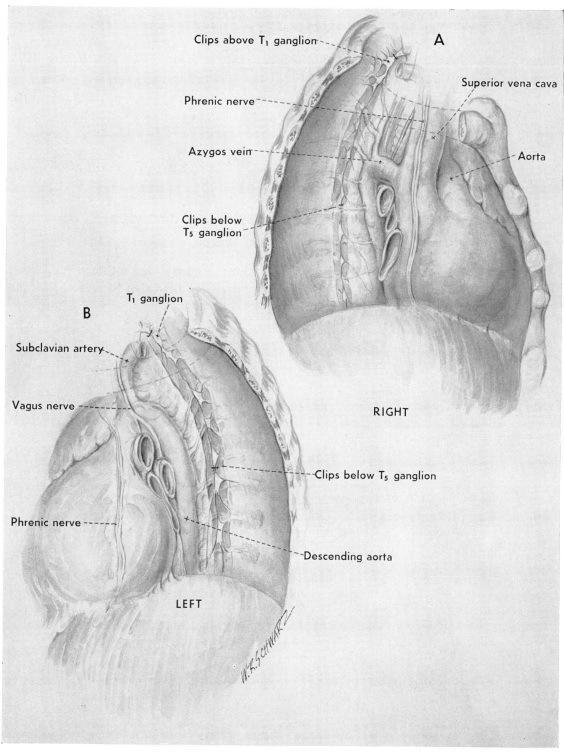

Clips above T₁ ganglion

Phrenic nerve

Azygos vein

Clips below
T₅ ganglion

A

Superior vena cava

Aorta

RIGHT

B

T₁ ganglion

Subclavian artery

Vagus nerve

Phrenic nerve

Clips below T₅ ganglion

Descending aorta

LEFT

W.R.SCHWARZ

Fig. 71. Thoracic sympathectomy. **A,** Lateral view of mediastinum and sympathetic ganglia (right). **B,** Lateral view of mediastinum and sympathetic ganglia (left).

235

level the ganglia of the thoracic chain are rather regularly segmental, with less variation than is encountered in the lumbar chain. The highest (greater) splanchnic nerve arises from about the level of the fifth to the ninth thoracic segments. With regard to cardiac innervation, the preganglionic sympathetic fibers either terminate in the upper thoracic chain ganglia or ascend to synapse in the cervical ganglia. Thus, upper thoracic sympathectomy, if it extends to the first dorsal vertebra, interrupts the preganglionic fibers to the heart. Afferent fibers, not part of the sympathetic system, may run in any of the so-called cardiac nerves, however. As in sympathectomy elsewhere, interruption of the sympathetic chain will not affect any sympathetic fibers that lie within the somatic nerves.

Closure

1. Place an anterior chest tube in the fourth intercostal space through a small separate stab incision.
2. Approximate the ribs with pericostal sutures.
3. Close the pectoral fascia, superficial fascia, and skin in layers.

Complications

Morbidity rate is as low as that of operations with less satisfactory exposure. Horner's syndrome does not occur unless the upper portion of the stellate ganglion or its rami are disturbed, and it is temporary.

Chapter 14

The upper extremity
and
superior mediastinum

This chapter describes only the surgical anatomy and approaches to the arteries of the upper extremity. The common diseases such as injury, emboli, or, more rarely, aneurysm are treated according to the principles discussed in previous chapters.

EXPOSURE OF BRACHIAL ARTERY IN ANTECUBITAL FOSSA

Exploration of the brachial artery and its bifurcation in the antecubital fossa may be necessary after trauma about the elbow joint. Exploration should not be delayed when the signs and symptoms indicate interference with the circulation to the forearm. Delay in decompression of the brachial artery may result in ischemia and irreversible fibrosis in the muscles of the forearm (Volkmann's ischemic contracture).

Exploration and decompression of the brachial artery alone may not restore circulation if distal thrombotic occlusion has taken place. Arteriography prior to or during surgical exploration is helpful. Thrombi are removed by arteriotomy and, if there has been distal propagation, with a small Fogarty balloon catheter or by retrograde flushing via the radial artery at the wrist. Patch angioplasty is essential in small arteries such as the distal brachial (Fig. 57). In these small arteries the best patch is a piece of vein because of its smooth intimal lining and flexibility.

Procedure

1. Place the arm in the outstretched position.

2. Begin the incision on the medial side of the arm about 10 cm. above the elbow. Locate the position of the brachial artery here by palpation of the groove between the biceps muscle and the long head of the triceps muscle. Carry the incision downward to the crease of the antecubital fossa and then across the

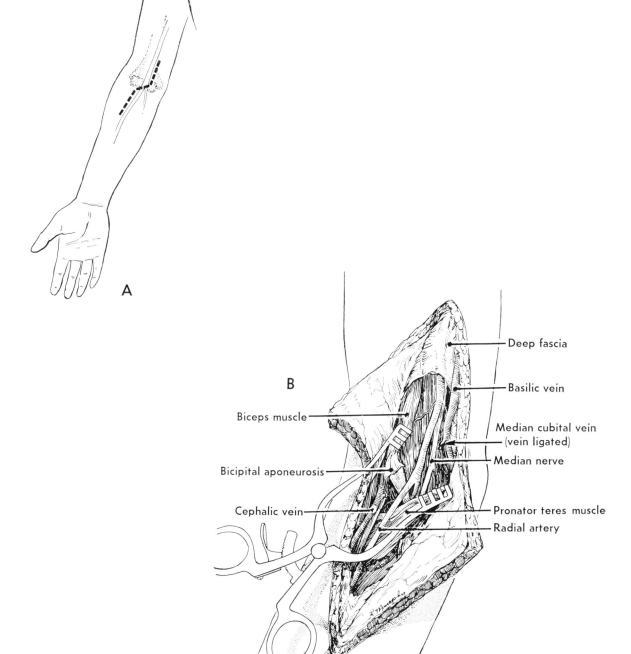

A

B

Deep fascia

Basilic vein

Biceps muscle

Median cubital vein
(vein ligated)

Median nerve

Bicipital aponeurosis

Cephalic vein

Pronator teres muscle

Radial artery

Fig. 72. Exposure of brachial artery in antecubital fossa. **A,** Incision. **B,** Relations of brachial artery.

skin crease to the lateral side of the arm. Now carry the incision again downward and slightly medially, following the medial border of the brachioradialis muscle and other flexors of the forearm. (See Fig. 72, A.)

3. Reflect the skin flaps superiorly and inferiorly.

4. Divide the median cubital vein.

5. Divide the deep fascia over the brachial artery just medial to the biceps muscle. Follow the artery to the midpoint of the antecubital fossa, and divide the thick insertion of the biceps tendon into the deep fascia of the forearm (bicipital aponeurosis) (Fig. 72, B).

6. Reflect the brachioradialis muscle laterally to expose the distal portion of the brachial artery.

EXPOSURE OF BRACHIAL ARTERY IN UPPER ARM
Introduction

A frequent indication for exposure of the brachial artery in the upper arm is retrograde injection for vertebral arteriograms or retrograde catheterization for arteriograms of the aortic arch. The details of retrograde catheterization with the Seldinger technique are given in Chapter 2. The percutaneous route using the brachial artery at the antecubital fossa, is preferable for arteriography.

The brachial artery may be needed for retrograde flushing of propagating thrombus from emboli in the axillary region if balloon catheters are ineffective. Such "tail" thrombus may be removed by inserting a large (No. 15) cannula into the exposed artery and flushing the vessel in a retrograde direction with warm heparinized saline solution (10 mg. or 1,000 units of heparin per 100 ml.).

Anesthesia

Local anesthesia, brachial plexus block, and general anesthesia are all satisfactory.

Procedure

1. Place the arm in the outstretched position with the palm turned upward. If retrograde catheterization of the artery is the purpose of exposure, wide draping should be employed.

2. Identify the groove between the biceps muscle and the long head of the triceps muscle.

3. Make an incision approximately 6 to 8 cm. long (Fig. 73, A) in the midportion of the arm over the groove just identified. Deepen the incision through the skin, subcutaneous tissue, and superficial fascia. When the deep fascia is reached, the brachial artery can be identified by its pulsations (Fig. 73, B).

4. Carefully incise the deep fascia over the groove between the long head of the triceps muscle and the biceps muscle. The basilic vein and medial cutaneous nerve of the arm are retracted posteriorly to expose the artery (Fig. 73, C).

5. If local anesthesia has been employed, identify and infiltrate the median nerve.

6. Dissect carefully around the brachial artery. Exposure is improved by a small self-retaining retractor (Fig. 73, B and C). At about the midportion of the forearm, the median nerve crosses superficial to the brachial artery but is easily

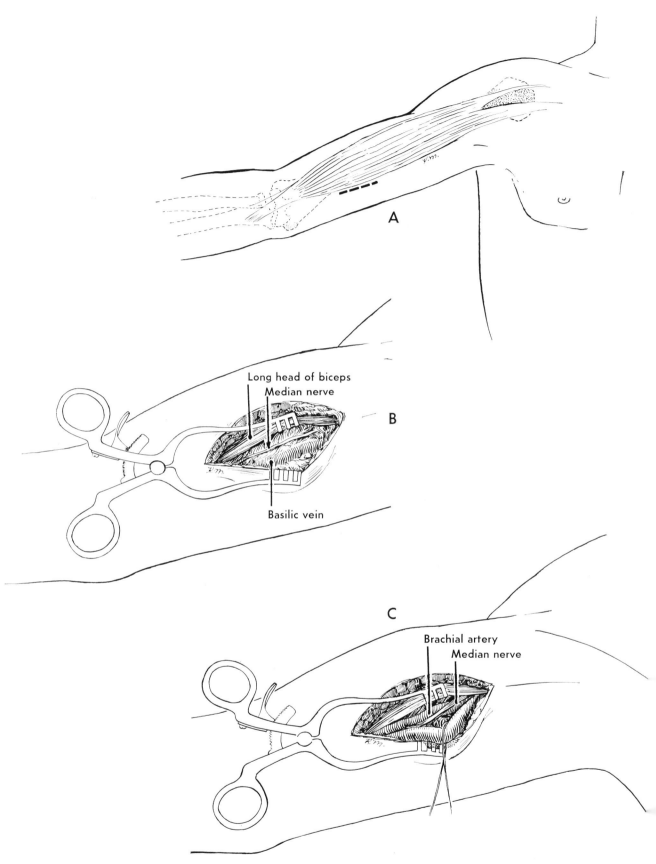

Fig. 73. Exposure of brachial artery in arm. **A,** Incision. **B,** Exposure of neurovascular bundle in midarm. **C,** Exposure of brachial artery in midarm.

retracted anteriorly. Occasionally there is a high division of the brachial artery into two branches, and sometimes the median nerve lies behind the brachial artery.

Discussion

The arteries of the arm seem susceptible to spasm. Therefore unnecessary dissection or excessive stretching should be avoided. Of course, sufficient lengths of artery should be exposed for satisfactory control of bleeding. If the purpose of the operation is insertion of a needle or catheter for arteriography, access to the front of the artery is sufficient and bleeding after withdrawal of the needle is controlled by gentle pressure or perhaps by a single stitch in the adventitia. For arterial injuries, however, proximal and distal control is achieved before approaching the injury and a sufficient length of brachial artery is readily mobilized for end-to-end anastomosis or vein graft reconstruction.

EXPOSURE OF AXILLARY ARTERY
Anesthesia

Because of the proximity of numerous large nerve trunks of the brachial plexus, general anesthesia is recommended.

Procedure

1. Place the arm in an abducted position with the palm upward.

2. Make an incision beginning in the arm along the medial side of the deltoid muscle and extending upward along the deltopectoral groove to the lateral border of the clavicle and along the clavicle for a short distance (Fig. 74, A).

3. Reflect a moderate-sized skin flap in the arm.

4. Incise the insertion of the pectoralis major muscle over the short head of the biceps muscle, and reflect the origin of the pectoralis major muscle medially and inferiorly to bare the contents of the axilla (Fig. 74, B).

5. Usually the tendinous insertion of the pectoralis minor muscle must be divided on the coracoid process. If, at this time, it is necessary to follow the axillary artery into the neck, the midportion of the clavicle is resected subperiosteally with a Gigli saw. The anatomy is amply illustrated in Henry's book.* The clavicle need not be replaced, but the periosteum may be closed loosely and the tendons resutured.

Wide exposure of axillary and subclavian vessels

When extensive exposure of the axillary artery and distal subclavian artery is required, Lexer's approach may be suitable. With this method the incision starts at the midportion of the clavicle, extends medially to the sternoclavicular junction, then downward over the costal cartilages of the second and third ribs, and again laterally toward the apex of the axilla (Fig. 75, A). The clavicle is divided or disarticulated medially and divided in its midportion with the Gigli saw but remains attached. The incision is then deepened through the subcutaneous fascia, the deep fascia, and the pectoralis muscles. The entire flap, including the pectoralis major and minor muscles and the medial one-half to two-thirds of the

---

*Henry, A. K.: Extensile exposure, Baltimore, 1958, Williams & Wilkins Co.

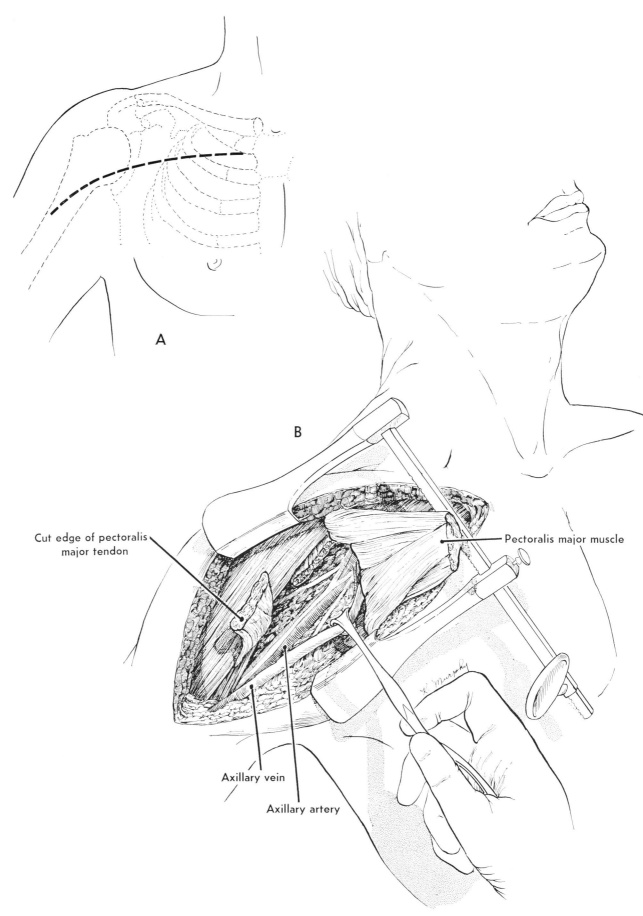

A

B

Cut edge of pectoralis major tendon

Pectoralis major muscle

Axillary vein

Axillary artery

Fig. 74. Exposure of axillary artery. **A,** Incision. **B,** Relations of axillary artery.

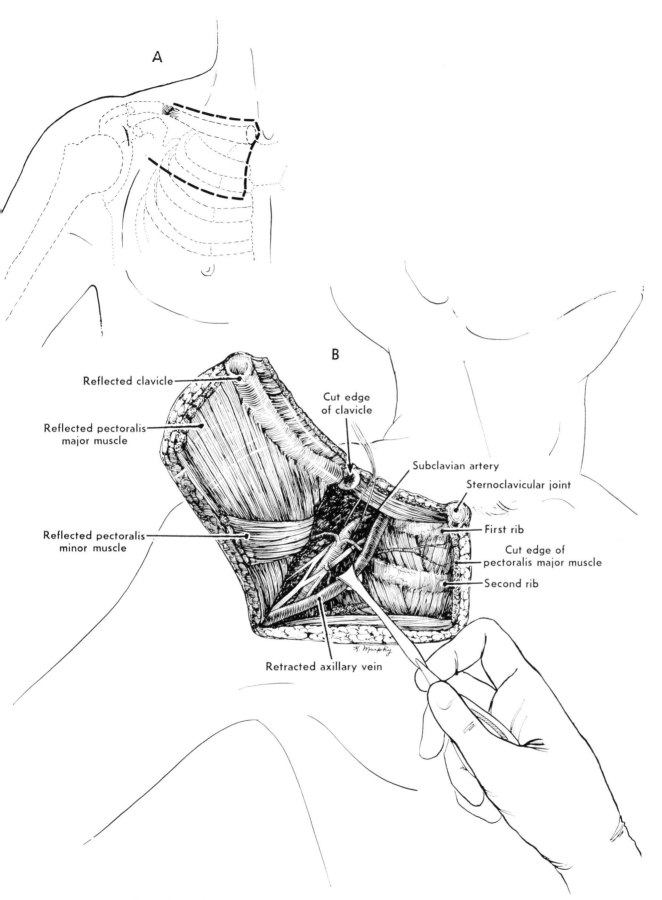

A

B

Reflected clavicle

Reflected pectoralis
major muscle

Reflected pectoralis
minor muscle

Cut edge
of clavicle

Subclavian artery

Sternoclavicular joint

First rib

Cut edge of
pectoralis major muscle

Second rib

Retracted axillary vein

Fig. 75. Wide exposure of axillary and subclavian vessels. **A,** Incision. **B,** Relations of axillary and subclavian arteries.

clavicle, is lifted up and reflected laterally to expose the upper portion of the axillary artery and the subclavian artery (Fig. 74, *B*).

Useful variations are resection of the clavicle, and a short sternum-splitting incision with resection of a portion of the first rib to widen exposure of the subclavian vessels.*

EXPOSURE OF SUPERIOR MEDIASTINUM
Introduction

Splitting the sternum gives access to the superior mediastinum for operations on the innominate artery or the proximal carotid or right subclavian arteries and for operations on the vertebral artery in a person who has a short neck. Arterial injuries, aneurysms, and lacerations of the great veins are rare, but all require surgical treatment.

Proximal control of the origin of the left subclavian artery or of the innominate artery is readily achieved by an anterolateral approach through the third interspace. This incision may be extended easily by splitting the sternum transversely or vertically as needed. Sternal incisions are seldom needed for treating occlusive diseases of the great vessels in the superior mediastinum because the bypass procedure described in Chapter 10 is preferable to endarterectomy.

The following description of the approach must be supplemented by reference to anatomy textbooks.

Procedure

1. Begin the incision at the midpoint of the sternal notch, and continue it vertically downward to the third intercostal space and then laterally through the appropriate intercostal space. Superiorly the incision may follow the upper border of the clavicle or may be extended upward along the sternocleidomastoid muscle in the neck (Fig. 76, *A*) according to the distal exposure needed.

2. Reflect the skin flap laterally.

3. Incise the deep cervical fascia between the sternal heads of the sternocleidomastoid muscles in a transverse direction. Continue this incision to the side and divide the insertions of the sternocleidomastoid muscle. Isolate and divide the sternothyroid and sternohyoid muscles. Beware of the great veins beneath.

4. Separate the contents of the upper mediastinum from the posterior surface of the sternum, using careful blunt dissection.

5. Begin the sternum-splitting incision with the Lebsche knife in the space of Burns. When the third intercostal space has been reached, carry the incision into it in a slanting direction. When necessary, the sternum can be split into the left third interspace also. The sternal closure is more stable if the transverse incision is V shaped (Fig. 76, *A*).

6. When the sternal incision has been made, spread the cut edges of the sternum by inserting a self-retaining sternum retractor (Fig. 76, *B*). For further exposure, divide the clavicle with a Gigli saw and/or divide the ribs attached to the flap. A portion of the first rib may be resected. These procedures allow the sternal edge to be moved farther laterally.

---

*Mannsberger, A. R., and Linberg, E. J.: First rib resection for distal exposure of subclavian vessels, Surg. Gynec. Obst. **120**:578-579, 1965.

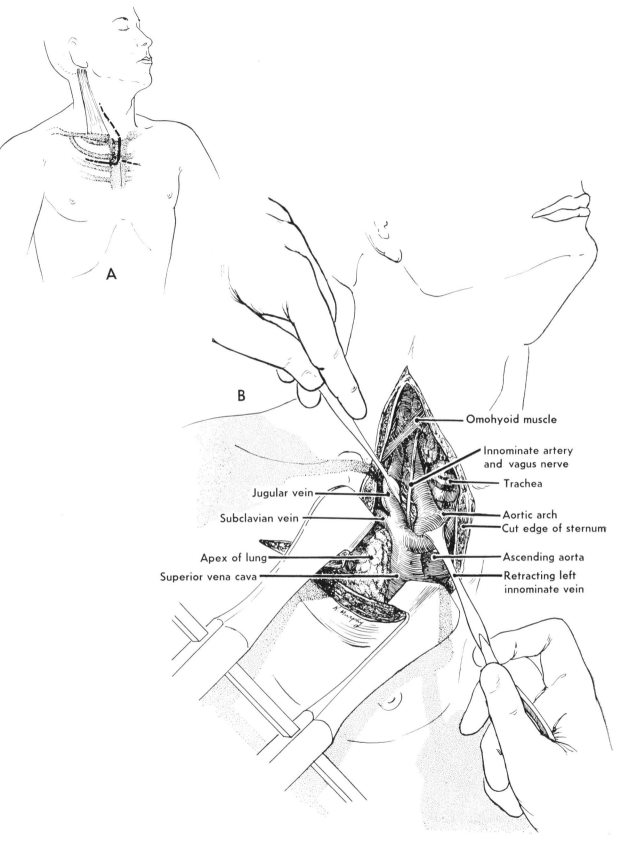

Fig. 76. Exposure of innominate artery. **A,** Incision. **B,** Anatomy of right anterior superior mediastinum.

Omohyoid muscle

Innominate artery and vagus nerve

Trachea

Aortic arch

Cut edge of sternum

Ascending aorta

Retracting left innominate vein

Jugular vein

Subclavian vein

Apex of lung

Superior vena cava

7. After the operation, the sternum must be reapproximated with stainless steel wire because even the stoutest silk may fray and break. The stout needles and attached wires supplied for sternotomy closure are most useful for this.

Comment: *The fourth or even lower interspaces may be used for the lateral limb of the skin and sternum-splitting incisions to obtain lower exposure. If exposure remains difficult, either the first rib or the clavicle, both of which effectively brace the sternum, may be divided as noted previously.*

Chapter 15

Surgery of the veins and thrombophlebitis

DIAGNOSTIC PROCEDURES FOR VARICOSE VEINS

The surgeon must determine if varicosities are secondary to other disease such as deep phlebitis, pregnancy, pelvic tumor, or arteriovenous fistula. The diagnosis is usually made solely on the basis of history and physical examination, although phlebography may be helpful. If the varicosities result from diseases of the deep veins or other causes, the prognosis and treatment are different. Varicosities may accompany multiple congenital arteriovenous fistulas. These are noted in young persons. The varicosities may have an unusual distribution, are often unilateral, and cause the affected limb to grow larger than the normal one. The anomalies may involve skin, muscle, or bone. Port-wine stains or cutaneous nevi are frequent manifestations. Various combinations of these signs and symptoms have various eponyms such as the "Klippel-Trenauney syndrome," etc. We prefer to call these rarities *congenital angiodysplasias* without further subclassification. Multiple tiny arteriovenous fistulas are found.

The vast majority of superficial varicosities of the leg represent the result of dilation and valvular incompetency of the superficial system of veins. The deep veins of the calf or thigh are probably not involved. The condition usually first affects the long saphenous vein and progresses to the short saphenous vein and the communicating veins. The results of adequate operation are excellent.

Postphlebitic syndrome

The patient suffering from the consequences of old phlebitis of the deep veins of the leg usually gives a history of pregnancy, a fracture, or a serious illness. The original episode of acute phlebitis may have been overlooked, and complications are frequently not severe for many years. The symptoms of the postphlebitic syndrome are edema, pigmentation and induration, dermatitis, ulcer, enlarged superficial veins, and congestive leg pain. Recanalization of the acute thromboses usually occurs gradually. Valves may be damaged, however, by less severe attacks of phlebitis, and the final result is valvular incompetence, reflux, and stasis. Superficial veins may dilate early to serve as venous collaterals. Later they may become varicose as pressure is transmitted to the superficial system via incompetent communicating veins.

If the phlebitis is mild, only a few perforating veins may be incompetent, and stasis ulcer may appear without superficial varicosities.

Rarely, occlusion of the deep veins does not recanalize, and the complications of stasis appear early and are unusually troublesome. For such patients, surgical excision of the superficial venous collaterals is useless and even hazardous. Phlebography is necessary for diagnosis.

Physical examination

The physical examination should be conducted in good light with the patient standing erect. Visible varicosities are marked with gentian violet. When the continuation of a vein is not obvious to visual inspection, palpation will usually reveal its location. Nests of varicosities are, as a rule, the wormlike tortuosities of a single vein rather than several veins. The short saphenous vein should always be sought by palpation, since this vein is frequently not visible in the upper one-half or two-thirds of the lower leg.

Incompetency of greater saphenous system

The Brodie-Trendelenburg test is performed to test the function of the venous valves.

1. The patient lies down and elevates the affected leg.
2. A tourniquet is applied high on the thigh.
3. The patient stands.
4. Interpretation is as follows:
    (a) If the varicosities fill rapidly, blood is flowing into them through incompetent communicating veins.
    (b) If the varicosities do not fill within about thirty seconds, release the tourniquet. Sudden filling of the varicosities from the greater saphenous vein above the tourniquet demonstrates that the valves of the greater saphenous system are incompetent and reassures the examiner that there are probably no seriously incompetent communicating veins. Incompetence of some perforating or communicating veins is difficult to localize without cinephlebography.

Incompetent communicators

Incompetent communicating veins are one of the most frequent causes of recurrent varicose veins and are an important cause of stasis dermatitis and ulceration. Most incompetent communicating veins are found below the knee, important locations being just above the ankle, medial and lateral, and at the lower end of the adductor canal. The more advanced the varicose veins have become, the more likely it is that incompetent veins will be communicating between the deep and superficial systems. In some patients the location can be apprehended without a dynamic test by observing a nest of varicosities and palpating a small defect in the deep fascia at the site of perforation. Many of these perforating veins have only a tortuous or indirect superficial communication with the saphenous system. The modified Trendelenburg procedure is the usual test for localizing communicating or perforating veins. Lately we are using phlebograms on most patients. The cinephlebograms visualize and permit marking of the incompetent perforating veins to guide the surgeon.

Modified Trendelenburg procedure

1. Elevate the leg.
2. Apply three torniquets: one below the knee, one just above the knee, and one about the thigh.
3. Have the patient stand.
4. Observe and palpate the filling of the superficial veins and varices. Rarely, all segments will fill independently. First release the most distal tourniquet. If filling that was not previously observed is now noted, the assumption is that the lesser saphenous vein is incompetent. Now release the middle tourniquet. Filling of superficial veins that were previously empty will occur if there are incompetent veins communicating between the deep and superficial systems in the thigh. The purpose of the highest tourniquet is to prevent downward reflux of blood in an incompetent greater saphenous system. By repeating the test and varying the position of the middle tourniquet or by placing a tourniquet around the calf, more precise localization of incompetent perforating veins can be attained.

Perthes' test

Perthes' test is the standard examination to determine the state of deep venous return. It may be difficult to interpret.

1. Collapse the superficial varices with a snugly applied elastic bandage.
2. Have the patient walk for five to thirty minutes.
3. If the patient suffers with increasing discomfort or cramplike pain during the period of exercise, he will not be materially benefited by stripping of the superficial veins.

Modified Perthes' test

A modification of Perthes' test is performed by having the patient elevate the leg and applying a tourniquet around the thigh. The patient is instructed to walk with the tourniquet applied. If the superficial veins collapse and remain empty, it is assumed that deep venous return is adequate. If superficial veins under these conditions remain engorged, the cause may be either obstruction in or reflux from the deep veins via incompetent communicating veins.

Venous pressures

Measurement of venous pressure while the patient walks (walking erect venous pressure) is a quantitative demonstration of the tests just described. It is useful in difficult diagnostic problems. The venous pressure in the saphenous system is measured with a long manometer connected to a Rochester needle or plastic catheter in the saphenous vein or one of its tributaries. Pressures are compared while the patient is standing and walking in the erect position with and without occlusion of the saphenous vein.

When doing venograms, the walking venous pressure is conveniently done through the same vein as the venogram. Actual ambulation is unnecessary, for the patient may perform walking movements of the foot and calf in an almost-upright position on the fluoroscopic table footrest.

By this method the venous pressure in the foot when the patient rests in the erect position is almost identical with the distance from the foot to the right auricle. In normal persons the pressure falls about 50 cm. on walking without saphenous occlusion. In persons with simple varicose veins, the fall in pressure is only 25 cm., but the decrease in pressure is normal while walking with digital or tourniquet occlusion of the saphenous vein. When the valves in the deep veins are incompetent or obstructed, there is little or no fall in the venous pressure while walking, and the pressure may even increase.

The method of measuring venous pressures while the patient walks furnishes physiological data and is useful in evaluating patients who have had deep phlebitis.

Discussion

If varicose veins fill from above only, no further examination is necessary and the surgeon may assume that this is a case of primary varicose veins and that there is no involvement of the deep circulation. If filling is through incompetent veins connecting the deep and superficial systems, an attempt must be made to localize those veins. Normally all flow is from the superficial toward the deep system. Reversal of this flow may or may not be associated with occlusion or incompetency of the deep system. A decision regarding phlebography of the deep veins usually can be reached through consideration of the history. The value of Perthes' test is limited. Phlebography is recommended for all patients with previous phlebitis or previous vein surgery. It reveals perforating veins in unusual locations, permits their ligation with small incisions, and has made the subfascial exploration and ligation of perforators unnecessary.

For the ordinary case of varicose veins, the diagnostic value of numerous dynamic tests has been overemphasized and overrated and the simple procedures of inspection and palpation have not been sufficiently emphasized.

PHLEBOGRAPHY OF LEG
Introduction

Phlebography is needed to visualize the deep veins whose condition can otherwise only be inferred. Phlebography is most useful in distinguishing between obstruction and incompetence of the deep veins of the leg. Injection is usually made into a vein of the foot, and passage of the opaque medium into the superficial veins is prevented by a tourniquet at the ankle. The functional capacity of the valves must be tested by observations of the patient in the semi-erect or erect position. The precise localization of incompetent perforating veins is best revealed by the cinetechnique with television image intensifiers. Phlebography may be used for the more precise diagnosis and localization of acute phlebitis.

Clear visualization of the iliac veins and the inferior vena cava is best obtained by injection of the saphenous or femoral veins at the groin. Obliteration of the iliac veins is frequently noted in postphlebitic syndrome.

The long cassette and the tunnels used for multiple exposures during arteriography are very useful and furnish a map of the deep veins of the leg. The direction of flow and the function of the venous pump mechanism can be observed and recorded in the image amplification techniques with the television monitor and spot films or cinetapes. The newer contrast media such as Conray are safer and less irritating, and complications are rare even during acute phlebitis.

TILTING (ASCENDING) PHLEBOGRAPHY OF LEG

The ascending phlebogram furnishes a map of the deep veins and supplies functional information about the venous pump of the lower leg.

Position and anesthesia

No anesthetic is necessary. Place the patient in a supine position on the tilting fluoroscopic x-ray table with the feet 30 to 40 degrees lower than the head. Place a tourniquet about the ankle. An ordinary piece of rubber tubing or Penrose drain will do.

Choice of site of injection—intracalcaneal or dorsal vein of foot

A dorsal vein on the foot is usually accessible for injection.

The intracalcaneal injection is useful for patients with edema that obscures the foot veins. We used this intraosseous injection in more than fifty patients, but it caused more discomfort and offers no advantages for most patients. Rarely, osteomyelitis has been reported following intraosseous injections.

Technique of intracalcaneal injection

1. With the patient in the supine position, prepare and drape the foot. Inject a dermal wheel of 1% Xylocaine one inch distal to the tip of the *lateral* malleolus and three-fourths of an inch posterior to it. Infiltrate the subcutaneous tissue and periosteum.

2. Introduce a No. 17 Rosenthal needle or a Turkel sternal biopsy needle through the skin and to the periosteum. The needle can then be turned like a drill and advanced into the marrow one-half to three-fourths of an inch.

3. Aspirate blood freely from the marrow. Then inject 3 to 4 ml. of 1% Xylocaine slowly. Inject 5 to 10 ml. of Conray 600 and take one film to ascertain the position of the needle and to be certain there is no extravasation.

4. Tilt the table 40 to 60 degrees from the vertical, with a footrest attached. Take a series of x-ray films or cinephlebograms as described later. Inject slowly over a three- to four-minute period so that pain is not excessive. A tourniquet above the malleolus will be necessary only if there is an incompetent perforator in the foot. To detect other incompetent perforators higher in the leg, the dye must be kept out of the superficial veins by the tourniquet.

5. Withdraw the needle upon completion of the procedure, apply a pressure bandage over the foot with an elastic bandage, and keep the foot elevated for several hours to avoid extravasation.

Technique of intravenous injection

1. Enter any prominent vein on the foot percutaneously or by "cut down" and insert a small catheter or needle connected to a length of plastic tubing and an assembly consisting of two syringes and a three-way stopcock for contrast medium and saline solution (Fig. 10, *H*). Infuse saline solution slowly to keep the needle open.

2. The foot of the table should be 60 degrees lower than the head. The feet rest on the footboard attached to the x-ray table.

3. Inject 40 ml. of Conray 600 slowly during one minute and make the first x-ray exposure. This film will show the veins in the calf and the popliteal area.

4. Prepare another film higher up in the leg. Remove the tourniquet and have the patient raise himself up and down on "tip toes" several times. Make two exposures of the calf and thigh during the next thirty to sixty seconds. A film covering the pelvic region may also be exposed to record the iliac veins. The injection of contrast medium at the groin may be needed to reveal full details of the pelvic and iliac veins.

5. Infuse saline solution to clear the contrast medium from the veins, and tilt the table to the horizontal position.

Technique of venous pressure determination in foot

Determination of venous pressure in the foot may be done in conjunction with phlebography in the leg whenever a vein is cannulated.

Purpose

The procedure is performed to test competence or function of the "venous pump" of the leg and the valves of the superficial veins of the leg.

Indications

Determination of venous pressure in the foot is an excellent physiological demonstration for the students but is seldom needed in clinical practice. The phlebograms reveal the mechanism and sites of reflux and are more useful.

Technique

1. Use the plastic cannula or needle that has been inserted into a foot or leg vein for phlebography.

2. Connect it to a plastic venous pressure monitoring set with manometer tube and infusion bottle.

3. Tape the venous pressure manometer and centimeter ruler to the side of the intravenous stand with the top slightly higher than the level of the heart. It can be lowered if necessary to keep the pressures on the scale.

4. Fill the manometer and tubing while the patient is standing.

5. Open the connection of the manometer to the foot and permit the fluid to rise in the manometer until the level is stationary. Repeat several times and record the pressure as the SVP (standing venous pressure) in centimeters of water. Consider zero to be at the floor level.

6. Measure and record the WVP (walking venous pressure) by having the patient rise up on tiptoes, repeating once per second for ten seconds.

These walking motions may conveniently be done "in place" on the foot board of the tilted fluoroscopic table and do not require actual walking. Measure the decrease in pressure by observing the manometer, and record the decrease as a percentage of the standing venous pressure. Using the percentage instead of the actual decrease in centimeters takes into account automatically the variation that might otherwise be induced into the figures by differences in the patients' heights and/or by the slight slant of the fluoroscopic table.

Interpretation of ascending phlebograms

The ascending phlebogram performed as just described furnishes a map of the veins and some functional information about the "venous pump" of the lower leg.

Normally, superficial veins will be seen easily on the roentgenogram to the height of the tourniquet. Above this level superficial veins should not be visible, since blood flow has been directed into the deep circulation by the tourniquet. The valves of normal communicating veins allow flow into the deep system but not in the reverse direction. Communicating veins may be visualized above the tourniquet. If communicating veins are incompetent, reflux into superficial veins is seen. Retrograde filling of communicating veins as far as the fascia is normal. Occlusion of the deep veins is evident by collateral circulation around the obstructions. Nonvisualization of the anterior tibial veins may result from tight tourniquets at the ankle.

Phlebography assists in locating incompetent perforating veins and ascertains the patency of deep veins. More precise localization of the incompetent perforators is obtained by the cinetechnique described in the next discussion. In phlebograms of good technical quality, saccular dilatations representing the valves of the deep system can be readily discerned. When recanalization of the deep system takes place following deep thrombophlebitis, these valves appear abnormal or are absent from the roentgenogram. Clearing of contrast medium from the leg following repeated contraction of the calf muscles suffices to demonstrate valvular competency below the knee, but the competency of valves in the femoral vein is not so readily demonstrated. Do not, however, rely on radiographic findings without knowing exactly how the procedure was performed. Phlebograms should be performed frequently to learn proper technique and interpretation.

CINEPHLEBOGRAPHY (ASCENDING PHLEBOGRAPHY) WITH IMAGE INTENSIFIER

When a television monitor and facilities are available, cinephlebography is the most satisfactory technique. The observation of the flow and the television tape and spot film records are not possible with other methods. Cinephlebography supplies additional information about the venous pump and the perforating veins. Loose tourniquets or other errors are seen and corrected immediately, and spot films can be repeated to verify doubtful findings.

Preparation of leg in radiological suite

1. The dorsal vein of the foot has been cannulated or the intracalcaneal needle is already in place.

2. Tape lead numerals on the skin of the anterior aspect of the leg 3, 6, 9, 12, and 15 cm. superior to the tip of the lateral malleolus.

3. Tape a lead marker on a cotton ball over the center of any ulcer or indurated area.

4. Incline the table 45 to 60 degrees from the vertical after the footrest is attached. The patient will bear weight on the opposite leg so that the leg being examined can be rotated.

253

Injection of dye and identification of communicating veins

1. Place a Penrose drain tourniquet tightly about the ankle below the malleoli to prevent filling of the superficial veins. If the tourniquet fails to prevent direct filling of the superficial veins, stop the injection and remove the unwanted dye by exercise or elevation of the leg. Reapply the tourniquet more tightly and continue the injection. It may be necessary to reapply the tourniquet just above the malleolus or at the top of an ulcer.

2. Inject Conray 600 at a rate as slow as 5 to 10 ml. per minute.

Comment: Avoid overfilling of the superficial veins in the early part of the examination. Otherwise superimposition of many superficial veins confuses the identification of deep veins.

3. View the contrast material flowing in the deep veins by observing the television monitor, and govern the volume and rate of injection by the abnormalities observed. Watch for retrograde flow from the deep into the superficial veins via the communicating veins.

Comment: Normal communicating veins may fill at rest. The communicating veins are abnormal only when retrograde flow into the superficial veins is observed. This is revealed by the cine technique. Series of static films at intervals are incomplete records of the flow. Start the cine recording early at 7.5 or 15 frames per second. Some take as much as 60 feet of film per patient.

4. Rotate the leg internally and externally so that any opacified superficial veins do not overlie the deep veins and may be more readily distinguished.

Comment: Sometimes transverse or circumferential skin veins appear to connect the deep and superficial systems, but rotation of the leg identifies these readily. The deep veins are displaced very little during rotation of the leg. By referring to the anterior lead markers, posterior veins are readily distinguished because they move in the opposite direction during rotation.

5. Mark on the skin with a radiopaque ballpoint pen the location of any incompetent communicating vein. The films during rotation of the leg show that the vein and the tip of the pen coincide, and pressure with the tip of the pen partially empties the vein being marked.

6. Take spot films for reference in the operating room. The level of each perforator is seen on the films because of the lead markers. Fill the deep veins slowly but adequately so as not to overlook any incompetent perforators.

Comment: Note if deep veins are obliterated. The anterior tibial vein may not fill readily and another tourniquet below the knee may be needed to be certain that nonvisualization means occlusion.

7. When dye is plainly visible in the popliteal and femoral veins, inspect these for the presence of valves. To fill all the veins, 50 ml. of Conray 600 may be needed. *Test the function of the valves of the deep system.*

8. Remove the tourniquet and have the patient stand on tiptoes five to ten times and observe the clearing of dye from the leg and film it. The cine is still running.

Comment: When the deep veins are normal, the dye moves upward rapidly and clears in a few minutes. Several abnormalities of flow may be noted:

(a) The normal veins empty, but dye remains pooled in varicosities.

(b) Dye may move up the leg with exercise but reflux down again when muscle contraction stops. The Valsalva maneuver may force dye back down the popliteal or femoral vein.

(c) Reflux into the superficial system at rest may be followed by flow from the superficial to the deep system during exercise.

Interpretation of cinephlebograms

As in all phlebograms, good technique is essential. The main advantage to the surgeon is the identification of the perforating or communicating veins and detection of incompetence of their valves. Incompetent perforators should be ligated. The tourniquet test of Trendelenburg does not localize these veins as well as the films.

The location of indirect perforating veins is quite variable. The direct perforating veins described by Cockett are fairly constant, but there may be others, particularly if the leg has been operated on before. The lowest perforator medially is posterior to the malleolus, and if it is incompetent the tourniquet may have to be placed above the malleoli to prevent flooding of the superficial system via this lowest perforator.

Perforating veins causing stasis or reflux are also noted far above the area of the induration or ulceration. Dye may be observed flowing up the deep veins out the perforator and down the superficial vein toward the ulcer. With the use of the cinetechnique, the localization of incompetent perforators will not require the exploratory long incision in the fascia and subfascial ligation procedures of Cockett or of Linton.

STRIPPING OPERATION FOR VARICOSE VEINS
Completeness of operation

The operation described has supplanted previous techniques. Removal of the varices prevents stasis, relieves symptoms, and improves the appearance of the leg. Varicosities may recur after incomplete operations or because an underlying disease is not recognized and treated. For example, varicosities may develop or recur in tributaries of untreated, incompetent perforating veins.

Varicosities of the lesser saphenous system are difficult to detect but often appear within a few years unless these veins are stripped also. Overlooking a tributary in the groin or an accessory saphenous vein is a preventable cause of recurrence.

Deep phlebitis with incompetence of the deep veins does not contraindicate removal of the superficial varices for cosmetic and functional reasons. Obstruction in the deep system, however, contraindicates removal of the superficial veins, which can be regarded as collateral circulation. With or without stripping, patients with deep phlebitis require lifelong attention to prevent edema of the leg. In difficult cases, support with a pneumatic boot is advised.

Preoperative care

When there is ulceration, marked swelling, induration, or dermatitis, a preliminary period of bed rest is desirable. Great improvement will follow bed rest and adequate elastic support of the limb. Disappearance of the dermatitis and edema and healing of small ulcers before operation improve postsurgical healing and prevent many complications.

Choice of procedure

The most complete procedure is the best procedure. Adequate operation includes the following:

1. Ligation of the greater saphenous vein at its entrance into the femoral vein with interruption and ligation of all tributaries near the fossa ovalis
2. Stripping of the greater and lesser saphenous system
3. Local ligation or interruption of incompetent communicating veins
4. Local excision of large nests of varicosities through which the stripper cannot be passed

Anesthesia

Spinal or general anesthesia is suitable.

Other preparations

On the evening preceding the operation, examine the patient in the erect position. Mark visible and palpable veins of the long and short saphenous systems and other large varicosities with gentian violet or ferric chloride–pyrogallic acid solution or by superficial scratches. Instruct the patient to scrub thoroughly with antiseptic soap such as pHisoHex. Blot the legs dry without rinsing to leave an antiseptic film on the skin.

Procedure

High ligation of great saphenous vein

1. Place the patient in the supine position.

2. Suspend the leg so that the leg and foot can be cleansed and prepared completely.

3. Drape the legs so that they may be lifted or flexed at the knee.

4. Make the groin incision about 10 cm. long, parallel to the inguinal ligament, with about one-third of the incision lateral and two-thirds medial to the fossa ovalis. This incision should be relatively high and should extend far enough medially to locate an anomalous external pudendal vein entering the medial superficial femoral vein (Fig. 77, A). The medial superficial femoral vein is usually a branch or continuation of the lesser saphenous vein in the medial side of the thigh and is also known as the medial accessory saphenous vein.

5. Deepen the incision through the subcutaneous fat and the subcutaneous fascia. This fascia is the first landmark. Any of the tributaries beneath the fascia lead to the greater saphenous vein. Do not search for the vein until the superficial fascia has been incised.

6. Pass a heavy suture or tape under the vein and place a small, self-retaining retractor to separate the incision. Follow the saphenous vein upward, and as branches are encountered, carefully free, ligate, and divide them. The number of tributaries may vary from a few to six, seven, or eight.

7. Lift the saphenous vein sufficiently to tent up the saphenofemoral junction slightly. Enlarge the fossa ovalis by incision of the femoral sheath 2 cm. superiorly and inferiorly. Identify the common femoral vein and ascertain that there are no additional subcutaneous tributaries entering the saphenous or femoral veins.

8. Ligate the saphenous vein flush with the femoral vein with a heavy silk ligature, followed by a transfixion suture. Divide the saphenous vein from the femoral vein, irrigate, and cover the incision.

256

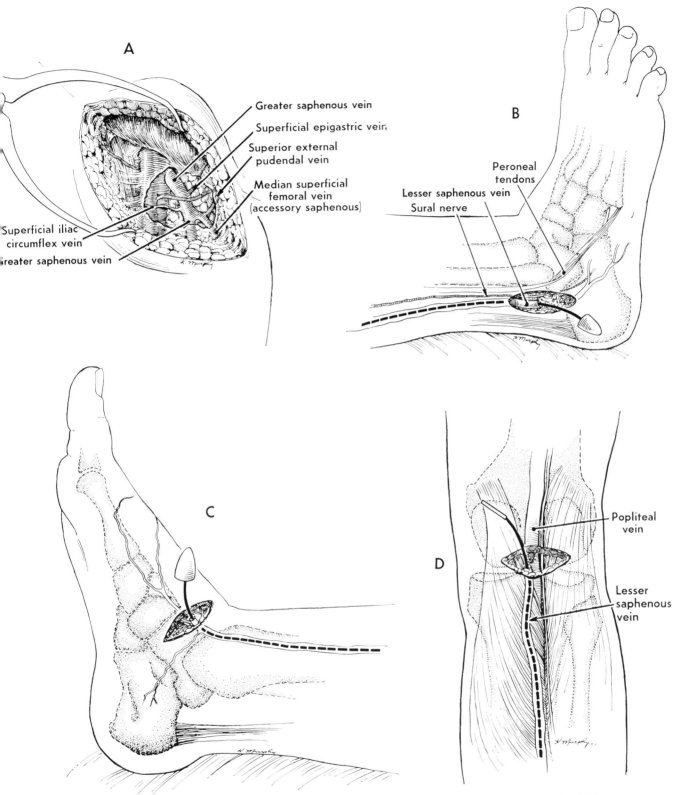

A

Greater saphenous vein
Superficial epigastric vein
Superior external
pudendal vein
Median superficial
femoral vein
(accessory saphenous)

Superficial iliac
circumflex vein
Greater saphenous vein

B

Peroneal
tendons
Lesser saphenous vein
Sural nerve

C

D

Popliteal
vein

Lesser
saphenous
vein

Fig. 77. Stripping operation for varicose veins. **A,** Groin incision and exposure for high ligation of greater saphenous veins. **B,** Ankle incision and exposure for stripping of lesser saphenous vein. **C,** Foot incision and exposure for stripping of greater saphenous vein. **D,** Popliteal incision and exposure for ligation and stripping of lesser saphenous vein.

Continued.

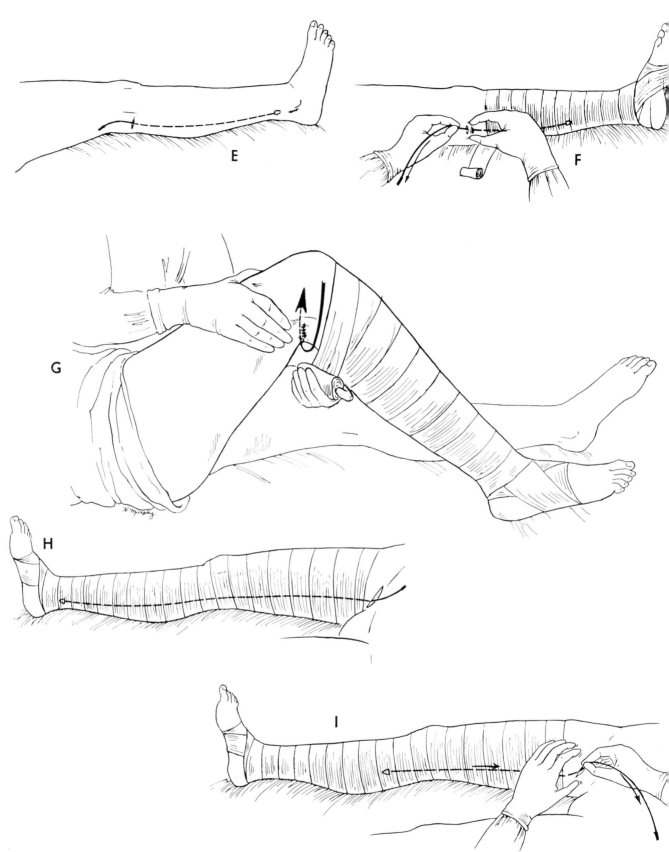

Fig. 77, cont'd. Stripping operation for varicose veins. **E,** Vein strippers in place and incisions closed below knee. **F,** Lower leg wrapped and stripper withdrawn from lesser saphenous vein. **G** and **H,** Entire leg wrapped. All incisions closed below groin. **I,** Stripper withdrawn from greater saphenous vein.

Stripping of long and short saphenous veins

1. Make an incision anterior to and just below the medial malleolus (Fig. 77, *C*). Isolate the greater saphenous vein. If the vein is prominent on the dorsum of the foot, it may be identified and stripped from there. Tie the vein distally with 2-0 or 3-0 chromic catgut, divide it, and pass the flexible intraluminal stripper upward through the veins. In many patients the stripper reaches the groin at once. However, sometimes the stripper is arrested by large and tortuous varicosities and accessory incisions are necessary. Through the accessory incision a perforating vein may often be found and ligated, and the same or another stripper can be passed up the rest of the saphenous vein to the groin.

2. The lesser saphenous vein is approached by tilting the table, flexing the knee, and rotating the thigh. It is cumbersome and unnecessary to turn the patient unless prominent popliteal varicosities require wider exposure.

3. Make an incision just behind the lateral malleolus (Fig. 77, *B*). The lesser saphenous vein is located in the groove between the tendo Achillis posteriorly and the tendons of the peroneus longus and brevis anteriorly. The sural nerve lies deep to the vein. Divide the vein and ligate it distally with fine catgut. There are numerous tributaries that should also be ligated.

4. Pass the stripper upward to the popliteal fossa and palpate with the knee flexed. Keep in mind the following anatomical variations of the lesser saphenous system if the stripper follows an unusual course:

   (a) The lesser saphenous vein may penetrate the deep fascia in the midcalf.

   (b) The lesser saphenous vein penetrates the deep fascia in the popliteal fossa, and a branch of varying size (accessory saphenous) ascends into the medial portion of the thigh.

   (c) The lesser saphenous vein may continue beyond the popliteal fossa into the medial thigh, joining the greater saphenous system at a higher level. There is a communicating branch to the popliteal vein in the popliteal fossa.

5. With the thigh and knee flexed and the thigh externally rotated, make a small incision in the popliteal fossa (Fig. 77, *D*). A sitting position is advantageous for the surgeon. Palpate the stripper. Ligate and divide either the lesser saphenous vein or its branch entering the popliteal vein at this site.

Comment: *Longer popliteal incisions are necessary in patients with many popliteal tributaries and large lesser saphenous varices. The longer incision permits meticulous ligation and interruption of these tributaries in the popliteal fossa. If the long popliteal incision is necessary, the legs should be draped so that the patient can be turned on his side. Annoying herniation of fat will occur unless the popliteal fascia is carefully closed.*

6. Excise any large nests of varicose veins locally. Ligate any previously located incompetent perforating or communicating veins. Below the knee all ligations should be accomplished with fine chromic catgut. Close these incisions.

7. Place the appropriate-sized olive tips on the distal ends of the vein strippers. Start them under the skin for a short distance (Fig. 77, *E*). Close the distal incisions. Apply sterile dressings and pad the ankle, dorsum of the foot, and subcutaneous edge of the tibia. Wrap the leg with a sterile foam rubber–coated elastic bandage or with a sterile self-adherent ("Peg"*) elastic bandage (Fig. 77, *F*).

---

*Becton-Dickinson & Co., Rutherford, N. J.

Withdraw the stripper from the lesser saphenous vein and close the popliteal incision (Fig. 77, G) when the wrapping has reached the knee.

8. Wrap the remainder of the leg so that the compression dressing is in place when the stripper is withdrawn at the groin—this reduces extravasation, swelling, and hematoma formation. Protect the knee with padding. Continue wrapping the leg with the elastic bandages until other incisions or the groin is reached (Fig. 77, H). Withdraw the strippers (Fig. 77, I), closing and dressing incisions as the wrapping proceeds.

The lower leg and ankle incisions, as well as the patella, Achilles tendon, and front of the foot, should be padded.

The elastic foam rubber and the self-adhering elastic bandages do not slip or wrinkle easily and minimize postoperative hematoma, swelling, and discomfort.

9. Close the groin incision in layers, using catgut for the subcutaneous fascia.

Comment: *The following method is expeditious when there are several assistants to work on both legs simultaneously.*

Place the appropriate-sized olive tip on the proximal end of the strippers and withdraw under the skin a short distance.

The surgical team simultaneously closes all incisions except at the ankle, where the ends of the strippers emerge. Place skin stitches in these ankle incisions but do not tie them until the legs are wrapped and the strippers are withdrawn.

Apply sterile dressings and pad all pressure points so that the leg can be wrapped snug with sterile elastic bandages. Use the 6-inch width to wrap the thigh and knee after the patella is padded. Use the 4-inch bandage to wrap the lower leg to the ankle after the tibia and Achilles tendon are padded.

Withdraw the strippers at the ankle. Tie the stitches previously placed. Then pad the dorsum of the foot and continue the bandage down over the ankle and foot.

Postoperative care

The following day, the patient should walk five minutes every hour. Sitting is not allowed. When not walking, the patient must lie in bed with the foot of the bed elevated.

Groin sutures are removed in one week. However, incisions lower in the leg, particularly if made through edematous and pigmented skin, may heal more slowly. Elastic bandages or elastic stockings are worn until edema and discomfort have ceased.

Foam rubber–lined or self-adhering elastic bandages provide better support than ordinary elastic bandages because they do not slip. In wrapping the foam rubber–lined bandage, care must be taken to avoid excessive tension. These bandages may easily be applied too tightly by those accustomed to applying stretchable cotton bandages. Because of the degree of pressure exerted, padding, as indicated in the preceding description, is essential beneath the bandage.

Complications

The most common complication of vein stripping is hematoma. External pressure obtained by wrapping the legs prior to stripping, as previously described, prevents troublesome subcutaneous hemorrhage.

Deep phlebitis is relatively rare if the postoperative regimen of early and frequent ambulation, snug wrapping, and elevation of the legs is followed. For the first few postoperative weeks, the patient is cautioned against long periods of sitting with the legs in a dependent position.

Complications in the groin incision are unusual. Careful preoperative cleansing, hemostasis, irrigation, and careful closure of the incision in layers prevent the collections of serum and lymph that predispose to infection.

RESIDUAL VARICOSITIES

Women who desire treatment of varicose veins for cosmetic purposes frequently desire further eradication of smaller veins that are not removed at a stripping operation. They may be eradicated by an electrocautery instrument.* In the electrocautery method, the instrument is introduced under the skin through a small incision. Cautery is applied to the undersurface of the vein, not to the skin. This method is applicable only to small veins and must not be used on the major veins of the leg. Small residual veins may be segmentally and carefully injected.

ELECTROFULGURATION OF VARICOSE VEINS

Purpose

Electrofulguration is used to obliterate small varicosities and small perforating veins, thus avoiding multiple incisions.

Principle

Both saphenous trunks are stripped and large perforators are ligated by the usual method. The remaining smaller veins can be reached and fulgurated with the special probe* through a few tiny stab incisions.

Procedure

1. The vein strippers are in place. The veins and perforators have been marked. The patient is in the Trendelenburg position so the veins are empty, and all veins to be obliterated by this method must therefore be carefully marked in advance.

2. Choose the site of the incisions so that the probe can be passed in several directions to reach the veins. Make a small stab incision with a No. 11 blade to pass the 11-gauge fulgurating probe beneath the skin. The incision should be at least 2 inches from the first point of electrocoagulation.

3. Pass the electrode subcutaneously along the vein and coagulate the vein at 1 cm. distances by pressing the trigger on the probe handle. Depress the handle so that the tip of the probe elevates the skin slightly.

Comment: *The duration of current is preset for 0.7 second. Set the current output at 8.5 for the larger electrode and 3 for the smaller electrode. There will be an audible sound with each "shot." The tip of the probe must not be too superficial or a blister and small burn will appear. Use caution in coagulating veins overlying bone, since periosteal and cortical bone necrosis may result when the tip of the probe is too close to the bone.*

---

*Vein Eraser, Medtronic Inc., Minneapolis, Minn.

4. The smaller electrode (16-gauge) is used where the skin and subcutaneous tissue are thin (for example, on the feet or popliteal area, over bone, at the ankle, and over the tibia) and also for the cosmetic eradication of small intradermal angiectases or venules. The generator output is set at 3.0.

5. The stripping is completed as previously described. The fulguration incisions need no closure.

6. Postoperative care is the same as that given following stripping. An occasional blister or burn needs no special treatment, but the small eschar may persist several weeks. If a few veins remain they may be fulgurated under local anesthesia on an outpatient basis. Fulguration is far superior to the sclerosing injections formerly used for this purpose.

Some numbness or paresthesia may occur and remain several months. However such peripheral neuritis is not troublesome.

SUBFASCIAL LIGATION OF COMMUNICATING VEINS

A small proportion of patients with numerous varicose veins and many incompetent perforating veins require a more extensive incision with ligation of the perforating veins beneath the deep fascia. These patients have usually had previous operations, recurrent varicosities, and ulceration from old thrombophlebitis. The advantages of subfascial ligation are better visualization of the perforating veins and better healing of the skin than after multiple incisions or more superficial skin flaps. Some of the patients will have had many previous incomplete operations. Phlebography is indicated to ensure patency of the deep veins of the calf before subfascial ligation is performed. Cinephlebography permits marking the incompetent perforating veins before operation.

The use of cinefluoroscopy can eliminate the need for this extensive procedure, which should be reserved only for patients with severe recurrent varicose veins and ulceration.

Anatomy

Communicating veins connect the superficial and deep systems of veins in the legs. The usual sites of penetration of the deep fascia are (1) just medial to the subcutaneous border of the tibia, connecting to the long saphenous system, (2) the calf on the posterolateral aspect of the leg, and (3) the anterior portion of the calf just lateral to the anterior tibial muscle.

Preoperative preparation

Bed rest with elevation of the leg, skin grafts, and preliminary vein stripping must all be employed as indicated, so that cellulitis, dermatitis, and ulceration have either healed or improved greatly before subfascial ligation is undertaken. For details of the stripping procedure, refer to pp. 255-260. For skin grafting, refer to pp. 264 and 265.

Procedure

1. Prepare and drape the leg so that the thigh and knee can be flexed.

2. Make a longitudinal incision along the course of the long saphenous vein from just below the knee toward the medial malleolus. Incise the fascia in a longitudinal direction slightly anterior to the greater saphenous vein.

3. Elevate the anterior flap of skin, subcutaneous tissue, and fascia to the edge of the tibia.

4. Ligate and divide all veins penetrating the fascia.

5. Elevate the posterior flap of skin, subcutaneous fat, and fascia as far as the midline posteriorly, and ligate all other veins penetrating the fascia.

6. If it still remains, identify the subfascial portion of the lesser saphenous vein in the popliteal fossa. Ligate this vein near the popliteal vein. The anatomical variations of the lesser saphenous vein have been reviewed in the preceding pages.

7. Identify the sural nerve as it accompanies the lesser saphenous vein and penetrates the deep fascia somewhat lower than the vein. Incise the deep fascia on both sides of the lesser saphenous vein. Exposure is obtained by flexing the knee and retracting the calf muscles. Remove a strip of fascia 0.5 to 1 inch wide from the popliteal space well down the posterior aspect of the calf. The strip may be narrowed toward the ankle.

Comment: *The purpose of fasciectomy is to remove a possible barrier to future development of communication between the deep and superficial lymphatic vessels of the leg. If lymphatic drainage does not seem to be a problem, it is probably better to allow the fascia to remain intact. The envelope of deep fascia about the calf muscles is an integral part of the venous pumping mechanism of the leg. It has been suggested that when the fascia is loose, indeed, that venous return may be restored by tightening the fascial compartments, but we have had no experience with the procedure. Firm elastic support should accomplish the same end.*

8. Complete any stripping, local excisions, etc. that have been done. Close the medial incision in the deep fascia with 3-0 chromic catgut. Close the skin incision with nonabsorbable suture material. Splint the foot, ankle, and leg with a well-padded compression dressing.

Distal subfascial ligation of communicating veins

Ulcers superior to one or both malleoli may be fed by incompetent perforating veins just above the malleoli, but in some cases the cinephlebograms show reflux from incompetent perforating veins higher up in the leg or on the opposite side of the leg. Sometimes superficial varicosities are minimal. These perforating veins may be interrupted and ligated beneath the fascia so as to avoid undermining indurated skin.

1. Make a longitudinal incision 1 inch posterior and parallel to the posterior border of the tibia. The incision starts 1 to 1½ inches above the medial malleolus and 1 inch posterior to it. The medial incision must be slightly longer.

2. Divide the deep fascia.

3. Identify the perforating veins beneath the deep fascia. With small ulcers there are usually only two or three perforating veins. Incompetent perforators are larger than normal veins and may be 3 to 10 mm. in diameter.

4. Divide and ligate these veins.

5. Close the fascia and skin with interrupted sutures.

6. Elevate the leg and apply snug elastic dressing from toes to knee.

Comment: *This operation is most suitable for small ulcers, particularly if there are no superficial varicosities. In such patients stripping of the superficial* *veins or the more radical excision and grafting are unnecessary. Occasionally stasis ulcers anterior to the lateral malleolus are fed by veins that course inferior to the malleolus and enter the lesser saphenous system posterior to the lateral malleolus. Cinephlebography using the image intensifier and repeated small injections of contrast medium are extremely useful in locating these veins. See technique on pp. 251-255. When the offending perforating veins are precisely located and marked in this manner, subfascial exploration is unnecessary.*

Postoperative care

Healing tends to be prolonged and indolent. Keep the leg elevated for seven to ten days, changing the dressing when necessary. Walking and weight bearing are allowed when the incisions are well healed and the limb is not edematous. A stout knee-length, open-toe, closed-heel elastic stocking is worn for six to twelve months after the operation.

EXCISION AND GRAFTING OF STASIS ULCER
Indications

Ulcers that cannot be healed by more conservative measures should be excised and grafted. A preliminary period of bed rest, lasting for several weeks, with elevation of the legs and frequent dressings, helps to clear local infection, relieve edema, and ensure rapid healing. Many ulcers can be healed by a regimen of conservative treatment consisting of bed rest followed by external elastic support.

When stasis in superficial varicosities is the main etiological factor, the veins should be stripped. If there has been a previous stripping, it is likely that incompetent communicating veins have been overlooked. Excision of the ulcer may reveal underlying veins and permits their ligation and interruption. A search for other incompetent perforators should also be made (see p. 263). The fascia beneath the ulcer is also affected by stasis and must frequently be removed to furnish a healthy bed for the skin graft.

Differential diagnosis

Other types of leg ulcers must be considered in differential diagnosis, including the ulcers associated with arteriosclerosis, blood dyscrasias, hypertensive ischemic ulcer, and leg ulcers associated with rheumatoid arthritis and erythrocyanosis. Carcinoma may develop in chronic stasis ulcers.

Anesthesia

Local anesthesia, spinal anesthesia, or general anesthesia may be employed.

Procedure

1. Prepare the entire leg on the affected side or both legs if the procedure is to be bilateral.

2. Drape the leg. Remove a split-thickness skin graft from the lateral thigh, where the skin is somewhat thicker. This should be taken with the dermatome set at 0.015 to 0.02 inch. Dress the donor site. Preserve the graft in a sponge dampened with Ringer's solution.

3. Outline the area on the leg to be excised with gentian violet or some similar marking fluid. The extent of excision is determined not by the area of

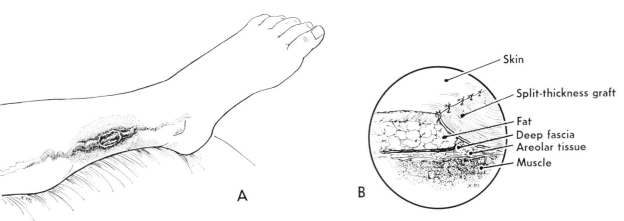

Fig. 78. Excision and grafting of stasis ulcer. **A,** Stasis ulcer above medial malleolus. **B,** Cross section of edge after excision and graft of stasis ulcer.

ulceration alone but by the amount of induration and dermatitis still surrounding the ulcer after a period of elevation or elastic support. Lymphatic vessels have not regenerated in indurated areas. Such areas must be excised. Otherwise, edema will prevent satisfactory "take" of the graft. The incision may be made through pigmented skin but not through the indurated area. (See Fig. 78, *A*).

4. Incise down to and through the deep fascia. The skin may be beveled. Along with the skin, remove the deep fascia. The bed for the graft is the areolar tissue overlying the periosteum and muscle. Do not follow fascia into the muscle septa.

5. Ligate the perforating veins as they are exposed.

6. Apply the split-thickness graft. Sew the edges of the graft to the fresh skin edges (Fig. 78, *B*). Interrupted or continuous sutures are suitable for this procedure. Do not allow the graft to overlap normal skin. Instead, try to secure edge-to-edge contact of skin and skin graft (Fig. 78, *B*). Make a few small holes in the graft to allow drainage of any serum that may accumulate beneath it.

7. Cover the graft with Xeroform or petrolatum gauze, topped by a generous bulky pressure dressing of machinist's waste. Apply an elastic bandage. A splint for the foot may be needed.

Postoperative care

The leg must not be dependent at any time during the immediate postoperative period. If it is, the skin graft will not adhere. Bed rest must be encouraged for the first ten to fourteen days.

Dress the wound on the fifth day or before. Remove the old dressing carefully so as not to disturb the graft. Trim any dead skin at the edge of the graft. At the first dressing some areas of the graft will appear pink and healthy, whereas others may be darkly colored. Darkly colored areas should not be removed, since they are usually viable. The superficial layers of skin will peel off—a condition that should not be mistaken for death or loss of the graft. Make a tiny hole in the graft over any small blister or accumulation of blood or fluid that may have appeared. Reapply a bulky pressure dressing. Remove the sutures between seven and ten days.

After the initial period of bed rest for seven to ten days and after take of the

265

graft seems ensured, observe the appearance of the graft while the leg is dependent. Allow ambulation for five to ten minutes each hour, but only with strong elastic support. Gradually increase the periods of dependency and increase ambulation. The patient must wear an elastic support and must have careful supervision for three months or until there is no edema in the limb. In patients with venous obstruction, lymphatic obstruction, or severe edema, the "Aeropulse" pneumatic legging* may control edema and maintain healing of the graft when all other forms of elastic support fail.

THROMBOPHLEBITIS

Thrombophlebitis may involve the superficial or the deep veins or both. If the superficial veins are involved, the diagnosis is obvious. In the deep veins of the calf, the diagnosis of thrombophlebitis is usually not difficult. The onset and initial symptoms may, however, be insidious and the clinical manifestations may be so mild as to pass unnoticed. Indeed, the first manifestation can be pulmonary embolism.

The physician must be watchful and suspicious of fever, pain, or discomfort in the legs of patients during early postoperative periods or in patients with fractures or other illnesses or injuries requiring bed rest. Slight distention of the pretibial vein, slight cyanosis, or edema may develop when the clots become obstructive. Pain and tenderness appear when the thrombosis excites inflammation or vasospasm. Homan's sign is helpful in differentiating deep phlebitis and other causes of calf tenderness. Phlebograms frequently show that clots are more extensive than suspected.

Saphenous phlebitis

Although minor episodes are managed conservatively, extensive saphenous phlebitis can be quickly cured by excision of the affected vein. Conservative treatment is prolonged and is followed by recurrence and varicosities.

When the patient has had varicosities prior to the attack of phlebitis, high ligation of the saphenous vein, together with excision of the thrombosed segment, should be performed. Supplementary stripping can be performed later if necessary. The saphenous vein should be opened before the ligation because unsuspected thrombus may be present and should be removed with the techniques and precautions described for iliofemoral thrombectomy. Anticoagulants are unnecessary. Ambulation is begun the day after operation, and postoperative care is the same as for elective stripping of varicose veins. Incisions for removal of the inflamed and clotted saphenous vein may be quite long, but the period of disability is short.

Septic thrombophlebitis

Infected clots cause septicemia and metastatic abscesses to the lungs, brain, liver, or other organs. Septic thrombophlebitis is uncommon but may result from inlying plastic catheters, pelvic inflammatory disease, etc. The treatment is ligation of the veins and appropriate antibiotics. Anticoagulants are no substitute for venous interruption in the treatment of septic thrombophlebitis.

---

*Surgical Research Corporation, 703 N. Lakeshore Drive, Barrington, Ill. 60010.

Conservative management of deep phlebitis

The following measures are beneficial to patients with acute deep phlebitis:

1. Elevate the foot of the bed. Phlebograms show that this prevents venous stasis in the small pockets just behind the valves of the deep veins.

2. Begin anticoagulation therapy. Heparin is preferable for the first few days. Dosage of anticoagulants should be guided by coagulation times or prothrombin times. Heparin may be administered intramuscularly or intravenously via inlying plastic cannulas with rubber caps or Teflon needles with flexible plastic obturators. The adult dose is 50 mg. every four to six hours.

3. Maintain bed rest. This prevents edema, congestion, and stasis. Loosely attached thrombi are less likely to dislodge.

4. Apply a hot pack to the leg. Application of heat as hot wet packs enhances blood flow in the extremity and helps prevent the extension of thrombosis. Ambulation has been advocated to achieve this same result but is undesirable for patients with pain or edema. Elastic bandages are applied to divert venous return into the deep system after hot packs are discontinued.

5. Vigilant and frequent observation is essential. Small emboli may give no sign except a simultaneous rise in pulse, temperature, and respiration (Allen's sign). Pleuritic pain, chest pain, cough, and hemoptysis mean pulmonary infarction.

Discussion

Conservative treatment has failed if pulmonary embolism occurs. Embolism may occur despite improvement of the legs. In such situations, interruption of the superficial femoral vein, common femoral vein, or the inferior vena cava must be considered.

Techniques for enzymatic dissolution of clots are under investigation and may be practicable in the future.

Currently the status of dextran in the treatment of phlebitis is under investigation. Those products currently available commercially with molecular weights of about 70,000 have a modifying influence on blood clotting and may be given to patients with phlebitis. Thrombolytic properties have been claimed for dextran of lower molecular weight, not commercially available. However, the use of dextran, which alters the physical and flow properties of blood, is no substitute for the treatment, particularly adequate heparinization outlined previously.

We routinely advise a low-fat diet because of the effect on coagulation of small fat globules in the bloodstream.

Bypass operation for venous obliteration

When permanent common femoral or iliac vein occlusion has occurred, some relief can be obtained surgically by mobilizing the saphenous vein in the opposite leg and bringing it subcutaneously to the affected femoral vein below the site of obstruction, where it is anastomosed and will now function as a cross-leg femorosaphenous vein bypass. Since the ulceration that follows deep phlebitis frequently takes years to appear, some time must pass before the long-term end results of this new procedure are evident. As criteria for the operation, we recommend edema and/or discomfort of the affected limb persisting for over six months and radiographic evidence of competent unaffected valves in the deep veins of the calf along with a demonstrated obstruction at the common femoral level or above.

Massive venous occlusion (phlegmasia cerulea dolens)
Signs and symptoms

The onset of massive venous occlusion may be slow, following a smoldering phlebitis, or may develop rapidly in an ambulatory patient. The symptoms are massive tense edema, severe pain, and bluish discoloration of the leg, thigh, and even the buttock. The limb becomes cold. Peripheral pulses may diminish and disappear in the involved extremity. Gangrene may result even though the arteries are patent. Venous pressures in the affected leg are very high, ranging from 40 to 100 cm. of water compared to pressures of under 10 in the normal extremity (with the patient supine).

Treatment

Many of the clinical manifestations of venous thrombosis of this degree are caused by vasospasms of both the arterial and the venous systems. Edwards* has observed a consistent and gradual decline in venous pressure after sympathetic block by spinal anesthesia and recommends a short trial of conservative treatment, including sympathetic block, elevation of the legs, anticoagulation with heparin, and prompt replacement by balanced electrolyte solutions of the extracellular fluid lost into the massively swollen leg.

If symptoms do not improve rapidly, thrombectomy should be performed before the clot becomes adherent (that is, within twelve to forty-eight hours after onset). Thrombectomy has also been advised for phlegmasia alba dolens to restore normal flow† and thus prevent the long-term aftereffects of deep phlebitis and destruction of the valves.

The syndrome may be a complication of some grave underlying disease.

FEMORAL VEIN THROMBECTOMY
FOR ILIOFEMORAL THROMBOSIS
Preoperative preparation

The clotting time is determined preoperatively. Heparin and several pints of blood should be available in the operating room. The operator should be prepared to encounter variations in the anatomy of the femoral veins (Fig. 79). The entire leg should be prepared and draped.

Anesthesia

Local anesthesia is preferred. Spinal or general anesthesia is also suitable.

Procedure
Exposure

1. Make a vertical incision beginning at the midportion of the inguinal ligament or at the point where femoral pulsation can be palpated. Extend the in-

---

*Edwards, W. S.: Observations on the pathogenesis and management of massive venous occlusion, Surgery **43**:153-163, 1958.
†Haller, J. A.: Thrombectomy for deep thrombophlebitis of the leg, New England J. Med. **267**:65-68, 1962.

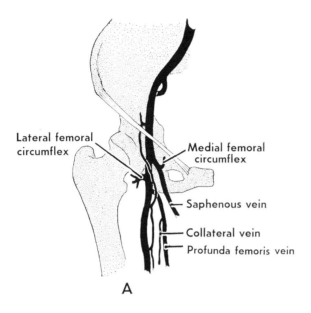

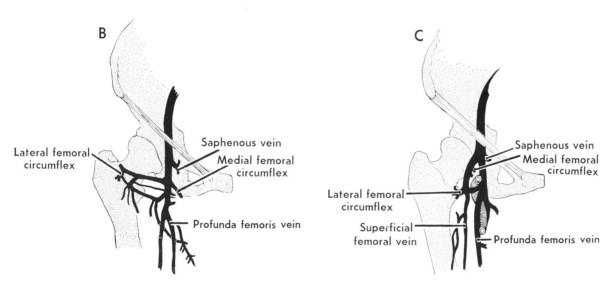

Fig. 79. Variations in tributaries of common femoral vein. **A,** Commonest pattern of veins at groin. **B** and **C,** Other variations. Note the progressively increasing size of the profunda branch and the corresponding decrease in size and importance of the superficial femoral vein in the changing patterns **A** to **C.** (Redrawn from Edwards, E. A., and Robuck, J. D.: Surg. Gynec. Obstet. **85:**547, 1947; by permission of Surgery, Gynecology & Obstetrics.)

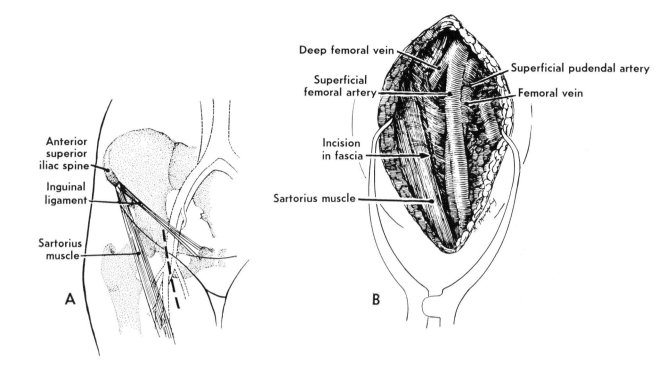

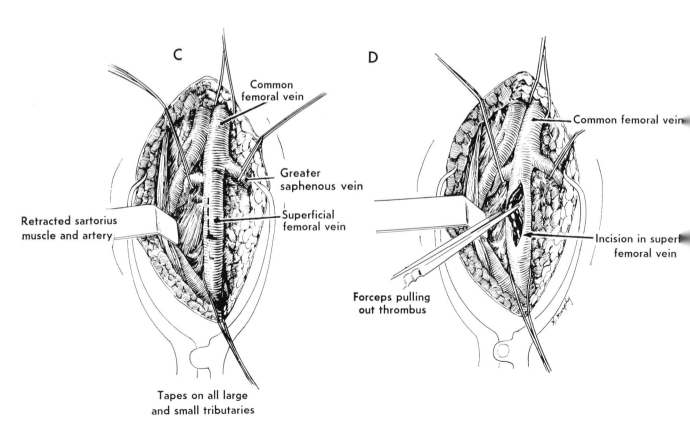

Fig. 80. Femoral vein thrombectomy. **A,** Incision. **B,** Exposure of veins and artery. **C,** Tapes in place for control of all tributaries during phlebotomy. **D,** Clot extrudes spontaneously under pressure.

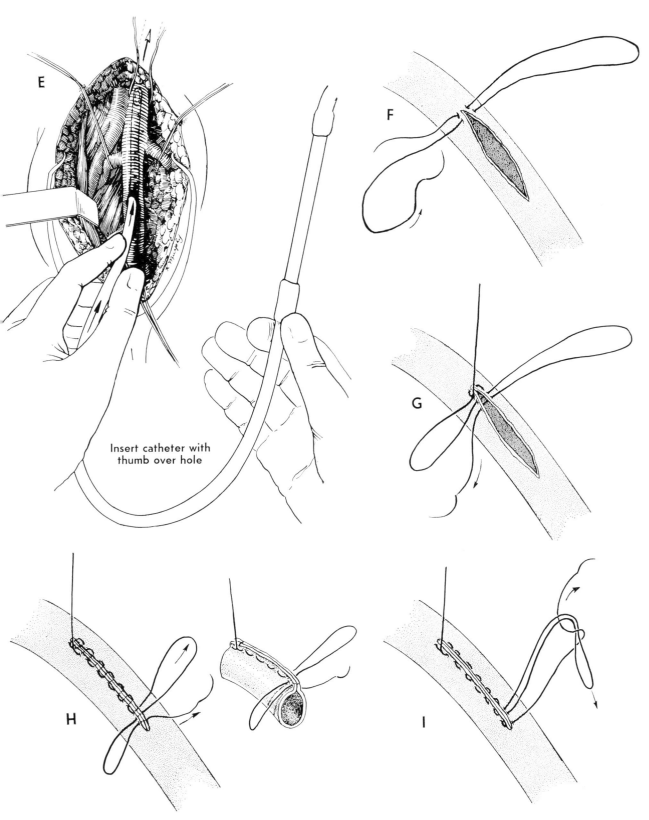

E

Insert catheter with
thumb over hole

F

G

H

I

Fig. 80, cont'd. Femoral vein thrombectomy. **E,** Removal of iliac thrombus with suction catheter. **F** to **I,** Closure of phlebotomy with continuous everting mattress suture.

cision four or five inches downward and medially following approximately the medial border of the sartorious muscle. (Fig. 80, A.)

2. Incise the deep fascia medial to the sartorious muscle, and retract the muscle laterally (Fig. 80, B). The tissue is edematous.

3. Incise the femoral sheath, beginning proximally, and carefully and gently isolate the femoral artery and vein. The diagnosis is confirmed by the tense bulging femoral vein, which appears thick walled, pale, and dull. Divide the superficial external pudendal artery as it crosses the femoral vein.

Proximal and distal control

Pass tapes about the common femoral vein proximally, about the saphenous vein, and about the common or superficial femoral vein distally (Fig. 80, C). The common femoral vein is preferable if the deep femoral vein is difficult to isolate. Variations in the anatomy of tributaries of the common femoral vein are illustrated in Fig. 79. All tributaries must be isolated and some provision (tape or clamp) made for their occlusion, or troublesome bleeding occurs after the incision in the vein.

Phlebotomy and thrombectomy

1. Traction on the tapes placed proximally and distally on the femoral vein and other tributaries controls bleeding. Tilt the operating table to elevate the patient's head.

2. Make a longitudinal incision about 1 to 1.5 cm. long in the vein, and the black gelatinous thrombus will extrude under pressure. The anesthetist should give 50 mg. of heparin intravenously at this time.

3. The peripheral portion of the thrombus is now removed by a combination of pressure and massage of the leg and thigh, suction, and introduction of Fogarty balloon catheters. These procedures should be continued until back bleeding is rather brisk.

Comment: *Vigorous massage starting distally is essential. Wet the leg so that your hands can slide on the skin.*

4. The proximal thrombus can usually be removed by a combination of suction with a long thin tip and forceful abdominal straining on the part of the patient. The suction tubing must have a side hole near the proximal end so that suction is controlled by the operator's thumb (Fig. 80, E). A rubber or plastic open-ended catheter is suitable. If general anesthesia has been used, the surgeon may apply manual pressure on the lower part of the abdomen. Also, particularly under general anesthesia, the Fogarty catheters may be employed for proximal thrombectomy. These procedures should be continued until blood flows freely from the vein proximally.

5. Hemostasis is obtained by elevation of the tapes rather than by application of clamps to the vein.

6. Irrigate the venotomy with dilute heparin solution.

7. Begin the closure with a mattress suture of 5-0 silk on an atraumatic needle (Fig. 80, F).

8. Suture is continued with small bites approximately 1 mm. apart as a horizontal running mattress suture, everting the edges of the vein until the end of the venotomy incision is reached (Fig. 80, G-I).

272

Regional heparinization

Regional heparinization is begun immediately through an inlying plastic catheter or needle inserted in the saphenous or other superficial vein in the foot. The Teflon needle has a sterile obturator which is removed to attach the syringe. From 20 to 30 mg. of heparin can be injected every three to four hours. Apply an elastic bandage to the leg above the ankle to occlude the superficial veins and to channel the heparin into the deep circulation. Continue regional heparinization for four days.

Discussion

All tributaries of the femoral vein must be identified and controlled. Failure to control a tributary results in massive bleeding and an obscure surgical field when the femoral vein is opened. Pertinent anatomical variations are shown in Fig. 80.

Thrombectomy as described can be done under local anesthesia with very little risk and is applicable to the very sick patient. Convalescence is rapid and the sequelae seem less severe than those following nonoperative treatment. Thrombectomy restores normal function of the venous system. In general, the indications for thrombectomy are massive edema and phlegmasia cerulea dolens secondary to massive iliofemoral thrombosis.

Regional heparinization is continued for three or four days, during which time the administration of bishydroxycoumarin (Dicumarol), warfarin, or a similar anticoagulant is commenced.

Iliofemoral thrombosis frequently originates in the proximal veins rather than in the calf. Early in the development of the disease and before extensive distal thrombosis has developed, there seems to be a time when thrombectomy may reasonably be expected to result in the complete return of normal anatomy and function. Prolonged follow-up will be needed to appraise the long-term results. The prompt relief of pain and edema after operation is gratifying.

Postoperative phlebograms are helpful in visualizing the results of thrombectomy.

LIGATION OF FEMORAL VEIN FOR THROMBOEMBOLISM

Ligation of the superficial femoral vein or the common femoral vein after removal of the proximal thrombus is sometimes advised because of previous embolization. In these instances bilateral exploration and ligation are necessary because emboli may arise from the asymptomatic side.

Proximal thrombi, when found, are removed before ligation by the method just described. Surgical exposure for ligation is the same as for thrombectomy. When ligation is elected, the veins should be doubly tied and divided.

Ligation of the common femoral vein almost always results in chronic and persistent edema. The common femoral vein may be ligated in bedridden patients with severe cardiac disease or if release of the occluding tape reveals no blood flow from the profunda femoris vein. Ordinarily, ligation is limited to the superficial femoral vein.

Superficial femoral vein interruption must be flush with the profunda femoris. Stagnant blood may clot if a pouch or diverticulum remains and can result in fatal embolism.

Vein interruption is effective for prevention of embolism when the level of interruption is high enough and operation is bilateral. The source of the emboli may not be clear, and ligation or partial occlusion of the inferior vena cava is a more certain prophylactic operation.

LIGATION AND PARTIAL OCCLUSION OF INFERIOR VENA CAVA

Introduction

Ligation or partial occlusion of the inferior vena cava is considered in the following circumstances:

1. Repeated pulmonary embolism associated with pelvic phlebitis or without an obvious source
2. Pulmonary embolism from ascending venous thrombosis that is not controlled by anticoagulants
3. Pulmonary embolism when anticoagulants cannot be employed.

When patients are operated on during anticoagulation treatment, the administration of anticoagulants should be reinstituted within twenty-four hours of the surgical procedure. Continuation of anticoagulation treatment for at least one more week is desirable. If much bleeding is encountered during the operative procedure, the wound should be drained.

In female patients with septic pelvic thrombophlebitis, the transabdominal route is used to gain access to the ovarian veins. These, as well as the inferior vena cava, must be ligated.

Ligation or partial occlusion of the inferior vena cava will prevent further pulmonary embolism except from those exceedingly rare emboli that may arise in the arm. Caval ligation is advised if anticoagulants are contraindicated or have failed and if emboli apparently arise above the common femoral vein.

The late sequelae of thrombosis or ligation of the inferior vena cava are caused mainly by the underlying thrombophlebitis. They are edema, varicosities, and ulcers. Careful postoperative care helps to prevent or control the edema and stasis.

Partial occlusion

Recently, several methods of partial occlusion of the inferior vena cava have been developed which prevent major pulmonary embolization and, at the same time, allow continued blood flow upward in the inferior vena cava. Plication with sutures or staples has been used, but we prefer the Adams-DeWeese clip, which is easily applied to the outside of the inferior vena cava as illustrated in Fig. 81. Clinical and experimental evidence shows that large emboli are arrested at the clip. Unless or until the passages through the clip are occluded by thrombi, the pressure in the inferior vena cava is not elevated and the postoperative course, edema, or thrombophlebitis seems less troublesome than that following complete ligation. Ligation, however, is necessary in the treatment of septic thrombophlebitis.

The availability and proved effectiveness of fenestrated clips should make physicians and surgeons more willing to offer partial occlusion of the inferior vena cava to patients who have had an episode of pulmonary embolism. If a

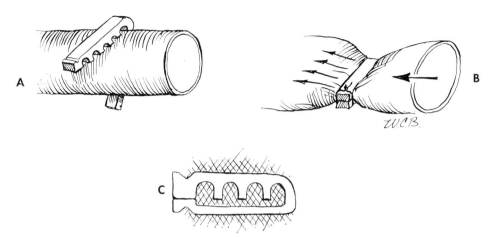

Fig. 81. Partial occlusion of inferior vena cava with DeWeese-Adams clip filters lethal emboli. **A,** Teflon clip applied to inferior vena cava. Smooth lower limb slips easily underneath vein. **B,** Flow continues, but significant emboli are "strained" from venous system. **C,** Cross section of clip.

major embolus is stopped by the clip, the patient's life has probably been saved. If no further embolism occurs, partial occlusion causes no stasis.

Anesthesia

General endotracheal anesthesia should be employed.

Surgical approach

The site for ligation or partial occlusion of the inferior vena cava is shortly above the confluence of iliac veins. In thin persons the supine position and a short transverse abdominal incision at the level of the umbilicus are satisfactory. In most patients the left lateral decubitus position similar to that employed for lumbar sympathectomy is preferable. The following surgical procedure is described using the lateral approach.

Procedure

1. Place the patient in the left lateral decubitus position, similar to that employed for lumbar sympathectomy. Employ the kidney rest to widen the space between the twelfth rib and the iliac crest. Flex the lower (left) leg, but extend the upper (right) leg. The left leg serves to stabilize the patient, whereas extension of the right leg puts tension on the psoas muscle, drawing it out of the operator's way. Place a pillow between the legs. This position is not identical to the position recommended for lumbar sympathectomy. (See Fig. 82, A.)

2. Make a transverse skin incision beginning 2 or 3 cm. to the right of the rectus muscles and at about the level of the umbilicus. The umbilicus is a landmark for the bifurcation of the iliac arteries and the confluence of the iliac veins. Carry the incision backward and slightly upward toward the twelfth rib. (See Fig. 82, A.)

3. Split the external oblique muscle, cutting directly across its fibers (Fig. 82, B).

275

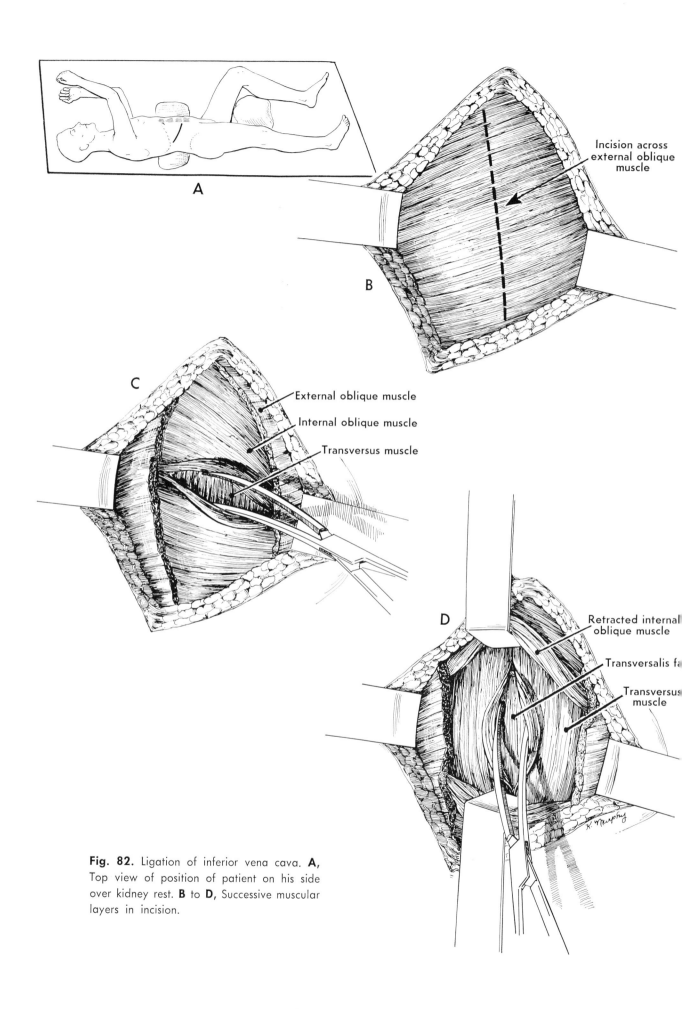

Incision across
external oblique
muscle

External oblique muscle
Internal oblique muscle
Transversus muscle

Retracted internal
oblique muscle

Transversalis fa

Transversus
muscle

Fig. 82. Ligation of inferior vena cava. **A,**
Top view of position of patient on his side
over kidney rest. **B** to **D,** Successive muscular
layers in incision.

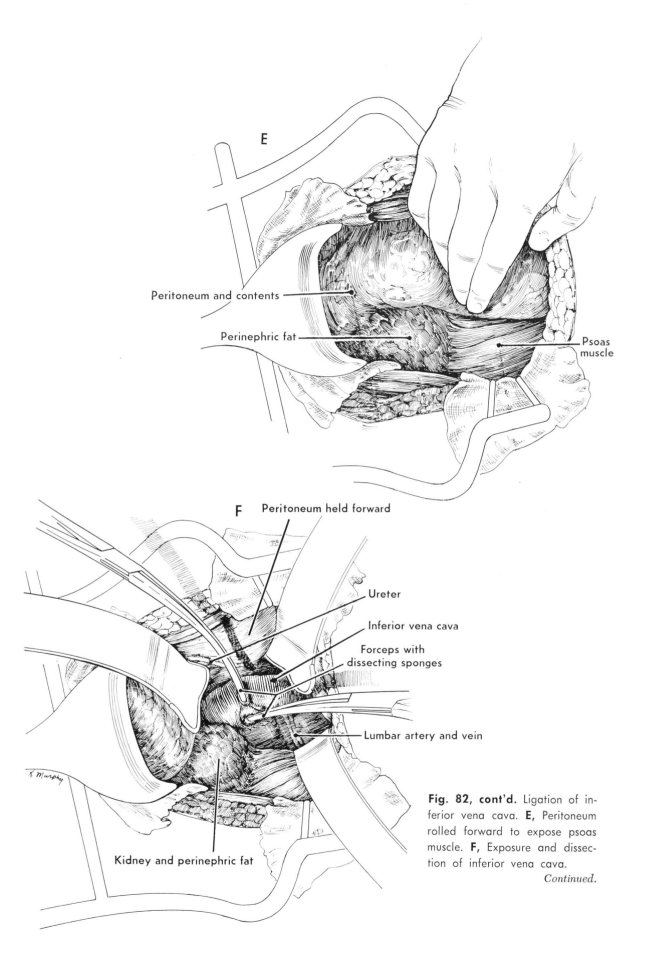

E

Peritoneum and contents

Perinephric fat

Psoas muscle

F Peritoneum held forward

Ureter

Inferior vena cava

Forceps with dissecting sponges

Lumbar artery and vein

Kidney and perinephric fat

Fig. 82, cont'd. Ligation of inferior vena cava. **E,** Peritoneum rolled forward to expose psoas muscle. **F,** Exposure and dissection of inferior vena cava.

Continued.

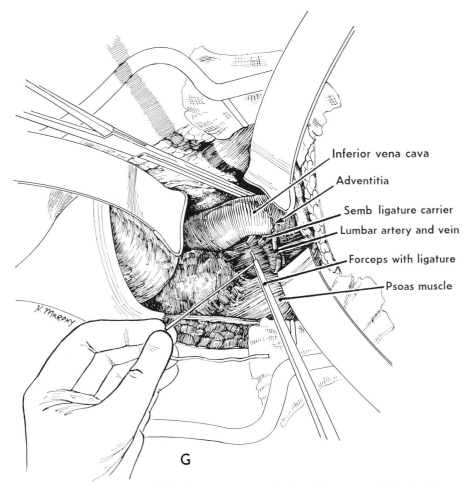

Inferior vena cava

Adventitia

Semb ligature carrier

Lumbar artery and vein

Forceps with ligature

Psoas muscle

G

Fig. 82, cont'd. Ligation of inferior vena cava. **G,** Pass ligature as illustrated here or apply DeWeese-Adams clip (Fig. 81).

4. The internal oblique muscle may be split in the direction of its fibers (Fig. 82, *C*). More ample exposure is obtained by dividing the muscle.

5. Split the transversus muscle in the direction of its fibers (Fig. 82, *D*).

6. Retract the wound widely (Fig. 82, *E*). In the plane of the properitoneal fat, roll the peritoneum and its contents anteriorly, using blunt dissection with gauze pads and sponge holders. The inferior vena cava is easily visualized deep and medial to the psoas muscle in the depths of the incision.

Comment: *Beware of thrombus in the inferior vena cava. In two patients we have found and removed thrombi which extended above the level of intended ligation and which might have been torn or released by ligation.*

7. Choose a convenient point on the inferior vena cava just above the iliac veins. Use two long clamps holding small rolls of umbilical tape as dissectors. Hold the vein to one side with one dissector, and with the other carefully roll the loose perivascular tissue away from the vein. Observe and avoid the lumbar veins. They are fragile and easily torn. A small pack of oxidized cellulose may be needed. (See Fig. 82, *F*.)

8. When the inferior vena cava is free, pass a heavy ligature of No. 2 silk

278

about it approximately 1 to 1.5 cm. above or below the lumbar vein and tie the ligature securely (Fig. 82, G). A great deal of pressure is not necessary because there is practically no hydrostatic pressure in the vein. Do not divide the inferior vena cava.

If a fenestrated clip is chosen, it is inserted at this time in place of the ligature. Clips with one smooth limb are preferred. The smooth limb slides under the inferior vena cava (Fig. 81). Tie the ends of the clip together.

9. Close the incision in layers.

Postoperative care

The main postoperative problem following ligation of the vena cava is edema. Prevention begins immediately by wrapping both thighs and legs with foam rubber–coated or self-adherent elastic bandages before the patient leaves the operating room. Postoperatively, the foot of the bed must be constantly elevated 15 or 20 degrees. Ambulation is begun early and is gradually increased unless swelling is troublesome. Prolonged elastic support* is necessary for several months. Intermittent use of heparin is advised for seven to ten days if there has been much edema before the operation.

---

*Supports for both legs to the waist are obtainable from the Jobst Institute, 1803 Jefferson Ave., Toledo, Ohio.

Chapter 16

Amputations, infections, and gangrene of the lower extremity

GENERAL PRINCIPLES OF AMPUTATION FOR VASCULAR DISEASE

In civilian medical practice more limbs are removed for chronic occlusive arterial disease than for any other cause. The disease is usually diffuse, involving arteries proximal to the proposed site of amputation. The sites and techniques of amputation therefore differ somewhat from amputations done for trauma or other reasons.

Only three levels of amputation need be considered for vascular disease in the lower limb. The low-thigh amputation is the best site to ensure healing when there is advanced arterial insufficiency. Amputation below the knee permits more rapid and more complete rehabilitation and a more normal gait. The transmetatarsal amputation will require no prosthesis, and the affected foot functions almost as well as a normal foot. After distal conservative amputations, healing may be slower and some patients will subsequently require reamputation at a higher level. Syme, Lisfranc, and other similar foot amputations are not usually suitable for patients with vascular disease.

The usual indications for amputation are gangrene, intractable infection, and severe intractable pain secondary to arterial insufficiency. More urgent problems, fortunately not too common, are uncorrectable arterial trauma or invasive infection that cannot be controlled by antibiotics or other conservative measures. The open amputations and drainage procedures for infections and gangrene of the neurotrophic feet of diabetic patients are special problems and are discussed on pp. 298 and 299.

Amputation as treatment for vascular disease is a semielective, definitive, closed, one-stage procedure. The aim is conservation of as much of the extremity as is consistent with good healing and rapid rehabilitation. The correct level for amputation is determined after consideration of the patient and his associated medical diseases, as well as evaluation of the limb. The absence of both pedal pulses or the more proximal pulses is a definitive and reliable sign of arterial occlusion. However, estimation of collateral circulation requires observation and judgment of the nutritional state of the limb as reflected in the skin, nails, toes, hair follicles, and muscle mass. Collateral circulation in diabetic persons without peripheral pulses is frequently excellent, and transmetatarsal or below-the-knee amputation may succeed even when popliteal and distal pulses are absent. When arterial insufficiency is further advanced, atrophy and dryness of the skin, muscle atrophy, and atrophy of soft tissues in the toes will be found.

Continuous pain on rest, improved somewhat by a dependent position of the foot, results in edema since the patient keeps the foot down almost constantly. Such a foot shows other signs of advanced arterial insufficiency such as skin and muscle atrophy. Transmetatarsal amputation will fail when pain on rest and dependent rubor are observed. Below-the-knee amputations frequently fail and should not be elected unless the signs of trophic change are mild and distal.

Special tests are usually not helpful for evaluation of collateral circulation. Arteriograms are advisable because they occasionally reveal a correctable arterial block and are sometimes helpful in the selection of the amputation level. Inability to visualize the collateral circulation in arteriograms may be caused by technical factors in the examination and should not be discouraging. Collateral circulation does not register on the oscillometer. More sophisticated methods of measuring blood flow in the limb are not available outside the laboratory. Clinical observation, including evaluation of the local response to several weeks of conservative treatment, is probably the most useful and reliable method for choosing the level of elective amputation. At the time of operation, pulsatile bleeding in the skin incision is always a good sign. The degree and amount of bleeding from muscular collateral circulation is more difficult to judge.

Conservative treatment and preoperative preparation for amputation should include management of associated diseases, antibiotics, rest, treatment and drainage of local infections, and skin preparation with an antiseptic soap (pHisoHex or similar preparation). The physiatrist should discuss and plan rehabilitation with the patient. The patient should not observe doubt or conflict among his physicians.

Careful and gentle surgical technique is essential, both to preserve blood supply and to minimize the opportunities for wound infection. Skin incisions are designed to conserve blood supply, and a circular incision without flaps should be used whenever applicable. The skin is elevated with the underlying fascia and is protected with moist packs. Crushing instruments and crude mass ligatures are avoided. Careful hemostasis will prevent hematoma. The incision may be closed without drainage. For the posterior portion of the amputation, a large sharp amputation knife is less traumatic than the small scalpel and prevents shredding of muscle tissue.

Many stump complications will be prevented by careful closure of the wound. Copious irrigations with saline solution remove bone dust and debris. In handling the skin, tissue forceps are avoided. There should not be excessive tension on the skin flaps.

Postoperative care must include correct positioning of the limb to avoid the tendency toward contracture. Sutures are removed in stages after ten to fourteen days, except for excessively tight sutures that are cutting into the skin, which may be removed earlier. Exercise and rehabilitation should be begun as early as possible.

Mortality after amputations, particularly those necessitated by extensive gangrene, is rather high. Many of the patients are elderly and have advanced coronary and cerebral atherosclerotic diseases. Careful medical supervision is essential to reduce postoperative mortality.

Some of the complications of the surgical procedure in amputations are avoidable. Infection can usually be avoided by preliminary drainage, by local treatment, by preserving the blood supply, and by avoiding hematoma and excessive surgical trauma at the time of operation. Phantom limb pain rarely persists unless amputation is long deferred and the pain pattern is established. Contracture of the hip, the knee, or the Achilles tendon is avoided by preoperative and postoperative exercises and correct positioning. Occasionally, amputation must be done above an established contracture. The redundant skin flaps at the sides of the limb after circular incisions for amputation will shrink and require no special treatment or revision. Early stump wrapping controls edema. As a rule, amputation neuroma is not symptomatic unless the lesion lies just under the skin or between skin and bone or is incorporated in the surgical scar. Progressive thrombosis sometimes requires reamputation at a higher level, and an occasional distal amputation will fail when collateral circulation is insufficient. Meticulous technique is necessary. Minor separation or infection may cause failure to heal when blood supply at the amputation site is barely sufficient.

The surgeon must evaluate the prospect of success and the expenses and hazards of failure in each individual patient when choosing the level of amputation. Unless a few of his conservative amputations fail, he is probably denying conservative amputation to some patients in whom a successful outcome might be anticipated.

ELECTIVE AMPUTATION ABOVE KNEE
Indications and choice of level

Amputation is performed through the thigh when the circulation is too poor to save the knee joint or when there is persistent contracture or other disease of the joint. The knee will be of little use to patients who will be unable to use a prosthesis. If such patients have serious heart disease, cerebral atherosclerosis, severe arterial insufficiency in the opposite leg, or blindness, the amputation should be above the knee when there is any doubt about the healing of a more distal amputation.

The optimum level above the knee is just above the distal expansion of the femur provided the common femoral and deep femoral arteries are open. The stump should be short enough to place the knee hinge of the prosthesis at the same level as the normal knee. Midthigh amputation, through the thicker portion of the thigh, is reserved for those limbs with less blood supply (that is, when the common femoral pulse is absent or weak and collateral circulation appears to be poor).

Preoperative care

Preoperatively, careful regulation and treatment of associated medical problems is mandatory, as is control of infection with drainage, antibiotics, and other conservative measures as indicated. Rehabilitation and adaptation to a prosthesis is aided by preoperative consultation with the physiatrist and indoctrination in

282

exercises, crutch walking, etc. Preoperatively, we recommend daily cleansing of the skin of the thigh and knee with an antiseptic soap (pHisoHex or similar preparation).

Anesthesia

Light general anesthesia or spinal anesthesia confined to the diseased limb is suitable.

Procedure

The patient is placed in the supine position with the leg extended. Amputation is performed from anterior to posterior, dividing successive layers as a cone (Fig. 83, *B*).

1. Make a circular incision in the skin several centimeters above the patella (Fig. 83, *A*).

2. The plan of operation, coning the successive layers, is shown in Fig. 83, *B*.

3. Divide the deep fascia, the patellar tendon, and the muscles anterior and lateral to the femur (Fig. 83, *C*).

4. Divide the tendinous attachments to the linea aspera. Pass a ribbon retractor beneath the femur. Retract the soft tissues remaining lateral to the femur. Divide and elevate the periosteum, stripping it distally. (Fig. 83, *D*.)

5. Hold the vascular bundle posteriorly with the ribbon retractor, and saw through the femur (Fig. 83, *E*).

6. Retract the distal end of the femur with a small retractor. Identify the popliteal artery and vein in the fat of the medial side of the popliteal fossa (Fig. 83, *F*). Clamp and divide these structures and ligate with a suture ligature.

7. Identify the sciatic nerve in the lateral aspect of the popliteal space (Fig. 83, *F*). Clamp the nerve and draw it downward for several inches (Fig. 83, *G*). Tie the nerve with a suture ligature as high as possible (Fig. 83, *H*).

8. Divide the sciatic nerve with a sharp knife, and allow it to retract several inches into the thigh (Fig. 83, *I*).

9. Straighten the leg. Place the amputation knife at the end of the proximal femur, and rapidly cut the muscles posteriorly (Fig. 83, *J*). Remove the amputated limb. Ligate the various bleeding points in the posterior muscle mass for complete hemostasis.

Closure

1. Inspect the stump carefully (Fig. 83, *K*). Meticulous hemostasis is important. Irrigate with saline solution. Elevate the stump on an inverted basin or a pack of towels.

2. Suture the fascial layer with 2-0 silk or chromic catgut, inverting the sutures so as to place the knot beneath the fascia (Fig. 83, *L*).

3. Suture the skin with fine silk (Fig. 83, *N*). A drain is usually unnecessary.

Postoperative care

Paint the skin of the thigh with tincture of benzoin. Apply dry gauze sponges over the end. Hold the dressing on the stump with stockinette rolled onto the stump. Avoid adhesive tape on the nearby ischemic skin. Do not elevate the stump on a pillow, since this encourages flexion contracture at the hip joint.

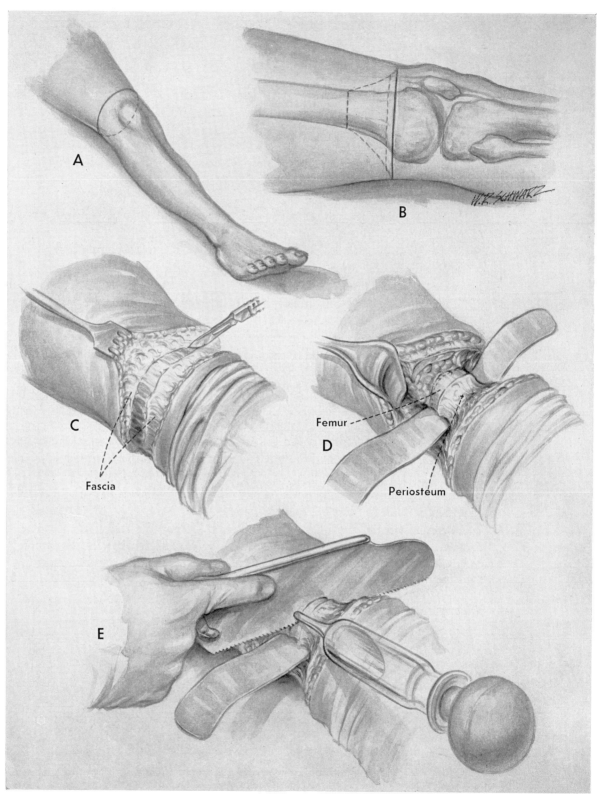

Fig. 83. Elective amputation above knee. **A,** Circular incision. **B,** Lateral view of incision. **C,** Incision in deep fascia. **D,** Incision on femur. Periosteum stripped distally. **E,** Saw femur.

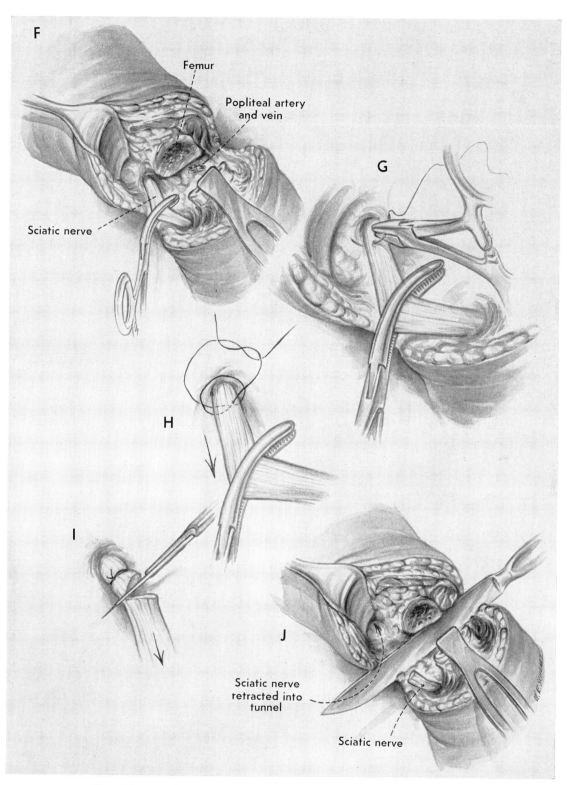

Fig. 83, cont'd. Elective amputation above knee. **F,** Identify sciatic nerve and draw it down. **G** and **H,** Suture ligature in sciatic nerve. **I,** Divide sciatic nerve under tension so that it retracts. **J,** Divide posterior muscles.

Continued.

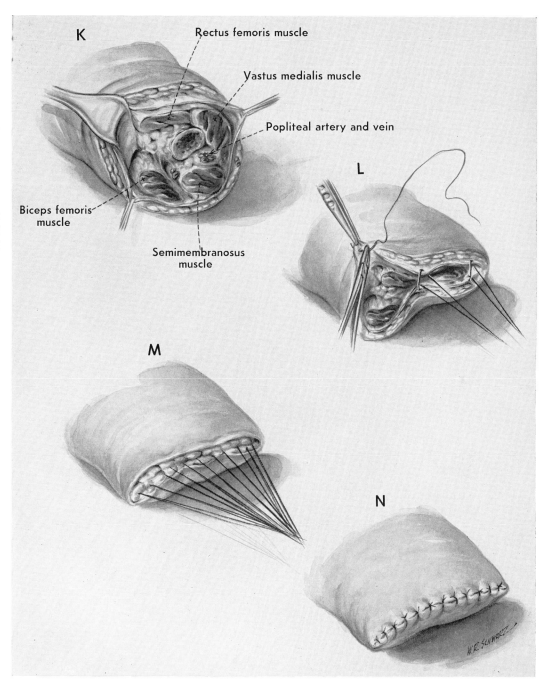

K, Rectus femoris muscle

Vastus medialis muscle

Popliteal artery and vein

Biceps femoris muscle

Semimembranosus muscle

L

M

N

Fig. 83, cont'd. Elective amputation above knee. **K,** Veins of open end of stump. **L,** Placement of sutures for closure of deep fascia. **M,** Closure of deep fascia completed. **N,** Closure of skin completed.

After five days the stump may be wrapped with an elastic bandage applied directly over the stockinette dressing. Redundant skin, the result of the circular incision, will shrink nicely. After the fifth day the patient must lie face down for short periods and hyperextend the stump. Later he may sit and may be up in a wheelchair. The physiatrist should visit before the operation and later, and exercises should be commenced as indicated. Patients may be trained with a temporary prosthesis without the intervening stages of crutch and wheelchair ambulation. However, temporary prostheses are an added expense.

Remove the sutures between the twelfth and fourteenth day.

AMPUTATION BELOW KNEE
Indications and choice of procedure

Below-the-knee amputation is performed when there is gangrene or arterial insufficiency distal to the ankle that is too severe to permit saving the foot.

Popliteal pulsation need not be present if collateral flow is adequate. The operation described makes the posterior flap long because the collateral flow is more abundant posteriorly from muscular branches of the peroneal arteries or the posterior tibial arteries when these are patent. Difficulty with healing is almost always at the center of the anterior flap, which should therefore be kept short and broad based. Circular incisions offer no important advantages in the calf, and placement of the scar is unimportant, although it should not adhere to the underlying bone. Other flaps and debridement of ischemic or damaged muscle, as described in orthopedic textbooks, are useful for acute occlusion of the popliteal artery, injuries, or other conditions in which cutaneous circulation is normal.

Contraindications

Definitive elective closed amputation below the knee should not be done when there is (1) invasive infection, (2) unstabilized arterial insufficiency after acute arterial occlusion, (3) pain on rest above the ankle, (4) other signs of severe arterial insufficiency, or (5) diabetic neuropathy with hypalgesia at the level of the skin flaps.

Preoperative preparation

Preoperative preparation has been discussed in detail on pp. 280 and 281. Supplementary procedures such as sympathectomy and refrigeration are rarely required.

Anesthesia

Spinal or light general anesthesia is suitable.

Procedure

1. The patient is placed in the supine position with the knee extended throughout the operation.

2. Mark the level of division of the tibia at a point 10 to 12 cm. distal to the knee joint (Fig. 84, A). Measure the circumference of the calf at this level with a silk suture. Divide the circumference measurement in half by cutting the suture. This piece of thread may then be used to measure the length of the flaps,

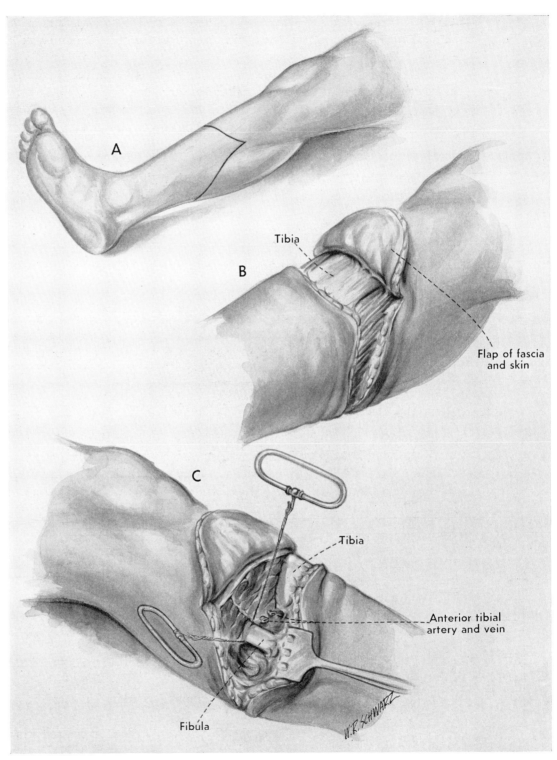

Fig. 84. Amputation below knee. **A,** Incision. **B,** Medial view of skin flap. **C,** Lateral view of division of fibula.

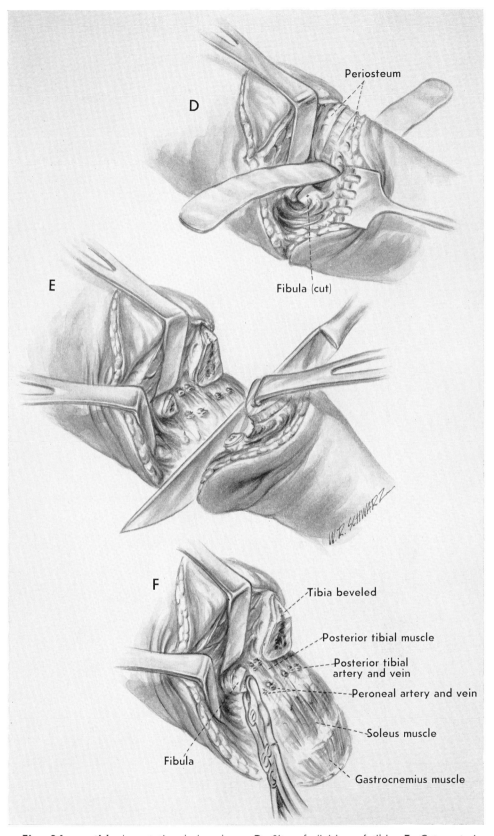

Periosteum

D

Fibula (cut)

E

F

Tibia beveled

Posterior tibial muscle

Posterior tibial
artery and vein

Peroneal artery and vein

Soleus muscle

Fibula

Gastrocnemius muscle

Fig. 84, cont'd. Amputation below knee. **D,** Site of division of tibia. **E,** Cut posterior muscles. **F,** Shorten fibula with double-acting rongeur.

Continued.

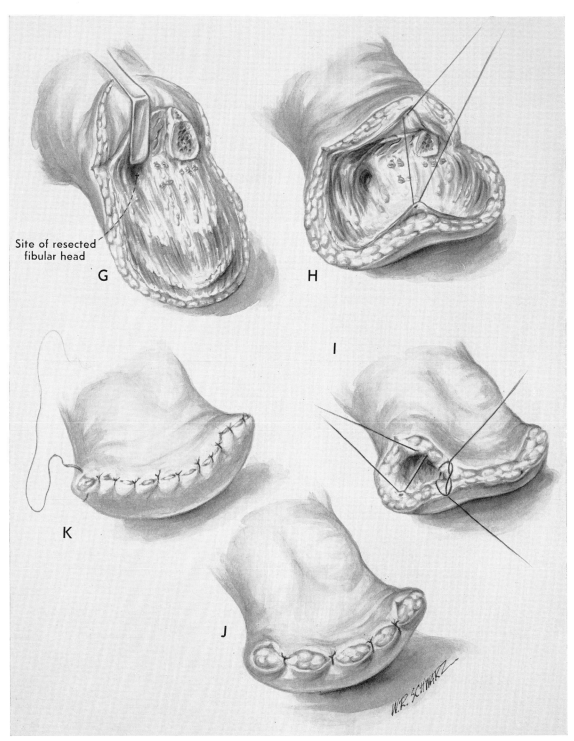

Site of resected
fibular head

G

H

I

K

J

W.R. SCHWARZ

Fig. 84, cont'd. Amputation below knee. **G,** Flaps prior to closure. **H,** Beginning fascial closure. **I,** Fascial closure completed. **J** and **K,** Skin closure.

the anterior flap being one-third and the posterior flap two-thirds of the thread's length. The tibia should be divided slightly above the junction of the two flaps.

3. Make the skin incision as measured and indicated in Fig. 84, A. Divide the deep fascia at a level slightly above the skin level. Reflect the anterior flap of skin and fascia (Fig. 84, B) and cover with moist gauze. Incise the anterolateral group of muscles down to the tibia and fibula. Evidence of stasis or lack of pulsatile bleeding from the muscle should suggest the need for amputation above the knee.

4. Retract and protect the soft tissues. Using the Gigli saw, divide the fibula as high as possible (Fig. 84, C).

5. Dissect free the muscles posterior to the tibia. Pass a ribbon retractor beneath the tibia. Incise the periosteum at the level selected for division of the tibia, and elevate the periosteum distally. (See Fig. 84, D.)

6. Before sawing directly through the tibia, make the anterior bevel cut just above the proposed line of division. Divide the tibia. Use the rasp or rongeur to reduce bony spurs.

7. Hold the distal divided tibia inferiorly. Use a sharp amputation knife to make a slanting cut through the posterior muscle mass of the leg (Fig. 84, E). Ligate the bleeding points in the posterior muscle flap.

8. Shorten the fibula by stripping periosteum away, retracting soft tissues upward, and dividing so that the fibula is at least an inch shorter than the tibia (Fig. 84, F).

9. Draw the nerves down with a hemostat, crush proximally with three hemostats, ligate through the crush with nonabsorbable suture, divide the nerve, and allow to retract.

Closure

1. Irrigate abundantly with saline solution and inspect for additional bleeding (Fig. 84, G). When amputation is done for vascular disease, bleeding is less than from limbs with a normal circulation. Hemostasis should be meticulous. Use no drains unless there is considerable ooze. If drainage is necessary, the drain should be removed within forty-eight to seventy-two hours.

2. Suture the fascia. Begin in the center (Fig. 84, H) and bisect the remaining sectors once or twice to ensure even distribution of tension (Fig. 84, I).

3. Place a few deep skin sutures rather far apart to close the skin and subcutaneous tissue (Fig. 84, J). Complete the skin closure with fine silk sutures, placed somewhat more superficially (Fig. 84, K). Avoid the use of tissue forceps on the skin. Skin closure should be accurate. Fig. 84, K, shows slight separation of the skin edges that we ordinarily would not tolerate.

Dressing and postoperative care

Apply a small dry dressing held in place with a sock of sterile stockinette. Tincture of benzoin applied to the skin of the leg and thigh will secure the dressing in place. Apply a small posterior splint to keep the knee extended.

Some details of postoperative care have already been given on pp. 283-287. If drains have been necessary, they are removed within the first few days. The first dressing should otherwise be done on the fifth day. A dusky anterior flap is usually a poor prognostic sign at this time. When healing seems assured, exercises and other rehabilitative procedures may be commenced.

TRANSMETATARSAL AMPUTATIONS

Indications

Transmetatarsal amputation is a useful conservative procedure when arterial insufficiency involves one or more toes proximal to a suitable level for transphalangeal amputations. Open transmetatarsal amputation is also useful for ulcerated or infected neuropathic feet and is described on p. 301. Considerable judgment is necessary in selecting patients for transmetatarsal amputation. However, the success of this procedure, which requires no prosthesis, is very rewarding.

Contraindications

Contraindications to transmetatarsal amputation are as follows:
1. Advancing infection in the foot
2. Necrosis or skin lesions proximal to the metatarsal-phalangeal joints
3. Insufficient collateral circulation for healing as evidenced by (a) pain on rest, (b) dependent rubor at the line of proposed skin incision, and (c) venous filling time of over one-half minute

Preoperative preparation

Preoperatively, a period of conservative treatment may be required to localize and stabilize necrosis, to arrest infection, and to encourage and evaluate collateral circulation. During this time the patient should be treated with bed rest, elevation of the limbs, antibiotics, local surgical drainage, and Buerger-Allen exercises. The period of preoperative preparation may require several weeks.

Anesthesia

Either light general anesthesia or spinal anesthesia is suitable.

Procedure

The operation is done with the patient in the supine position.
1. Make a dorsal skin incision straight across the foot at the same level as the proposed division of the metatarsals (Fig. 85, A). Do not undermine the skin proximal to the dorsal incision.
2. Hold the toes down, and cut through the tendons and soft tissues dorsally until the bone is reached (Fig. 85, B). Ligate the bleeders with fine plain catgut.
3. Make a plantar incision of sufficient length to close the wound (Fig. 85, C).
4. Now hold the toes up so that the flexor tendons will be stretched and, when incised, will retract proximally (Fig. 85, D). Leave all the soft tissue on the plantar flap, and do not trim the flap.
5. Dissect all soft tissue off the joints and metatarsal bones back to the proposed site of amputation (Fig. 85, E).
6. Divide the first metatarsal with the Gigli saw (Fig. 85, F). This bone is sturdy, and it fractures if divided with an ordinary bone cutter. Divide the first interosseous muscle with a sharp knife.

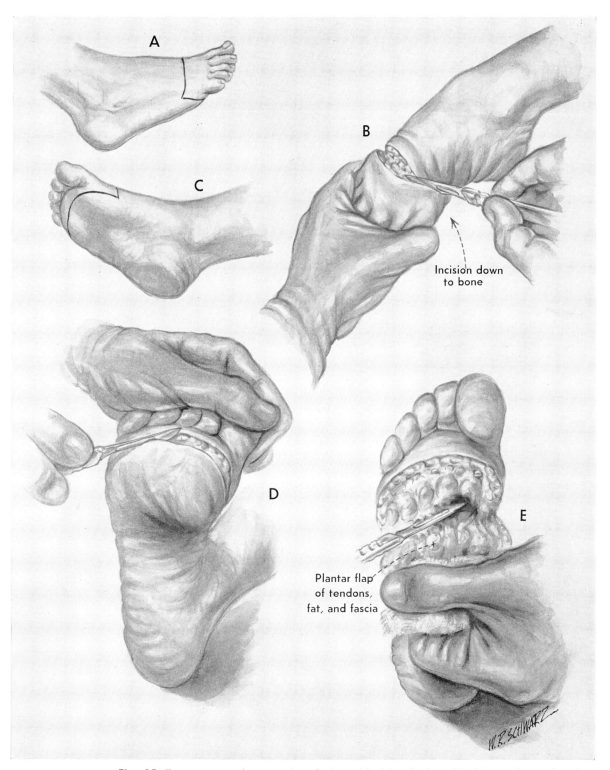

Fig. 85. Transmetatarsal amputation. **A,** Dorsal incision. **B,** Dorsal incision with toes flexed. **C,** Plantar incision. **D,** Plantar incision with toes dorsiflexed. **E,** Plantar flap, full thickness, dissected off metatarsal heads.

Continued.

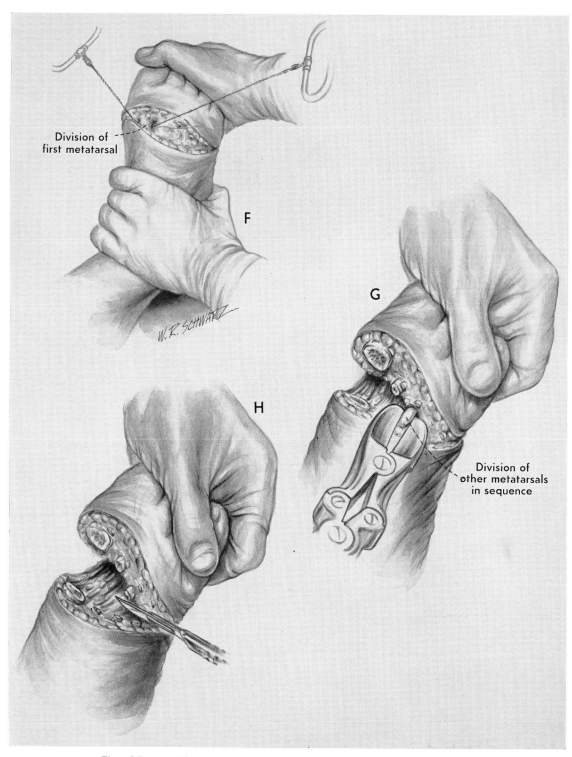

Division of
first metatarsal

F

G

H

Division of
other metatarsals
in sequence

W. R. SCHWARZ

Fig. 85, cont'd. Transmetatarsal amputation. **F,** Division of first metatarsal with Gigli saw. **G,** Division of other metatarsal bones. **H,** Divide interosseous soft tissue.

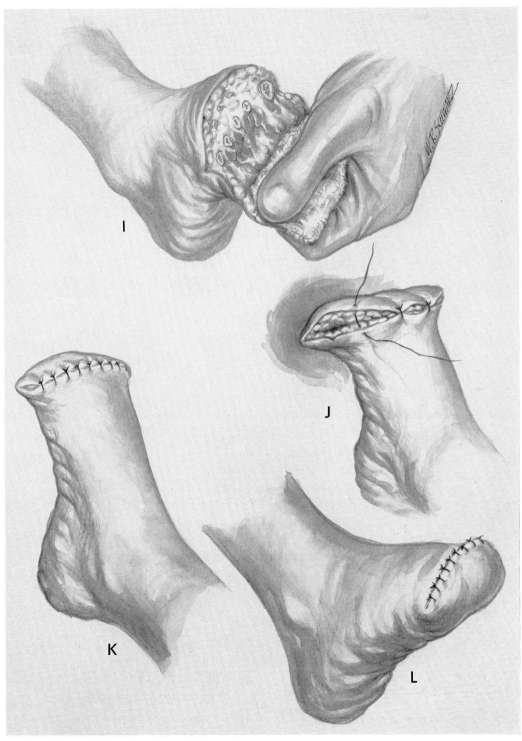

Fig. 85, cont'd. Transmetatarsal amputation. **I,** View of end of stump. **J,** Closure of skin flaps. **K** and **L,** Closure completed.

7. Divide the second metatarsal and the remaining metatarsals with the bone cutter (Fig. 85, *G*).

8. With a sharp knife divide the remaining interosseous muscles without loosening the proximal periosteum (Fig. 85, *H*). Remove the specimen. Change gloves and irrigate the wound with copious amounts of saline solution. Then smooth the irregular ends of the metatarsals with a rongeur.

Closure

Only the skin is closed.

The plantar flap is approximated to the dorsal incision with fine nylon or fine stainless steel wire. Be gentle. Do not use toothed forceps on the skin. Avoid an excessive number of sutures, and do not tie them too tightly. A drain is unnecessary (Fig. 85, *I-L.*)

Postoperative care

Apply a loose dressing to support the plantar flap and prevent tension on the sutures. Do not elevate the foot. The head of the bed may be elevated 6 inches to avoid blanching. If healing is in doubt, do not hesitate to splint the foot and the ankle.

Dressings are done on the fifth and tenth days. Remove the occasional suture that may have been placed too tightly and is cutting into the flaps. Ordinarily the sutures can be removed about the fourteenth day. Buerger-Allen exercises are begun about the tenth day, and exercises for crutch walking may also be begun early. However, prolonged early dependency of the foot that has been operated upon is avoided. Weight bearing is allowed in three to five weeks. When the patient is walking, the toe of the shoe is filled with lamb's wool.

ELECTIVE AMPUTATION OF TOES
Transmetatarsal amputation of fifth or first toe

Either the fifth or the first toe may be amputated at the metatarsal level through a racquet-shaped incision. The operation is indicated for ischemic lesions or infections in the proximal phalanx, but not if there is ischemia at the line of incision or in the interdigital creases. Lesions of other toes that extend to the interdigital creases of the first or fifth toe need complete forefoot transmetatarsal amputation. Open or drainage transmetatarsal amputation of the second, third, and fourth toes is discussed later. This operation is applicable only to neurotrophic feet in diabetic patients with relatively good circulation. Preoperative care is the same as for other foot amputations.

Procedure

Make a racquet-shaped incision (Fig. 86, *A-C*) so that the plantar flap is long and may be folded up to cover the cut ends of the bone (Fig. 86, *D* and *E*). Do not undermine the dorsal skin incision. Leave all soft tissue on the plantar flap, and cut the metatarsal obliquely at the level of the dorsal skin incision. Because the second metatarsal joint is close, cut close to the first joint.

Postoperative care

The same principles of surgical technique and postoperative care apply as for more extensive amputations of the foot.

296

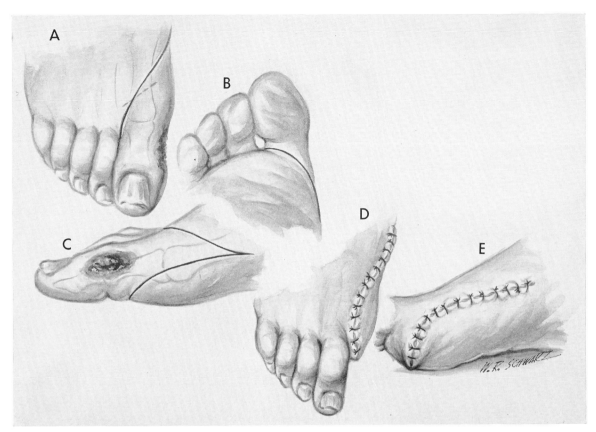

Fig. 86. Transmetatarsal amputation of fifth or first toe. **A** to **C**, View of "racquet" incision. **D** and **E**, Views of closure.

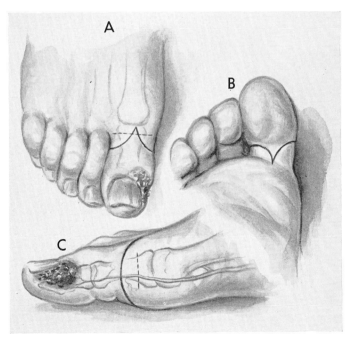

Fig. 87. Transphalangeal amputation. **A**, Dorsal view of skin flaps and site of division of bone. **B**, Plantar view of skin flaps. **C**, Lateral view showing digital artery at tip of flap.

Transphalangeal amputation

Transphalangeal amputation is indicated for deformity, infection, or ischemia in the tips or midportions of the toes. More proximal amputations have been discussed previously. Open amputation for drainage will be discussed below. For the first and fifth toes, transmetatarsal amputation (Fig. 86) is preferable and, as a rule, heals with less difficulty.

Procedure

Incisions should be made so that the digital vessels are divided at the tips of the lateral flaps (Fig. 87). There is no need for plantar skin over the end of the toe. Anterior and posterior flaps have less blood supply and heal more slowly.

Make the incisions for the flaps down to the bone, and turn the flaps back. The site elected for division of the proximal phalanx is close to the metatarsal-phalangeal joint. Divide the bone at the base of the flap, leaving only a button of proximal phalanx, without entering the joint. Close the incision with a few interrupted fine nylon sutures.

DRAINAGE AND DÉBRIDEMENT FOR INFECTIONS AND GANGRENE IN FOOT ASSOCIATED WITH DIABETES

Metabolic abnormalities appear to make diabetic patients unusually susceptible to infections and gangrene. In some instances arterial occlusion involves only smaller vessels, collateral circulation is good, and conservative treatment and minor amputations may be successful. The feet of diabetic patients are frequently involved in certain distinctive ulcers and infections that require surgical procedures. In each individual the degree and admixture of atherosclerosis and diabetic neuropathy vary. Accompanying the diabetic neuropathy, there is analgesia of the limb. Various minor infections therefore can proceed to abscess formation and osteomyelitis without causing warning of pain or discomfort.

Calluses, bunions, hammer toes, corns, blisters, and other minor foot disorders can lead to infection with major complications in the diabetic patient. Directions for care of the feet are included in the Appendix.

Infection of deep plantar space

Dangerous invasive infection deep to the plantar fascia and among the flexor tendons of the foot can result from a break in the skin almost anywhere on the foot or toe. From a "corn" or a "hammer toe" infection travels via the lumbrical canal (Fig. 88) directly into the plantar space. Web space infection between the toes invades the plantar space between the digital extensions of the plantar fascia. The flexor tendon sheaths lead infection into the plantar space from infected bunions, calluses, or ulcers over the heads of the metatarsals.

Sepsis in the deep plantar space is difficult to diagnose but must be suspected when there is any infection of a toe or the forefoot, particularly when there is severe systemic reaction, difficulty in control of diabetes, edema of the dorsum of the foot, or edema behind the medial malleolus. On examination the plantar surface of the foot is thick but frequently shows no redness or fluctuation. Pus is confined beneath the thick plantar fascia, which is a closed space. Sepsis in the plantar space may cause thrombosis of the digital arteries with wet gangrene of the toes.

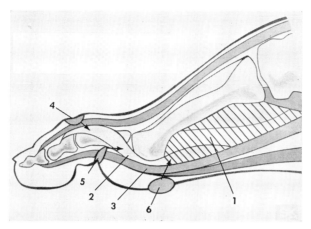

Fig. 88. Sources and routes of entry of plantar space of abscess. **1,** Plantar space abscess. **2,** Lumbrical canal. **3,** Flexor tendon sheath. **4,** Infected callosity. **5,** Web space infection. **6,** Mal perforant. (Courtesy Smith, Kline & French, Philadelphia, Pa.)

The diagnosis of plantar space sepsis is made by thorough examination, including removal of eschar, trimming of infected calluses, and opening of the skin to appraise the extent of infection and to permit probing of wounds. X-ray examination will occasionally reveal osteomyelitis that is not apparent on physical examination.

The operative treatment for plantar space sepsis is drainage and débridement. This is best accomplished by open amputation of the infected toe, drainage or débridement of the attached infected tendon, and incision extended into the plantar space for drainage. The required amputation may be transphalangeal, transmetatarsal, or wedge amputation according to the extent of débridement that is necessary.

Mal perforant

Mal perforant is a typical manifestation of diabetic neuropathy and is characterized by chronic painless ulcer on the plantar surface of the foot over a pressure point. As a rule, the ulcer appears over the first or fifth metatarsal head. The initial manifestation is a callus, which soon becomes infected. When the feet are neglected, necrosis under the callus results in the characteristic ulcer with overhanging edges, which is painless. Infection spreads into the underlying joint and proximally into the plantar space. Such complications may be avoided by proper care of calluses and of the feet, early treatment of minor infections, and the use of corrective shoes or arch supports. Open amputation of the toe and metatarsal head may be necessary for débridement and drainage.

Suppurative thrombophlebitis

Suppurative thrombophlebitis is occasionally observed in diabetic patients. If it becomes subfascial, incision and drainage, including fasciotomy, are required in addition to proximal ligation of the involved vein and ligation of the perforating veins.

299

AMPUTATION FOR DÉBRIDEMENT
AND DRAINAGE

Guillotine amputation for débridement and drainage is occasionally necessary when incision and drainage and antibiotics do not control the infection. The best level in the lower leg is just above the ankle. After the guillotine procedure, a second definitive closed amputation below the knee is performed at a later date. When the guillotine amputation is required above the knee, it should be performed as low as possible. Revision of the stump and secondary closure may be necessary later.

Open amputation above knee

Open amputation above the knee is rarely necessary. The procedure results in prolonged morbidity. However, healing by second intention will occur if adequate collateral circulation is available. Elective definitive amputation at a higher level may be impossible, but secondary closure in stages is occasionally helpful. Skin traction is difficult and uncomfortable and may even be hazardous to the skin in patients with diabetes or an ischemic limb. The procedure should be performed with a circular incision at a level that is as low as possible consistent with adequate blood supply and good healing. The amputation may be done below a sterile tourniquet of stout rubber tubing to permit more rapid operation without excessive blood loss.

Open amputation below knee

Open amputation below the knee is usually done in an effort to control invasive infection that has not been successfully managed by simple drainage or by antibiotics. Semielective guillotine amputation may be performed for necrosis or for major bone or joint sepsis about the ankle. Fortunately, such procedures are seldom necessary. The best level for débridement procedures below the knee is just above the malleoli. Little bleeding is encountered here, and it is not necessary to divide a great deal of soft tissue. All tissue planes and tendon sheaths should be left open for drainage. Open amputation at the level of election for below-the-knee amputation and the development of flaps in open amputation should be avoided. In patients with vascular disease, slow healing leads to more prolonged morbidity than a two-stage procedure, and it is usually advisable, after adequate drainage has been established, to perform a subsequent elective definitive amputation at a higher level.

Guillotine amputation at ankle

The patient is prepared preoperatively by conservative measures, antibiotics, and the other measures previously described for elective amputations wherever they are applicable. Spinal or light general anesthesia is suitable. A sterile tourniquet should be applied to the midcalf.

Procedure

1. Make a circular incision down to the bone at the thinnest part of the leg just above the ankle malleoli. Clamp and divide the major vessels.
2. Divide the tibia and fibula just above the malleoli.
3. Apply petrolatum gauze over the surgical wound, and hold the bulky

300

soft gauze dressing in place with tube gauze or tubular stockinette held to the skin with tincture of benzoin.

4. Apply a posterior splint.

5. Plan an elective second-stage amputation when infection has been controlled.

Open amputation or drainage amputations in foot

Open amputations in the foot are usually indicated for suppurative infection and gangrene in conjunction with diabetes. These infections frequently involve the bone or the metatarsal-phalangeal joint and invade the plantar space along the flexor tendon. Operation must be designed to remove the infected toe along with the tendon and bone complex. Fortunately, patients suffering from diabetic neuritis frequently have pedal pulses and adequate circulation.

Preoperative preparation consists of minor débridement, incision, and probing of drainage tracts. Such preoperative investigation is usually painless and assists greatly in appraising the problem and in planning the operation.

Open transmetatarsal amputation

The incision used for elective transmetatarsal amputation of the entire forefoot is not adequate to drain flexor tendon sheaths, even if the flaps are left open. Open transmetatarsal amputation, however, can be done when there is extensive plantar space abscess if the plantar flap is widely undermined. This requires an extensive incision along the medial side of the foot. In severe cases the abscess frequently extends to the tarsal bones. As a rule, only one or two tendon-joint complexes are involved, and a wedge type of amputation may be employed.

Wedge amputation of toe and metatarsal

Wedge amputation is indicated for infection and gangrene involving the proximal phalanx, a web space, or a metatarsal-phalangeal joint along with the metatarsal bone.

Anesthesia

Spinal or light general anesthesia is suitable.

Preoperative preparation

Preoperative preparation is conservative and as described previously (pp. 280-282).

Procedure

1. Place the patient in the supine position.

2. Use a V-shaped incision (Fig. 89, A). The dorsal skin may overhang the end of the bone somewhat. Extend the incision as necessary along the sole of the foot (Fig. 89, B) in order to drain the deep plantar space and the associated flexor tendon sheath. One plantar incision will also suffice if two adjacent toes with metatarsal heads are to be resected.

3. Cut between the metatarsals with the knife blade directed against the joint to be resected, thus avoiding opening into the neighboring normal joint only a few millimeters away.

4. Transect the flexor tendon.

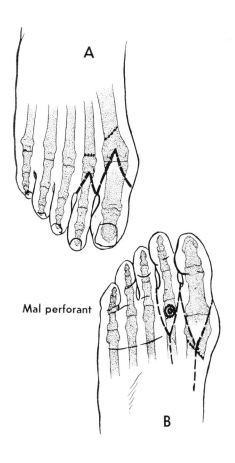

Mal perforant

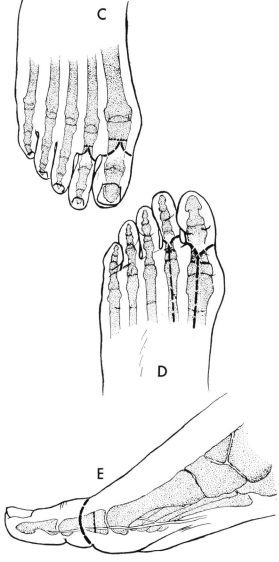

Fig. 89. Wedge amputation of toe and metatarsal. **A** and **B**, Incisions for transmetatarsal amputation of toes. **C** to **E**, Incisions for transphalangeal amputation of toes.

5. Cut the metatarsal bone, beveling the edge, so that drainage is not obstructed (Fig. 89, *A*). In the big toe use the Gigli saw to divide the metatarsal. Also resect the sesamoid bones in this location.

6. Pack the open wound lightly with dry gauze or iodoform gauze. Do not suture.

7. When the wound is clean and healthy, packs are removed or lessened and the foot is bandaged so that the sides of the defects created by the surgical procedure are coapted. Healing is by secondary intention.

Transphalangeal toe amputation

Suppurative infection with gangrene of the toe, which has not extended proximally, may be controlled by open transphalangeal amputation (Fig. 89, *C-E*). Such a procedure is frequently elected for infected hammer toes, corns, and wet gangrene of the tips of the toes. The surgical technique is identical to that used for elective closed amputation except that the incision is packed open. The incision may be extended proximally onto the plantar surface of the foot for drainage (Fig. 89, *D*) of associated tendon sheaths that may be invaded.

Appendix

BUERGER-ALLEN EXERCISES

Buerger-Allen exercises attempt to increase circulation in the pulseless foot by alternately emptying and distending the blood vessels with the aid of gravity.

Indications

Pain at rest caused by ischemia may be relieved somewhat by Buerger-Allen exercises. The edema that results from prolonged and persistent dependency may also decrease. The visible changes in the feet and the indoctrination and habits developed remind and encourage the patient to give his extremities proper care.

Position 1—draining old blood out (Fig. 90, A)

While lying in bed the patient elevates his feet and legs until the skin is blanched. This may take from ten to sixty seconds. Elevation must not be continued long enough to cause pain.

Position 2—letting fresh blood in (Fig. 90, B)

The patient sits up with his legs hanging over the side of the bed and moves his feet slowly. Color returns, the veins fill, and when maximum rubor has returned, the patient assumes Position 3. This usually requires two to three minutes. Slow rhythmic movements of the feet (Fig. 90, C) are also performed while the feet are dependent.

Position 3—resting (Fig. 90, D)

The patient lies supine to complete the five-minute cycle and then begins again with Position 1.

Comment: *In some patients, faithful use of these exercises alleviates pain, and improvement will also be noted by a more rapid filling time. In other patients the main value may be as "occupational therapy."*

Discussion

The whole cycle requires five minutes, in some instances ten minutes. The times in Position 1 and Position 2 are determined by observation of the particular patient. The time at rest in Position 3 is merely to round out the cycle to the convenient period of five or ten minutes. Instruct the patient to begin each cycle on the even five-minute or ten-minute reading on a watch or clock. Normally, thirty-minute sessions are performed four times daily.

The patient is given instructions and thereafter performs the exercises himself. No equipment is necessary except a chair, pillow, and watch.

DIRECTIONS FOR CARE OF FEET

Small difficulties and trivial infections and injuries can lead to serious difficulty. The following directions will help prevent injury and infections, as well as blisters, corns, calluses, and other conditions that might lead to complications.

1. *Cleanliness.* The patient's feet should be washed carefully each night with soap and warm water, dried thoroughly, rubbed gently with 70% rubbing alcohol, and dried again. The skin should then be rubbed with toilet lanolin so that it is soft and moist but not sticky or greasy. The lanolin should be applied especially to any cracks, calluses, or rough or dry areas.

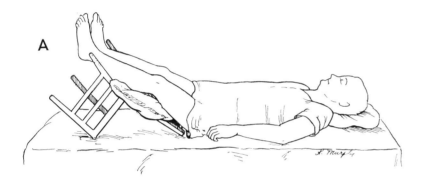

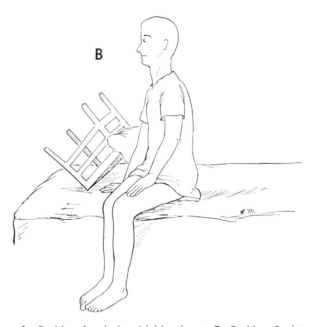

Fig. 90. Buerger-Allen exercises. **A,** Position 1—drain old blood out. **B,** Position 2—let new blood in.

Continued.

305

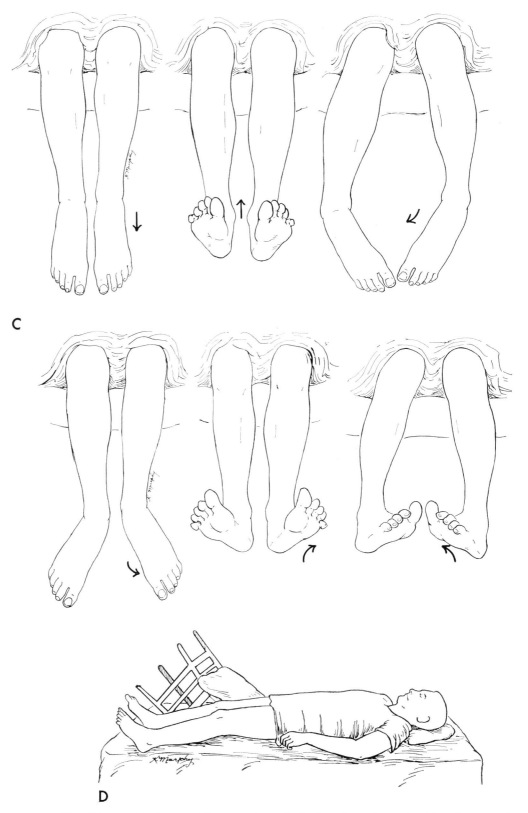

Fig. 90, cont'd. Buerger-Allen exercises. **C,** During dependency (position 2), move feet and ankles slowly as diagramed. **D,** Position 3—rest until time to repeat cycle with position 1.

VASCULAR EXAMINATION

Name:_____ Date:_____ Age:_____

Complaint, previous surgery, diagnosis, significant past and family history:

Subjective

	Right leg	Left leg	Right arm	Left arm	Hip
Cyanosis					
Pain					
Coldness					
Numbness					
Redness					
Claudication					

Objective

	Right leg	Left leg	Right arm	Left arm
Cyanosis				
Sweating				
Redness				
Dependent rubor				
Pallor on elevation				
Ulcer				

Pulses

	Right leg	Left leg	Right arm	Left arm	Right carotid	Left carotid
Dorsalis pedis						
Tibialis posterior						
Popliteal						
Femoral						
Radial						
Ulnar (Allen test)						
Carotids						

Other signs

	Right leg	Left leg	Right arm	Left arm
Oscillometer				
Blood pressure				
Saline wheal (sec.)				
Skin temperatures				
Swelling (cm.)				

Bruits

	Right	Left
Femoral		
Carotids		
Abdomen		
Chest		
Aorta		

2. *Clothing.* Exposure to cold, particularly wet cold, must be avoided. The patient should wear clean woolen socks and, if necessary, long underwear or slacks. In the summer, clean cotton socks are sufficient. Shoes should be of soft leather and should fit well. Occasionally, special shoes may be prescribed.

3. *Injury.* The patient should cut the toenails only after they have been softened by a footbath. A good light should always be used. When the nails are trimmed, they should be cut straight across—the corners should not be cut back. In some cases it may be necessary for you to trim the nails yourself or advise the patient to consult a chiropodist. The patient should not cut corns or calluses himself. He should also refrain from using strong antiseptics or chemicals on the feet since the delicate skin can easily be injured. Sunburn of the feet, ankles, or legs must also be avoided, although gradual tanning is safe. Hot-water bottles, hot-water bags, and electric pads can be dangerous when applied to the feet. If the feet are cold in winter, loose-fitting bed socks are advisable.

4. *Circulation.* To improve the circulation, moderate exercise within the limits imposed by pain, fatigue, or cramps is helpful. Circular garters should be avoided. If the feet have a tendency to swell, instruct the patient to keep them in a horizontal position on a hassock or footstool whenever he is sitting. If the feet show marked changes in color, the exercises illustrated on pp. 305 and 306 will be beneficial.

5. *Help and supervision.* The patient should report all trivial signs of blistering, infection, ingrown toenail, or any difficulty with bunions, calluses, or athlete's foot. In some cases it may be necessary to ask a member of the family to examine the patient's feet daily and watch for warning signs.

6. *Smoking.* In some patients life-long abstinence from smoking is essential. This should be discussed with the patient.

VASCULAR EXAMINATION

The use of a short form (see p. 307) ensures the regular completion of a basic vascular survey.

Index

MEDICAL
OBSERVATIONS
AND
INQUIRIES.

By a Society of Physicians in LONDON.

VOL. II.

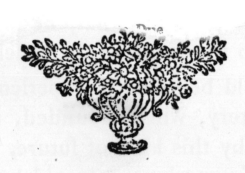

LONDON:

Printed for WILLIAM JOHNSTON,
in *Ludgate-street.*

MDCCLXII.